The Secret Malady

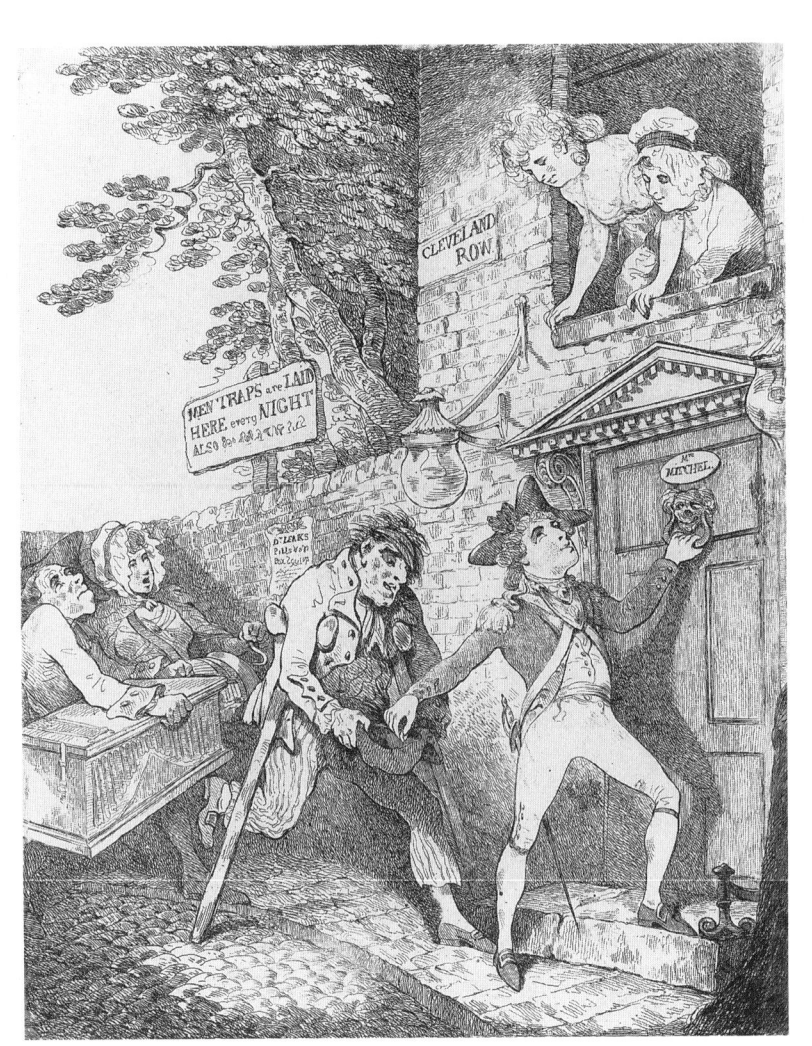

The Secret Malady

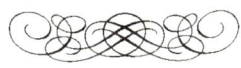

Venereal Disease in Eighteenth-Century Britain and France

LINDA E. MERIANS
EDITOR

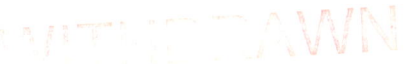

ITHACA COLLEGE LIBRARY

THE UNIVERSITY PRESS OF KENTUCKY

Frontispiece: "Charity Covereth a Multitude of Sins."
Courtesy of the Print Collection, Lewis Walpole Library, Yale University.

Copyright © 1996 by The University Press of Kentucky

Scholarly publisher for the Commonwealth,
serving Bellarmine College, Berea College, Centre
College of Kentucky, Eastern Kentucky University,
The Filson Club, Georgetown College, Kentucky
Historical Society, Kentucky State University,
Morehead State University, Murray State University,
Northern Kentucky University, Transylvania University,
University of Kentucky, University of Louisville,
and Western Kentucky University.

Editorial and Sales Offices: The University Press of Kentucky
663 South Limestone Street, Lexington, Kentucky 40508-4008

96 97 98 99 00 5 4 3 2 1

Library of Congress Cataloging-in-Publication Data

The secret malady : venereal disease in eighteenth-century Britain and
  France / Linda E. Merians, editor.
    p. cm.
  Includes bibliographical references and index.
  ISBN 0-8131-1989-8 (cloth : alk. paper).—ISBN 0-8131-0888-8
(pbk. : alk. paper)
  1. Sexually transmitted diseases—Great Britian—History—18th century.
  2. Sexually transmitted diseases—France—History—18th century.
I. Merians, Linda Evi.
RC201.6.G7S43   1997
616.956'100941'09033-dc20   96-20580

This book is printed on acid-free recycled paper meeting
the requirements of the American National Standard
for Permanence of Paper for Printed Library Materials.

Manufactured in the United States of America

Contents

List of Illustrations   vii

Acknowledgments   viii

Introduction   1
Linda E. Merians

Part One
Historical and Medical Contexts of Venereal Disease

1. The Pox in Eighteenth-Century France   15
   Susan P. Conner

2. From Courtesan to Prostitute: Mercenary Sex and Venereal Disease, 1730-1802   34
   Kathryn Norberg

3. "Laying Aside Any Private Advantage": John Marten and Venereal Disease   51
   Roy Porter

4. Exposing the Secret Disease: Recognizing and Treating Syphilis in Daniel Turner's London   68
   Philip K. Wilson

5. John Burrows and the Vegetable Wars   85
   Marie E. McAllister

6. "And blights with plagues the Marriage hearse": Syphilis and Wives   103
   Mary Margaret Stewart

7. The Problem of Syphilitic Children
in Eighteenth-Century France and England   114
Barbara J. Dunlap

8. The London Lock Hospital and the
Lock Asylum for Women   128
Linda E. Merians

**Part Two
Representations of Venereal Disease**

9. Decorums   149
Betty Rizzo

10. The Meaning of Venereal Disease
in Hogarth's Graphic Art   168
N.F. Lowe

11. Satiric Representation of Venereal Disease:
The Restoration versus the Eighteenth-Century Model   183
Rose A. Zimbardo

12. Pox and Malice: Some Representations of Venereal Disease in
Restoration and Eighteenth-Century Satire   196
Leon Guilhamet

13. Avoiding the Subject: The Presence and Absence of Venereal
Disease in the Eighteenth-Century English Novel   213
April London

14. Job's Curse and Social Degeneracy in Rétif de la Bretonne's
LE PAYSAN PERVERTI   228
Diane Fourny

15. Contagion and Containment: Sade and the Republic
of Letters   243
Julie Candler Hayes

Contributors   261

Index   263

Illustrations

Figures

1. "The King's Evil" 3
2. "Le transport des filles de joye à l'hopital" 29
3. Daniel Turner 69
4. The scenario of syphilis treatments 77
5. Daniel Turner's public appeal 79
6. "Mercury and his Advocates defeated" 86
7. Lock Hospital 130

Plates [follow page 184]

1. Antoine Watteau, *La toilette du matin*
2. François Boucher, *La toilette*
3. William Hogarth, *A Harlot's Progress,* Plate I
4. William Hogarth, *A Harlot's Progress,* Plate II
5. William Hogarth, *A Harlot's Progress,* Plate III
6. William Hogarth, *A Harlot's Progress,* Plate IV
7. William Hogarth, *Marriage à la Mode,* Plate I
8. William Hogarth, *Marriage à la Mode,* Plate II (detail)
9. William Hogarth, *Marriage à la Mode,* Plate III (detail)
10. William Hogarth, *Marriage à la Mode,* Plate VI (detail)
11. William Hogarth, *A Rake's Progress,* Plate III (detail)
12. William Hogarth, *A Rake's Progress,* Plate VIII (detail)
13. William Hogarth, *The Four Times of Day: Morning*
14. William Hogarth, *The Four Times of Day: Evening*
15. *La Vie d'un joli Garçon ou Le Paysan perverti*
16. *La Vie d'une jolie Fille à Paris ou La Paysanne pervertie*

Acknowledgments

THIS BOOK BEGAN TO TAKE SHAPE AT THE 1994 MEETING OF THE AMERICAN Society for Eighteenth-Century Studies when I chaired a session on social diseases. Professors Norberg, Rizzo, and Stewart have been kind enough to revise their papers into articles for this collection. The other articles have been written especially for this collection. I extend my deepest gratitude to all the authors. Their hard work and generosity have made my task as editor not only easy but enjoyable. I also extend grateful thanks to Elaine Durham Otto for her extremely careful and skillful copyediting.

I am indebted to Joan H. Sussler, curator of prints at the Lewis Walpole Library, and Toby Appel and Amy Sharon at the Harvey Cushing/John Hay Whitney Medical Library at Yale University for their generous advice and assistance in securing some of the illustrations for this book.

Friends and colleagues in the East-Central Region of the American Society of Eighteenth-Century Studies and at my own institution also deserve special thanks. T.E.D. Braun helped me find authors, and Elizabeth Lambert helped me polish my prose. At La Salle University, Gervasio T. Ramirez proved himself to be the most patient desktop publishing specialist on the planet, and Zane R. Wolf, professor of nursing, was kind enough to read a draft of the introduction. Francine Lottier made it possible for me to meet my deadline. James A. Butler and Kevin J. Harty were generous with their encouragement and support. Finally, Gabriel Fagan, F.S.C., has accepted with unfailing graciousness a particular burden of friendship with me, that is, being asked to read rough draft after rough draft of almost everything I write.

More than anyone else, however, Betty Rizzo has been a wise and supportive advisor as I have put this volume together. It is to her and her husband, Ray, that I dedicate this volume.

Introduction

THE SUBJECT OF VENEREAL DISEASE IN EIGHTEENTH-CENTURY BRITAIN AND France is characterized by startling and compelling ironies. Venereal disease existed in epidemic proportions, yet it was the great secret malady of the time. Men and women who acquired venereal disease often wished to keep knowledge of their infection secret from their own sexual partners and families or from society at large. Despite having to endure painful periods of treatment, many regarded the disease as an expected consequence of partaking in sexual activity and sometimes even spoke with great bravado about being afflicted. Swaggering language was also adopted by legitimate and illegitimate medical practitioners who, while often promising to cure their patients of the disease, had very little correct understanding of it.

Whatever one called it—the French disease, the pox, the clap, the gleet, the Italian disease, *le mal de Naples, la chaude-pisse, la maladie vénérienne, la vérole, la grande vérole, morbus gallicus, lues venerea*—one could find it everywhere. As several articles in this collection demonstrate, dissertations and representations of venereal disease appear in visual art, operas, plays, poetry, novels, scientific essays, periodical essays, and private letters and journals. Whether one lived in Paris or London, the existence of venereal disease was evident on the streets and in the business of everyday life. Literal and figurative references to venereal disease would have been evident to the eye of any beholder. Jean Astruc complains in his *De morbis venereis libri sex* about the number of quacks selling their false remedies in Paris (1736, 1740 in Latin; 1737, 1754, 1755, 1770, 1787 in English; 1755, 1777 in French). In London, men and women walking along Goose-Alley would have seen a golden ball hanging over the back door entrance to Liveth G. West's surgery. Both cities were, of course, hosts to a seeming legion of writers and publishers who were responsible for myriad texts on venereal disease.

The culture of venereal disease also supported related industries. Lawrence Stone points out in his *Family, Sex, and Marriage in England, 1500-1800* that advertisements of cures for venereal disease accounted for more column space in the eighteenth-century English periodical press than any other product.[1] Indeed, as did many of his competitors, the self-proclaimed "Regular

Surgeon" Liveth G. West advertised his practice in *The General Advertiser* (28 January 1747). There he promised to cure "all the various Symptoms of the FRENCH DISTEMPER, whether fresh contracted, or of long Continuance, by a new speedy and sure Method; and a RECENT CLAP, in a few Days, without Confinement, Hindrance of Business, or the Knowledge of a Bedfellow."

Venereal disease entered the political arenas of both nations. Members of the royal families as well as those in aristocratic and parliamentary circles were touched by the disease personally and politically. The satiric print "The King's Evil" (fig. 1, dated 28 September 1786) demonstrates how the worlds of venereal disease and politics intersected in the public discourse. Here the Prince of Wales, crotch-centered, stands in the foreground as his mistress, Mrs. Fitzherbert, sits amidst vials of medicine with a knife or letter opener in her hand pointing in a suggestive direction, and a note that reads, "To the part affected." Her state of undress and her outspread legs emphasize further the relevance of why what is on the top of the table is necessary. The Order of the Garter that hangs above her head has written on it, "evil to them that evil thinks." Is it a coincidence that the garter's shape suggests a noose or that the two upside down pistols point at the prince's head?

Venereal disease ended public careers, and it also influenced the writing and the enforcement of laws that served to increase the oppression of women in particular. By the end of the eighteenth century, political and social leaders in Britain and France perceived venereal disease to be, in real and imagined ways, an extremely serious threat to the political, economic, and spiritual well-being of their nations.

In both countries venereal disease was often used, literally or metaphorically, to represent the utterly corrupt, the unromantic, the unpatriotic, the ungovernable, and the "other." For example, sometime in 1746, the year of the English massacre of Scots at Culloden, a pamphlet appeared entitled *The Highlanders Salivated, or the Loyal Association of M—ll K—g's Midnight Club: with a serious Address of the Ladies of Drury, to the batter'd strollling Nymphs of their Community."*[2] In France during the last two decades of the eighteenth century, debates about politics and sexuality often merged. As Lynn Hunt and others have shown, the "political pornography" produced during this time, be it in the form of tracts against Marie Antoinette or others, often made the claim that "sexual degeneration went hand in hand with political corruption."[3] In his 1986 *Le Mal de Naples* (translated and republished in English in 1992 as *The History of Syphilis*), Claude Quétel writes that "nothing is more revealing of a society than the history of its diseases, particularly the 'social' diseases," and he adds that syphilis was "the one which has terrorized people the most . . . it was the disease which caused the most, and the blackest, ink to flow."[4]

Introduction 3

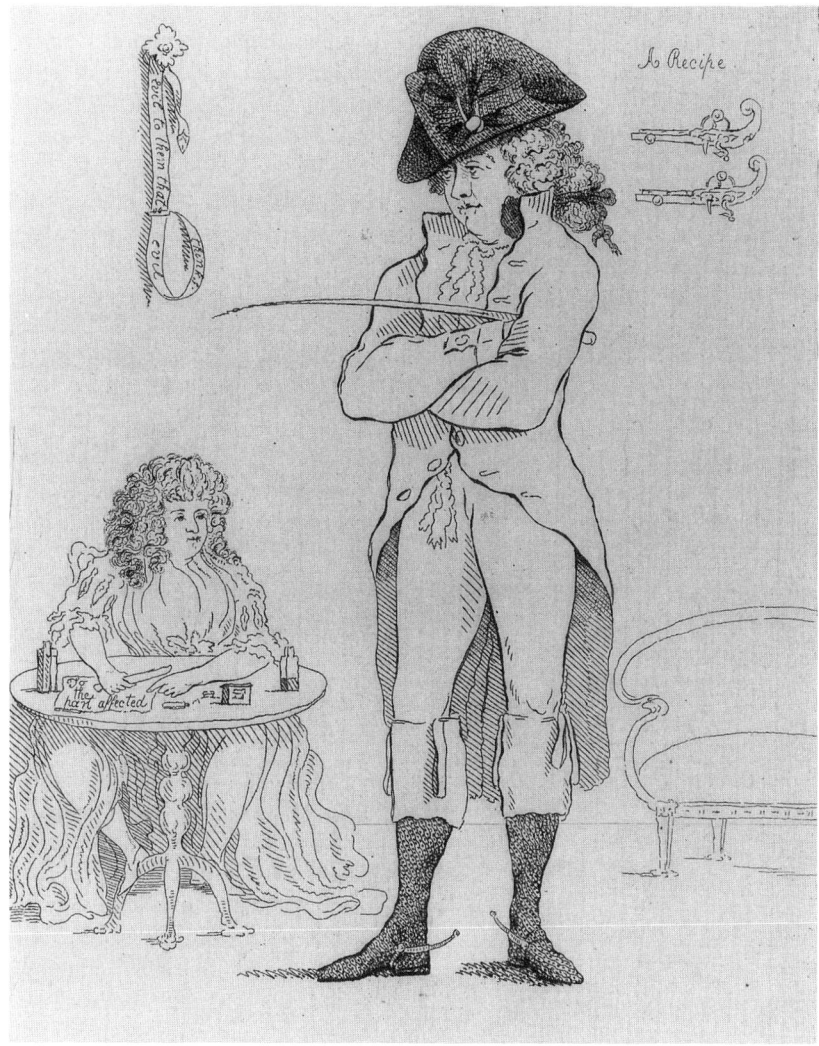

Fig. 1. "The King's Evil." No. 6986 in M. Dorothy George's *Catalogue of Prints and Drawings in the British Museum: Political and Personal Satires.* Courtesy of the Print Collection, Lewis Walpole Library, Yale University.

Interestingly, in Restoration and eighteenth-century Britain and France, the disease was initially regarded as something to joke and boast about. Playwrights placed witty remarks about it in the mouths of their most rakish characters, and poets and pamphleteers often used it as a metaphorical vehicle to satirize or insult someone or something else. That venereal disease had a "light side" is an indication of the exuberant and robust nature of life and sexuality in the eighteenth century. That the "dark side" of venereal disease would be what was carried into the nineteenth century suggests a shift in the disease's reception that is inextricably linked to the more restrictive constructions of self and society that emerged during the 1780s and 1790s.

The prevalence of venereal disease forced both the French and the British to create medical and nonmedical institutions that could combat the disease for the individual as well as for the society's greater good. It was no secret that venereal disease was an economic as well as a medical problem for the middle and lower classes. In London a charity society began work in July 1746 to found a hospital devoted to treating only venereal disease cases, and by the end of January 1747, the London Lock Hospital admitted its first patients. In 1780, the Vaugirard Hospice was established in Paris to treat children with venereal disease. French adults, however, would have to wait a little longer. Throughout much of the eighteenth century the Parisian poor afflicted with venereal disease received treatment (and died) in wards at the prison-hospitals of Bicêtre and la Salpêtrière. In 1792, the Hospice des Vénériens opened its doors to patients, and survival rates began to increase. A significant number of the secondary cities in both countries also erected charity and municipal hospitals during the eighteenth century, and most of these establishments would eventually agree to treat those afflicted with the disease.

To discuss representations of venereal disease without raising issues related to eighteenth-century ideas about sexuality, family, and nationhood is impossible. In regard to Britain, many scholars have found, in the increased religiosity inspired by Methodism and Evangelicalism, the seeds for the late-eighteenth-century shift away from the "relaxed and permissive attitude to sexual behaviour" ushered in by the Restoration.[5] That some of Britain's leading Evangelicals were among the most active governors of the Lock Hospital and Lock Asylum for Women is most suggestive. Whoever or whatever the cause, by the end of the eighteenth century the idealization of the maternal woman had taken hold in the collective British imagination. Ruth Perry has written that "in the eighteenth century, maternity came to be imagined as a counter to sexual feeling, opposing alike individual expression, desire, and agency in favor of a mother-self at the service of the family and the state."[6] This new ideology ensured the demonization of the sexual woman, and consequently the figure of the prostitute came under special fire. She was seen as the agent of contamination. Indeed, in both France and Britain, prostitutes would find themselves under increasing moral and legislative attack by the start of the nineteenth century. Venereal disease became a subject these two societies preferred to eschew, but as its prevalence made this impossible, the ruling voices (official and cultural) in both nations found other ways to address the problems it caused. Nineteenth-century French and British culture needed the secret malady to remain a secret.

Eighteenth-century medical researchers and writers were not able to uncover many of the mysteries of venereal disease. One secret about venereal disease that remained intact during the eighteenth century concerned how it came to Europe in the first place. European countries had been in the clutches of a syphilis epidemic since 1495, and despite the fact that historical, religious, and literary texts document gonorrhea in Europe before that year, it was mistakenly linked to syphilis when the epidemic overtook the Continent. Pre-eighteenth-century writers and eighteenth-century authorities believed that syphilis was brought to Europe by the sailors who returned with Columbus in 1493. The theory was that they had been infected by the women of "the new world." Astruc and others believed that the indigenous people of Hispaniola and those in other "torrid zones" had venereal disease because of a "disposition to impurity, and the same propensity to a promiscuous copulation."[7]

What was certain was that the army led by France's Charles VIII, which marched through Italy in 1493-94, caused the disease to spread throughout Europe. By 1497, separate decrees had been signed in Paris that obligated infected residents and nonresidents with venereal disease to move to specific locations in the St. Germain des Prés suburbs or to quit Paris altogether and to pay a fine of sixty livres. Syphilis also arrived in England and Scotland by 1497. In Scotland the disease was perceived as being such a threat that in September 1498, James IV signed a decree ordering all those suffering from syphilis to leave Edinburgh.[8] Only a few eighteenth-century authors believed that venereal disease was present in Europe before the discovery of the "new world." William Becket (1684-1738), a surgeon at St. Thomas's Hospital in London (Southwark) and a well-known antiquary of his day, wrote three articles arguing this point, but they and he would be attacked sharply by Jean Astruc and others.[9]

The mistaken link between gonorrhea and syphilis led most to believe that they were manifestations of the same disease albeit in different stages. Throughout the eighteenth century in both France and Great Britain, the unicist (one disease) theory was held by the general public and by the majority of those who wrote about the disease. Astruc makes the unicist claim throughout his *De morbis venereis libri sex* (1736), and a mistake made in 1767 by John Hunter, one of Britain's most prominent surgeon-anatomists, seemingly demonstrated the validity of the theory. Hunter injected himself with pus from a patient he mistakenly thought had only gonorrhea, but when he later developed symptoms of syphilis, he saw this as proof that the two were the same disease. In the first part of his *Treatise on the Venereal Disease* (1786), Hunter writes that "the matter produced in both is of the same kind, and has the same properties; the proofs of which are, that the matter of a gonorrhoea will produce either a gonorrhoea, a chancre, or the *lues venerea*, and the matter of a chancre will also produce either a gonorrhoea, a chancre, or the *lues venerea*."[10]

There were some, however, who argued a "dualist" view. The three major proponents of this view were Francis Balfour *(Dissertation medica inauguralis de gonorrhoea virulenta*, 1767), Andrew Duncan the elder (*Observations on the operation and use of mercury in the venereal disease*, 1772), and Benjamin Bell (*A Treatise on Gonorrhoea Virulenta and Lues Venerea*, 1793). Their correct instincts were confirmed in the nineteenth and early twentieth centuries. In 1837, Philippe Ricord, a physician at l'Hôpital du Midi in Paris, recognized John Hunter's mistake. In 1879 Albert Neisser found the gonococcus that is the causative agent of gonorrhea, and in 1905 Fritz Schaudinn at the Berlin Health Institute isolated *Treponema pallidum*, the spirochetal bacterium that causes syphilis.

Although the pathology of venereal disease remained a secret throughout the eighteenth century, the topic was frequently and loudly debated in the printed press by physicians, surgeons, quacks, and hacks. In both countries, a lack of credentials, training, and clinical experience did not often restrain a person from arguing his or her own theory about venereal disease or from promoting a method of cure. As W.F. Bynum points out, literate men and women in Great Britain could inform themselves about the secret malady and varieties of treatment from well over one hundred works.[11] There were some works that did presume to be exhaustive and scholarly in approach. Astruc's *De morbis venereis libri sex* (1736) is a good example of a text that worked hard to establish its own authority. Other works seemed to have a particular audience in mind. As Mary Margaret Stewart explains in her article in this collection, Dr. John Profily's *Easy and Exact Method of Curing the Venereal Disease* (1748) seems to be aimed at a female audience, paying special attention to women and the problems they have in relation to venereal disease. The majority of the texts, however, were often devoted to excoriating certain kinds of treatment while detailing alternative treatments that would prove far more beneficial. There were men and women, like John Burrows, who advocated "natural" cures and published works advertising their special approaches. Actually, many of those who treated venereal disease cases mixed and matched modes of therapies, using drugs internally and externally (applied with poultices or by friction), with supplementary courses of bleeding, fumigation, baths, and the drinking of medicinal liquids.

For a variety of cultural and physiological symptoms, women afflicted with venereal disease faced a most difficult challenge. Generally, by the time women realized they were infected, they would be in a more advanced stage than their male counterparts, and thus the chances of a complete cure were less certain. Seeking treatment often meant breaking the secret, and most women, be they wives, unmarried women dependent on their lovers, or young prostitutes, were not in a position to do so. Certainly, many women who had the economic means to be treated and cured never sought to do so, or they hesitated before engaging "reliable" surgeons or physicians. Also, women afflicted with venereal disease were often accused by the men who shared in their infections of having given them the dreaded malady on purpose.[12] It would not be engaging in overstatement to say that venereal disease must have played a significant role in raising the level of misogyny during the eighteenth century.

The most controversial therapeutic question centered on the use of mercury, which could be administered as ointments, pills, injections, and liquids. Astruc, Hunter, and others agreed that mercury had no effect on gonorrhea but was an effective cure for what they identified as chancre and *lues venerea* (syphilis). Undergoing a course of "salivation" treatment, which entailed rubbing a mercurial ointment into the body in progressive stages and then wrapping the body in flannel, guaranteed at least a six-week period of misery. Mercury cures also had the capacity to exact a price years after treatment, when the effects of mercury poisoning would begin to appear in other parts and organs of the body. In the case of a gonorrheal infection, the modern truism "the cure is worse than the disease" has merit. Gonorrhea was generally a localized medical infection, and it was not fatal.

The telltale symptoms of gonorrhea in men quickly became apparent. Within days of being infected, they would often experience uncomfortable discharges of semen and burning sensations when urinating. Boswell immortalized in his *London Journal* that on 12 January 1763, he was "five times . . . fairly lost in supreme rapture," but six days later he would begin "to feel an unaccountable alarm of unexpected evil: a little heat in the members of my body sacred to Cupid, very like a symptom of that distemper with which Venus, when cross, takes it into her head to plague her votaries."[13] Boswell had nineteen bouts of urethritis (and probably gonorrhea) during his lifetime, and he endured a variety of treatments to be cured of the disease.[14] As in the case with Boswell, the initial symptoms of gonorrhea were painful enough to induce most men to seek medical assistance. The symptoms of the disease would subside after a short time whether or not the men received treatment. If the gonorrhea moved from the front to the back of the urethra, more serious conditions could ensue.[15] Blockages in the urethra, prostate gland complications, bladder problems, sterility, and impotence could be the result of what became known as compound or complex gonorrheas. In many of these cases, surgery might have been performed to alleviate some of these secondary complications. For the more conventional cases, Astruc details three stages of treatment, beginning with bleeding and the ingestion of liquids that would cool "the heat of the parts" and serve to keep the bowels loose. The next stage entailed the ingestion of even more purging and other liquid medications as well as the application of poultices and external mercurial frictions to the genitalia, buttocks, and groin areas. The final phase of the cure would occur when the patient was free of symptoms, during which he/she would drink liquids, often made from balsams, milks, and china and sarsaparilla roots, to clean and heal any internal ulcers.

Women afflicted with gonorrhea were generally unaware they had the disease, and so they were often unknowing carriers of it. Although Astruc believed that women infected with gonorrhea suffered initially from "unusual moisture" and itching and burning sensations in their genitalia, he goes on to say that women "are apt to neglect any discharge."[16] Hunter found less fault with women, understanding that many women evinced no initial symptoms whatsoever or had such a "slight" inflammation that they could not know they were infected or that they could infect their partners.[17] His usual method for curing women of gonorrhea was to give them many of the same medicines he gave to his male patients.

For both men and women, syphilis was the more dangerous venereal disease. The first symptom of the primary stage of the disease manifested itself two to six weeks after infection in the form of a chancre (usually a single "painless" ulcer) appearing most often at the location where the bacterium entered the body. Chancres could thus be found on the mouth, genitalia, or buttocks of sexually active men and women, and on the mouth or fingers of nursing children. Women could also have internal chancres. Although chancres would heal after several weeks, Hunter and others tried to cure or destroy them. Generally, external mercurial dressings were applied if the chancre was located in an accessible location; otherwise, mercury would be given internally. Hunter would also sometimes try to remove the chancre, either by applying a caustic substance or by incision. Complicating matters even more, the lymph nodes closest to the chancre were often enlarged and in need of treatment.

The secondary stage of syphilis would generally appear months after the primary symptoms disappeared. External chancres could reappear along with other visible skin rashes and lesions. Also, one or more internal organs could be infected with the disease. The secondary stage of the disease also signaled that syphilis had the capacity to travel from the initial point of infection to other locations throughout the body. Sometimes a swelling and hardening of the glands (known as buboes) would occur, and fevers, aches in bones, warts, and other symptoms would present themselves. At this point, patients would receive some sort of internal and/or topical mercury treatment that was often accompanied by bleeding, induced vomiting, and surgery. Hunter, for example, discusses one patient who underwent a penile amputation.[18] Symptoms characteristic of the secondary stage of syphilis would disappear within several weeks, although they could reappear in untreated patients during the first two years of infection. If a person developed tertiary syphilis, which was often announced by symptoms similar to the second stage, he or she would most likely also develop the disease in his/her brain and throughout his/her cardiovascular system. Dementia and death would follow, but the process could be slow and extremely painful.

Children could be born infected with syphilis or gonorrhea, and they could also be infected after their birth by their mothers or wet nurses. Infants could also be carriers of the disease, and thus they could spread it to their wet nurses, who could then carry the disease to other children. The symptoms of congenital or acquired infantile syphilis were snuffles, rashes, skin lesions, eye problems, and venereal ulcers on the nose, mouth, lips, anus, or genitalia. Hunter describes children born with syphilis as sometimes emerging with blisters and spots on their skin. Even more symptoms could manifest themselves within months of the child's birth, but there were also many infected infants who showed no symptoms until years later. Gonorrhea in children often expressed itself as gonorrheal ophthalmia. It is interesting that the major works on venereal disease devoted little space, if any, to descriptions of venereal disease in children. Presumably, treatment administered to afflicted children was similar to the courses of therapy given to adults.

In the twentieth century, historians and literary scholars have tended to honor the secrecy of the secret malady, treating it tangentially as imagery or as anecdote. Within the last twenty years, such social and medical historians as Lawrence Stone, Roy Porter, and W.F. Bynum have begun to recognize and treat its presence and the role it played in family life and attitudes about sexuality in Britain. Venereal disease in France has been more thoroughly investigated. Works by Paul Delaunay, E. Jeanselme, and more recently by Erica Marie Benabou and Susan P. Conner have made important contributions.[19] Claude Quétel's *Le Mal de Naples* (1986) is the most important modern work devoted to the history of venereal disease in Europe from the late fifteenth to the late twentieth centuries.

Our collection of articles seeks to present a cultural history of the secret malady in Britain and in France during the eighteenth century. No collection can presume to be comprehensive, but we hope that the essays presented here will begin what is long overdue, that is, a scholarly conversation about venereal disease in the eighteenth century. We believe the consequences of the eighteenth-century venereal epidemic and the public and private responses to it need to be further investigated. How responsible was venereal disease for making sex and sexually transmitted diseases a taboo subject of private and public discourse? How did venereal disease serve to enforce the distinctions between the classes? How did venereal disease influence the construction of race? How did some of the more free-spirited eighteenth-century discussions of sex or venereal disease serve to inhibit later discussions of the same subject?

Finally, how did venereal disease, especially the late-eighteenth-century construction of it, serve to reinforce patriarchal systems to the detriment of women?

The two-part structure of this volume is designed to present first the historical and the medical contexts of venereal disease in Britain and France during the eighteenth century. To this end, the opening articles by Susan P. Conner and Kathryn Norberg focus on the medical and cultural situation in France generally and in Paris specifically. Roy Porter, Philip K. Wilson, and Marie E. McAllister then examine the perception and reception of venereal disease in Great Britain, particularly in the print and commercial wars it generated. Porter and Wilson focus on the careers of John Marten (d. 1737) and Daniel Turner (1667-1741), two of the most influential early-eighteenth-century (self-appointed) experts on the disease. McAllister looks at how venereal disease created its own school of alternative medicines and approaches, and the career enjoyed and endured by John Burrows serves as her case in point. Mary Margaret Stewart presents three case histories of wives who were infected by their husbands, and Barbara J. Dunlap focuses on syphilis in children in eighteenth-century France and Britain. My article discusses the establishment of the London Lock Hospital and the Lock Asylum for Women.

The second half of the collection is devoted to exploring how venereal disease was discussed in private conversations, letters, and journals as well as in literary forms and visual works of art. Betty Rizzo delineates some of the different eighteenth-century decorums for discussing venereal disease, focusing particularly on the lives of Lady Diana Spencer and Lord "Bully" Bolingbroke. N.F. Lowe explores the meaning of venereal disease in Hogarth's art. Rose Zimbardo, Leon Guilhamet, and April London examine references to and depictions of venereal disease in Restoration and eighteenth-century British drama, satire, and novels. Diane Fourny and Julie Candler Hayes focus on representations of venereal disease in eighteenth-century French literature, particularly in works by Rétif and Sade. In regard to the perception and representation of venereal disease, perhaps no two writers exist in greater opposition to each other as do Rétif and Sade. In her article, Julie Candler Hayes returns our discussion of infection and contagion to our own time, thereby showing us that contemporary discussions of pornography, for example, rely on some of the same assumptions and strategies that guided eighteenth-century discussions of venereal disease.

It makes great sense that the last article in this collection returns us to present-day discourse. It is, after all, impossible to read and write about venereal disease in the eighteenth century without thinking about AIDS and those who live and die with it today. As Susan Sontag notes in her *AIDS and Its Metaphors*, "More than cancer, but rather like syphilis, AIDS seems to foster ominous fantasies about a disease that is a marker of both individual and social

Introduction

vulnerabilities."[20] In this regard, I hope that the articles in this collection can help us to see where some of today's practices and rhetoric can take us.

NOTES

1. Lawrence Stone, *The Family, Sex, and Marriage in England, 1500-1800* (New York: Harper and Row, 1977), 600.
2. I am grateful to Jim May for this reference.
3. Lynn Hunt, "The Many Bodies of Marie Antoinette," in *Eroticism and the Body Politic,* ed. Lynn Hunt (Baltimore: Johns Hopkins Univ. Press, 1991), 119.
4. Claude Quétel, *The History of Syphilis,* trans. Judith Braddock and Brian Pike (Baltimore: Johns Hopkins Univ. Press, 1990), 2.
5. I am using Lawrence Stone's language here. See his *Family, Sex, and Marriage,* 648. See also Roy Porter and Lesley Hall, *The Facts of Life: The Creation of Sexual Knowledge in Britain, 1650-1950* (New Haven: Yale Univ. Press, 1995).
6. Ruth Perry, "Colonizing the Breast: Sexuality and Maternity in Eighteenth-Century England," *Eighteenth-Century Life* 16 (Feb. 1992): 188.
7. Jean Astruc, *A Treatise of the Venereal Diseases in Six Books Containing an Account of the Origins, Propagation and Contagion of this Distemper,* trans. William Barrowby, M.D. (London, 1737), 1:103.
8. See Dr. Iwan Bloch, "The History of Syphilis," in *A System of Syphilis,* ed. D'Arcy Power and J. Keogh Murphy, 2d ed., 5 vols. (London: Oxford Univ. Press, 1914), 1:2-39.
9. Becket's articles in order of appearance in the *Philosophical Transactions of the Royal Society* are "A Letter concerning the Antiquity of the Venereal Disease," no. 357 in 1718; "An Attempt to Prove the Antiquity of the Venereal Disease, long before the Discovery of the West-Indies," no. 365 in 1718; "A Letter to Dr. Halley . . . in Answer to Some Objections Made to the History of the Antiquity of the Venereal Disease," no. 366 in 1718. Astruc directly refutes Becket's theories in chapter 6 of *De morbis venereis libri sex* (1736).
10. John Hunter, *A Treatise on the Venereal Disease* (Edinburgh, 1787), 15.
11. See Bynum's "Treating the Wages of Sin: Venereal Disease and Specialism in Eighteenth-Century Britain," in *Medical Fringe and Medical Orthodoxy, 1750-1850,* ed. W.F. Bynum and Roy Porter (London: Croom Helm, 1987), 5-28. Bynum explains that of the over one hundred books he consulted, he counted a total of sixty-four "regular" authors of works on venereal disease. Of these, forty-five were surgeons and nineteen were physicians.
12. For example, Boswell and Andrew Douglas, his friend and surgeon, were both sure that Mrs. "Louisa" Lewis "could not but know" that she was infected with venereal disease, and thus knowingly passed it on to Boswell. Boswell's journal entry for 20 January 1763 records his suspicious and condemnatory thoughts about Louisa, part of which reads: "What! thought I, can this beautiful, this sensible, and this agreeable woman be so sadly defiled? Can corruption lodge beneath so fair a form? Can she who professed delicacy of sentiment and sincere regard for me, use me so very basely and so very cruelly? No, it is impossible. . . . But perhaps she was ignorant of her being ill. A pretty conjecture indeed! No, she could not be ignorant. Yes, yes, she intended to make the most of me" (*Boswell's London Journal, 1762-1763,* ed. Frederick A. Pottle (New York: McGraw-Hill, 1950), 155-56.
13. Ibid., 139 and 149.

14. I am using William B. Ober's figure and terminology. See his *Boswell's Clap and Other Essays: Medical Analyses of Literary Men's Afflictions* (Carbondale: Southern Illinois Univ. Press, 1979), 1-42.

15. Many surgeons published works detailing their particular methods for treating urethral problems. For example, the tenth chapter of William Bromfield's *Chirurgical Observations and Cases* (1773) presents many of his own case histories, providing in some instances descriptions of his use of the *bougie* (an implant designed to reopen the urinary tract).

16. Astruc, *A Treatise of the Venereal Diseases*, 1:248, 273.

17. Hunter, *A Treatise on the Venereal Disease*, 11.

18. Ibid, 249.

19. See Paul Delaunay, *Le monde médical parisien au dix-huitième siècle* (Paris, 1906); E. Jeanselme, *Histoire de la syphilis* (Paris, Doin et Cie, 1931); Erica Marie Benabou, "'La maladie antisociale': le 'danger vénérien' à Paris au XVIIIe siècle," in *La France d'ancien régime: Études réunies en l'honneur de Pierre Goubert*, 2 vols. (Toulouse: Société de démographie historique, 1984), 1:47-54. Susan P. Conner, "Politics, Prostitution, and the Pox in Revolutionary Paris, 1789-1799," *Journal of Social History* 22 (1989): 713-34.

20. Susan Sontag, *AIDS and Its Metaphors* (New York: Farrar, Straus and Giroux, 1989), 65.

One

Historical and Medical Contexts of Venereal Disease

Chapter 1

The Pox in Eighteenth-Century France

Susan P. Conner

Twenty-three-year-old Marianne was experiencing venereal disease for the first time. She was not a known prostitute, and on 7 July 1779 she was allowed to admit herself to a clinic known as la Petite Pologne in Paris. Medical practitioners who observed her entry into the clinic questioned her, probed and examined her, and finally categorized and confined her. According to their examination, she was "of good temperament, and ordinarily regular in her periods." That phrase unfortunately was the last of their good news. While her temperament was sound (a condition critical to a successful and expeditious cure), the symptoms of venereal disease in Marianne's body were massively present. The report of her examination then continued with an air of clinical detachment: her condition was characterized by "chancres and ulcerated pustules on the edges of her labia, an inflammation of the mucous membrane of the anus, rashes and swelling over every part of her body, and dry skin eruptions at the base of her breasts."[1] The disease was no stranger to her body; she was indeed *vérolée*. Marianne was pox-ridden.

For Marianne, her *visite* [medical and gynecological examination] and the therapeutic regimen of la Petite Pologne reflected the growing fascination of the eighteenth-century medical profession with venereal disease. She had, in fact, been chosen to be among the first patients on whom they would test a new drug. That concoction, called the *Tisane Caraïbe,* was allegedly a wonder drug that contained no mercury of any sort. Since "mercury was king" in eighteenth-century medical circles, Marianne's treatment was, at the least, an anomaly.[2] But her treatment also responded to demands made by sufferers and medical practitioners to find a remedy for venereal disease that was less devastating than the compounds and treatments made from mercury and its salts that conveyed serious, debilitating, and sometimes fatal side effects. Marianne's physicians—Saint Léger, de Horne, Bacher, and Roussel de Vauzesme—were attempting to find such a remedy. They oversaw the proceedings of her nonmercurial treatment, dosage, and schedule, and they later published their findings concerning her and nineteen other French men and women who had undergone the unusual cure. Their contribution to eighteenth-century cypridology or venereology joined a literature that included some three hundred other treatises and nearly two thousand medical atlases and publications that had been issued on venereal disease since its appearance in Europe two and a half centuries earlier.

According to the records, doctors at la Petite Pologne methodically traced the days of Marianne's life in the treatment rooms of their clinic. Was the *Tisane Caraïbe* yet another item to be placed on the list of false hopes, or would their patient bear the fruits of the Nègre de Mondragon's ill-smelling, boiled, filtered, and dried cloudy brown concoction? Even the name of the concoction and its creator had given them pause. Yet the Nègre de Mondragon's formula had been promoted by a prestigious member of the Académie des Sciences de Toulouse, and they had been assured of the gentleness and efficiency of the cure, unlike its rival mercury derivatives. Believing that mercury convulsed the system mechanically to expel the venereal poison, they were satisfied that the alkali-based tisane, which had been made from New World vegetable matter, affected the system solely in a physiological manner by "taming and redirecting the bodily humours."[3] Whether it proved to be a mechanical or physiological treatment, the physician-commissioners knew that the clues to its success would come from Marianne's body.

Case studies of French men and women like Marianne confirm what historians of medicine have traditionally argued: that the eighteenth century was obsessed with venereal disease.[4] It was, after all, the era of the condom, of the noseless Pangloss in *Candide,* and of efforts to combat a variety of epidemics, some of which had decimated even the royal court in the course of their virulence. According to Voltaire, who never missed an opportunity to describe the worst characteristics of his age, "Depend upon it when 30,000 men engage in pitched battle against an equal number of the enemy about 20,000 on each side have the pox."[5] According to his contemporary Hardy, for example, in *Mes Loisirs,* the obsession with venereal disease had gone so far that the lieutenant general of police of Paris had sent a request to all French curés to inform their parishioners of the epidemic, even though a discussion of venereal disease and its sexually explicit vocabulary might prove to be scandalous in the sanctuary.[6]

Serious scientific inquiry abounded in the eighteenth century, but charlatanism abounded as well. Animal, mineral, and vegetable concoctions were widely advertised, the crown granted lucrative patents for innovations, and individuals were encouraged to cure themselves. In that environment, advertised nostrums included everything from "virgin water" [*l'eau de pucelle*], which could not only cure but prevent venereal disease, to antisyphilic nectar and antivenereal chocolates, which would not interfere with a patient's schedule or lifestyle while the treatment was cleansing the internal organs and revitalizing the external body. A well-to-do or highly placed man, as the case might be, could even cure himself in the presence of his unsuspecting wife as he sucked upon what resembled a dessert each evening.[7] Whether treatments came from market vendors or from surgeons in the prison-hospitals and doctors in private clinics, the *contagion dépopulatrice*, as venereal disease came to be viewed, could not be avoided. It was *le mal de Naples, las bubas, la gross vérole*, a scourge, the antisocial "social disease," a cancer at the heart and skeleton of society.

In that context, this chapter explores a number of interrelated aspects of the venereal contagion, its carriers, and its policing in eighteenth-century France. We will consider the state of medical knowledge concerning venereal disease in eighteenth-century France and treatment at French prison-hospitals and clinics. What was venereal disease to eighteenth-century surgeons, physicians, and to the public? In other words, what were the diagnostic and popular definitions? What was the nosology of venereal disease? How did these definitions find practical application in the standard mercury treatment called the *grands remèdes*? We also will review recommendations for new treatments, the debate within the medical profession, and the widespread charlatanism that characterized French efforts. In the course of the discussion, we will return to people like Marianne. She was among the thousands of women and men who underwent various treatments for the "venereal poison." We will conclude by analyzing the work of Michel Cullerier, among others, and the Hospice des Vénériens where the most medically humane system of eighteenth-century French treatment was established at the end of the century. That humane treatment, however, was a mixed blessing, as revolutionary and Napoleonic officials incorporated *le contrôle sanitaire* into the lives and bodies of French men and women.

Although physicians and surgeons generally accepted that venereal disease had been transported from the New World to Europe by 1495, the French medical community could agree only in general terms on a common definition of the disease. That definition was clearly reflected in the midcentury writings of the widely published and well-respected J.J. Gardane of the Faculté de Médecine de Paris, who had provided French practitioners with a working, albeit flawed, definition. He had written: "The principal and unequivocal signs of a recent venereal contagion are chancres, pustules, lesions, pulpy reddish discharges, inflammations of the mucous membranes, various types of skin eruptions, rashes, and tumors, and pus or milky secretions from the vagina or urethra, while at the same time [the patient experiences] depression and syphilitic bone growths [exostosis]."[8] In his efforts to be inclusive and all-encompassing, what Gardane did not know was that he was describing not only symptoms of the first and second stages of syphilis but also full-scale tertiary syphilis.

In all, the nosology of sexually transmitted disease was still in a stage of medical infancy in which any one of the symptoms that Gardane described was viewed as a manifestation of one venereal infection, a unitary disease. Such proponents were, in fact, called unicists. Although some medical practitioners had begun to question this position, the profession in France was nonetheless dominated by unicists. Gardane's writings simply reinforced a long medical tradition based on a series of earlier works, including a lengthy treatise by Jean Astruc of the Faculté de Médecine de Montpellier. Astruc's work, which was considered a classic analysis in France, had summarized all of the symptoms of the venereal contagion that one might find both at the beginning and at the end of the disease, including gonorrhea or discharges, tumors, lesions of the genitalia, and rashes or warts.[9] There was little effort to separate the various symptoms, and in spite of the wealth of what appeared to be sophisticated and erudite theses and dissertations on venereal disease, study was far from accurate or complete. Gonorrhea, for example, was typically considered an external secretion of a syphilitic contagion, and skin diseases like scabies and psoriasis were often confused with third-stage syphilitic rashes, gummata, and nodules.[10] Furthermore, physicians showed little concern for the incubation period, leading to vast errors in treatment. Not until the nineteenth century did members of the medical profession clarify their serious definitional and therefore diagnostic errors.[11]

Although French physicians generally did not make a distinction between gonorrhea and syphilis, let alone the variety of other venereal conditions that existed, the vocabulary of the nonmedical community frequently did reflect a limited differentiation. For very visible cases of venereal disease à la Gardane's description, a broad portrait of the sufferers in the extreme might be painted. They were *gâtés, gangrènes, vérolés, pourris à la moelle* [decaying, gangrenous, poxed, rotting to the very core or bone marrow]. However, if symptoms were minor (e.g., a simple milky discharge from the urethra which today would probably be diagnosed as simple gonorrhea), males often used a less potent vocabulary to describe what had happened. They would note that a common indiscretion had brought such an unpleasant inconvenience; it was innocent *galanterie*. Whether the memoirist was Jacques-Louis Ménétra describing the rudely taken woman whom he had shared with members of his guild as a pseudoinitiation rite or whether the writer was among the lotharios who circulated on the fringes of court society, eighteenth-century libertines considered the frequent discharges and painful urination that they experienced as one of the curable facts of life for active men. In the litany of names, there was even a label for what priests might acquire: "la rhume ecclésiastique."[12]

Along with diagnostic and popular definitions of venereal disease, how venereal disease was acquired was an equally debatable topic in eighteenth-century circles. French medical science had long since separated this "Neapolitan disease" (it was not called the French disease in France) from diseases like Arabic and Greek leprosy and forms of elephantiasis, and medical practitioners no longer dealt in the kind of fanciful speculations about its origin that had included snakes, signs of the zodiac, and bestiality.[13] Yet, the medical profession's knowledge of the disease *qua* disease left a great deal to be desired, and ignorance of the vector of the disease was extraordinary. Only on the most limited scale were physicians correct, e.g., when it came to studies of infants. They noted that venereal disease could be transmitted congenitally from a mother to her offspring. But for the general population the disease vector was not so easily isolated. Unaware that the causative organism of syphilis was the *Treponema pallidum*, they also did not recognize that transmission of the disease was fundamentally through contact with an infected lesion. Once within the body, the infection became systemic, carried through the bloodstream into the organism.

Without that knowledge, theories of the transmission of the disease varied extraordinarily, described in colorful hypotheses. According to the theory of a doctor attached to the French navy, venereal disease was acquired only in the presence of a *fluide électrique* that was set off by certain types of movements: the rhythmic rubbing of coitus, the friction of kissing, even flickering eyelids. Obviously Le Bru, the author of the theory, had been influenced by Mesmer and the hotly debated but fashionable experiments with animal magnetism. Although his theory was widely known, it was not placed among the most credible theories of transmission.[14] Those more widely accepted theories included the presence of various types of parasites that brought on the disease, including "tiny living worms" that copulated, causing the spread of contagion, and minuscule corpuscles that penetrated the body and then disturbed the sensitive balance of the humours.[15]

What remained the most common explanation of the cause and spread of venereal disease was a belief that a corrosive acid or "virus vérolique" existed. According to *James's Medical Dictionary*, which Denis Diderot had translated in 1747, the virus in question was an "active, penetrating poison" that was "an extremely subtle sulphurous fluid, or . . . an ethereal and fermentative phlogistic principle, which by its communication infects the other fluids of the body."[16] According to the popular theory, the disease emerged from the mixture of differing semen in the woman's vagina. When another male engaged in intercourse with her, the action of their coitus created an acidic fermentation, making the coitus impure and ultimately diseased. Gnawing ulcerations, degeneration of the body, and ultimately putrefaction would result. At the base of the theory was also a general agreement that women's internal organs harbored the contagion.[17] As historian Erica Marie Benabou noted, "From there came the notion of women's corruption and major responsibility in the disease."[18]

Although the medical profession seemed obsessed with venereal disease, the treatment of venereal disease in eighteenth-century France posed serious problems. Among the approximately fifty hospitals and clinics in the city of Paris, for example, few treated pox-ridden subjects of the French kingdom. The options, in fact, were less than minimal: the *dépôts de mendicité* for the non-Parisian poor and marginal people; prison-hospitals like la Salpêtrière and Bicêtre for the Parisian poor, incarcerated, and miserable; and clinics for those on whom experiments would be conducted or for those who could afford the various treatment regimens.[19]

In the case of Paris, diseased women, including poor, insane, and criminal women as well as prostitutes, were sent initially to la Salpêtrière, an imposing prison bordering the Seine, southeast of the markets and the Place Maubert on the Left Bank. At la Salpêtrière, at any particular time, there could be from four to five hundred *femmes publiques,* felons, and petty criminals, some of whom were diseased and some of whom were not. Because of the closeness of their confinement, efforts were made to separate healthy women from diseased inmates, but little effort was made at la Salpêtrière to provide any treatment. Only the gynecological and medical examinations were conducted there. In the meanwhile, female inmates were regimented into confessions three times daily. If their behaviors and bearings were not appropriately penitent and contrite, they could also be whipped and beaten. There in the confines of the prison, women inmates were assigned to sleep six to a bed in beds actually constructed for four; they were shaved, given clogs and coarse tunics to wear, and fed bread, water, and occasional broths or several ounces of meat. The rooms, five feet in height, had no cross ventilation and remained humid and infected with the fetid odor of dirty linens year-round.[20]

For these *vénériennes* and for males who were poor, insane, mentally deficient, hopelessly untrainable, or criminal, or who carried the venereal poison, their final lodging for treatment was the prison-hospital known as Bicêtre. This institution stood on a hill near the Bièvre outside the barriers of Paris between Villejuif and Gentilly. From the late 1750s until 1792, venereal disease treatment was a leading responsibility of the staff of Bicêtre, which quickly became known as a "tomb of humanity," a vast *oubliette,* a place of fearsome unhealthiness and overcrowding. To memoirist Louis-Sébastien Mercier, Bicêtre was a "terrible ulcer on the body politic."[21] Its mortality rate in treating venereal disease reinforced that image: 15 percent for women and 13 percent for men.[22]

The conditions of treatment at Bicêtre varied dramatically depending upon a patient's circumstances of admission. Volunteer patients, for example, were housed on the ground floor and first floor in areas called the Miséricorde and the Salle des Remèdes. They were first on the registry for treatment, a system that admitted only fifty-six men and fifty women at two-month intervals. Although there was a formula for selecting each group of patients, including criteria such as voluntary admission, seniority, and severity of the disease, no one doubted that admission to the *grands remèdes* was manipulated by money and requests from highly placed friends.

Prior to the Revolution, it was customary for the inmates of Bicêtre to begin treatment with "moral purification." This moral purging, or whipping, was believed to allow the body to be opened to treatment. As Michel Foucault theorized in *Folie et déraison,* venereal disease had come into the Age of Enlightenment "more as impurity than as illness." The treatment, which was severe and administered severely, "was a medicine," Foucault continued, "which, all at the same time, fought disease at the expense of health and favored survival of the body at the expense of the flesh."[23] For the involuntary patient-inmates, in particular, punishment and cure were constructed to go hand in hand. Even for voluntary patients, the *grands remèdes* by themselves could be devastating.

Once patients had been admitted to the *grands remèdes,* they were bled, purged, and bathed for three days. Although bleeding and purging tended to weaken the patient, it was generally believed that the body, especially the digestive tract, needed to be cleansed before mercury could be administered. Common purgatives included potassium tartrate, jalap, and senna. A very light diet was recommended and stringently enforced once mercury treatments began. Forty-eight hours after the last cathartic and after a series of baths, the patient typically began oral (internal) consumption of various derivatives of mercury or applications (external) of various ointments of mercuric oxide.[24] The extent of external or internal use of mercury depended upon the temperament of the patient: external for an active, passionate person and internal for an inactive, calm person. Furthermore, the external application might take the form of rubs, plasters, fumigations, baths, or frictions while a patient consumed liqueurs or syrups containing mercury.

At Bicêtre, two treatments were used most often in combination, beginning with two spoonfuls of *mercure sublimé corrosif* [mercuric chloride] taken twice daily with milk or various syrup and marsh weed concoctions. On the following day, between the morning and evening ingestions of mercuric chloride, external application of an ointment made from crude mercury and well-washed pork lard began. On the first day of the external application, the ointment was rubbed on one side of the body from thigh to groin. The next day brought precisely the same treatment. Thereafter, the opposite side of the body received the rub, then an interval of a few days was observed, and the ointment was applied to other parts of the body. After the final treatment, the body was purged again and bled. According to instructions, only the stomach and the back did not receive the ointment. In sum, the treatment included four purgatives over a period of four weeks, and it employed three ounces of ointment and twenty-four grains of mercuric chloride.[25] The *grands remèdes* took approximately six weeks to conduct, but most patients spent far longer at Bicêtre awaiting the treatment and recovering from it.

The value of mercury treatment was certainly its effectiveness in curing venereal disease, but the costs of the cure in human suffering were high. The ingestion of mercuric chloride (favored by French practitioners), mercuric liqueurs, and various other drugs made from mercury caused side effects that were frequently consequential: eruptions in the mouth, nausea, vomiting, problems with eyesight, and ulcerations of the digestive tract. The ointments, because of the amounts of mercury contained in them, also produced massive salivation, which was designed to eliminate the venereal venom but which also destroyed the gums and teeth and frequently caused long-term dysentery.[26] Away from those Dantesque places like Bicêtre, it is not surprising that tested and untested alleged cures and blatant charlatanism abounded.

The advertisement proclaimed: "The public should take confidence in the success of a new 'vegetable' which has cured a multitude of persons and which has been favorably reviewed by some of the most distinguished practitioners of the medical art. This remedy purifies the blood in the gentlest, surest, and most prompt manner, and is the least costly. It is an infallible cure for all types of venereal diseases including the oldest, most inveterate, and even the allegedly incurable types." According to this notice, which appeared in the *Journal de Paris* and which was entitled simply "Antisyphilitic," the price of the antivenereal vegetable juice was three livres for a four-ounce bottle. Six bottles were sufficient for a recently acquired bout of venereal disease; eight were required for an inveterate case.[27]

This advertised antisyphilitic "vegetable essence" was but one of the many cures, some spurious and some serious, that were hawked, debated, and sold to individual patients, soldiers, and the administrators of poor houses, clinics, hospitals, and prisons during the eighteenth century. Therapeutic duels were frequent; lampoons could be found printed in everything from the press to medical scholarship. Whether it was the Nègre de Mondragon's vegetable-based treatment (which Marianne experienced), antivenereal aphrodisiacs, or prophylactic ointments, there was a wide market for any concoction that might cure venereal symptoms without side effects. The difficulty of monitoring this freewheeling but increasingly dangerous marketplace came from at least two sources: physicians, who tended to close the door to innovation particularly if it came from outside the *facultés de médecine,* and the public, which demanded better treatments. In both cases, the result was an open invitation to charlatanism.

A wealth of studies have chronicled the rivalries among physicians, surgeons, barber-surgeons, and empirics in the eighteenth century.[28] What is significant about that rivalry is the general detachment of physicians from clinical medicine, leaving a vast arena for experimental medicine. For example, physician Jean Astruc, famous for his classic work *De Morbis venereis* on venereal disease, had written a manual on obstetrics without delivering a single baby. Another physician, Philippe Hecquet, had written his *Traité de la peste* in 1722 without visiting a single victim of the plague.[29] The debate among the various ranks within the medical profession commanded most of the literature of the century and left the various contingents, particularly the physicians and surgeons, pitted against each other. In the meantime patients—who might be volunteers, pensioners, wards of the state, or inmates—were ultimately both under the care and at the mercy of French practitioners.

As physicians railed that only members of their august body had the right to deal with venereology and as surgeons reminded the public of their practical training, venereal disease treatments and drugs flooded the market. Experiments were ubiquitous, both on willing and unwilling participants, and medical literature carried some of the most vitriolic debates of the century. That debate on venereal disease, not surprisingly, was highly charged for a number of reasons. The contagion was well known to affect all portions of society from the newborn, to innocent wet nurses or wives, to aging dowagers, to common and well-placed males, to "les vénus des carrefours" and to their clients, who might be soldiers or other habitués of their rooms and brothels. The debate was also laden with controversy because of the medical reputations that could be made or broken and the financial rewards that could be reaped in a market avid for cures.

Among the offerings of the 1760s, for example, were antivenereal dilatants, guaranteed nonmercurial treatments, vegetable juices, and other easily used substances that allowed victims to care for themselves. Between 1772 and 1782, nearly fifty requests were filed with the monarch's representatives for permission to test new drugs and treatments. Not surprisingly, the most common place of experimentation was Bicêtre where, as one medical historian wrote, "the poor devils who had been conducted to Bicêtre because of their pox were stuffed with Keyser's drugs on one day, another day asphyxiated by Charbonnière, or poisoned by the Tisane Caraïbe of the gentleman de Mondragon."[30]

Fumigations, for example, which were identified early in the century with Charbonnière and later with Pierre Lalouette, required extensive monitoring of equipment, heat, and mercury vapors, which were taken into the pores and orifices of the body, allegedly curing the disease. Lalouette's patent, granted by the crown, authorized a saunalike fumigation box and pierced chair that left the head unexposed to the mercury vapors that would "pass easily through the pores of the skin and penetrate the blood stream." Four hundred patients ultimately paid Lalouette for their chance at health while seated inside his device. Although fumigation chambers were discussed extensively and were widely available in private clinics, percutaneous absorption of mercury showed little effectiveness.[31]

As far as the dilatant "candles" or *les bougies uréthrales antivénériennes* were concerned, they were supposed to work in a similar manner as fumigations but in more confined areas. Among the more interesting experimental items of the century, the dilatants were composed of a boiled and then dehydrated concoction of olive oil, red wine, and pigeon or chicken combined with beeswax, walnuts, spermaceti, diabotanum, and burned and powdered shoe leather. The concoction, spread on linen and rolled and cut to whatever size the maker desired, allegedly dilated and purified the urethral canal when used as directed.[32] The cure was far less dislocating or costly than appointments in a fumigation chamber situated within the private clinics of Paris.

The market was filled with further curious creations, including Guilbert de Préval's *eau fondante*, which protected men and women from venereal disease by changing color "at the simple nearness of the virus," and the most widely known alleged nonmercurial cure of the century, which came from a partnership of Paul Boyveau and Raffart de Marsilly. *Le Rob antisyphilitique de Boyveau-Laffecteur* was marketed in perhaps the most sophisticated manner of any offering. Its printed instructions bore the seal of approval of the Société royale de Médecine and described the process of the cure as a ceremonial, from administering the first warm laxative drink, to the choice of garments to wear, to the staging of possible bleedings and purgings. At twenty-four livres a bottle with two to three bottles recommended for a simple venereal discharge and eight to twelve bottles recommended to cure more inveterate syphilis, there was great wealth to be made from its successful sales.[33] The offerings did not stop there. Another purveyor of panaceas, named Le Fébure de Saint-Ildepont, publicized his treatment, alleging that each man could be his own doctor while taking his "chocolate aphrodisiacs which are as effective as they are pleasant to take." Playing on humankind's desires for simple cures for complex problems, the marketplace was becoming instead a very expensive consumer's nightmare. "The work of ingenious men," wrote Paul Delaunay in his study of the changing medical profession, "was to turn mercury into gold or silver."[34] It was not alchemy to which he was referring. Charlatanism reigned supreme.

In the decades before the Revolution, as alleged cures proliferated, so did experiments authorized by the royal authorities. The first medical practitioner to come under review was a former army surgeon-major named Royer. To prove the efficacy of Royer's antivenereal baths, two inmates from Bicêtre were chosen. In a virulent exchange of opinions after treatment failed to cure the selected patients, the government's representative, J.J. Gardane, labeled

Royer's efforts not only insufficient but dangerous.[35] Gardane asserted that to suggest that something was a cure when it was not, in fact, sent contagious individuals back into the life of the community. Such an act, he asserted, was both medically unsound and immoral. Royer replied that professional rivalry had doomed his invention. Even Keyser's drugs, which had become standard treatment in the military from the 1750s on, came under review, although they previously had been exempted from research because they contained mercury. Keyser, who had hoped to lessen the caustic nature of venereal treatments, recommended a solution of mercury meticulously diluted in acetic acid. When Keyser's drugs were placed on trial using four women at Bicêtre, the treatment was as devastating to the system as other mercury remedies: among the side effects were colic, diarrhea, fevers, nausea and vomiting, and ulcerated mouths to the point of gangrenous tissue. One of the four women suffered a miscarriage. Although the government did not charge Keyser with outright charlatanism, as had been the case with Royer, it could not ignore the rate of mortality. Keyser's drugs remained on the market but with serious caveats.[36]

While some voices demanded more monitoring of treatments, others demanded additional incentives for research and broader testing. Still others, knowing that mercury remained the most effective cure, wanted greater care in its further development so that side effects could be minimized. In a century of virulent debate, massive innovation, charlatanism, and inflammatory discourse, most physicians and occasional surgeons noted that the toll from mercury-based treatments was too high and that the numbers of victims continued to increase. If contemporary Jean Stanislas Mittié was correct, there were 200,000 *vénériens* and *vénériennes* in France. Something simply had to be done.[37]

In the last two decades of the eighteenth century, important changes took place in the treatment of venereal disease in France. Among those changes were the expansion of the number of private and public clinics caring for aristocrats, *haute bourgeoisie*, and the poor, the creation of the Hospice de Vaugirard for infected children along with the provision that pregnant women could receive treatment through the Hôpital-général, and the relocation of the prison *salles des remèdes* from Bicêtre to the Hospice des Vénériens. No longer could the extent of the scourge be ignored. The *contagion dépopulatrice* had to be tempered; its ravages against the French population had to be stopped.

In private and public clinics men like de Horne, who had followed the progress of Marianne at la Petite Pologne, maintained extensive practices. In the decade between 1776 and 1786, in fact, de Horne treated nearly two thousand nonincarcerated diseased French men and women, with only seventeen fatalities. At the government's request, he then published a comprehensive catalog of types of treatments, costs, results, and side effects, based on case studies, followed by recommendations concerning treatments.[38] A gangrenous disease was eating away at the health of France, he argued; it was not a disease solely of prostitutes but of "respectable people" as well. Remedies had to be made available—remedies that were not equally as devastating as the disease itself.

In the pages of de Horne's multivolume work, one meets the ultimately incurable Henriette whose tumorous and ulcerated condition was vile. After four and a half months of treatment including eighty-six antivenereal baths, six gros of mercurial pills, four gros of pills made from the popular compound of Belloste, and various amounts of lotions, calming drinks, and digestives, Henriette was released. Her ulcerated condition had healed to massive scarring and her bone growths were less pronounced, but the gummata remained untouched. There was nothing that could be done for her without imperiling her health further by subjecting her to a more severe regimen of mercury treatment that might also prove unsuccessful; in the end la Salpêtrière would probably be her home. Another patient was Marie, age twenty-six, who had just delivered a child. Within six weeks, after having taken four ounces of mercury into her body through frictions that were as gentle as possible because of her fragile condition, she was released as cured. Her child, however, was not so fortunate. Delivered with secretions in its eyes, its sight was severely damaged. Then there was a nineteen-year-old Parisian, Marie Elisabeth, who was battling her fourth bout of venereal disease. Although the symptoms were extensive, de Horne believed her case to be curable and recommended the use of mercuric chloride along with a regimen of purgings and moderate salivations. Her doses were carefully monitored to avoid side effects, and five weeks later Marie Elisabeth left the clinic. The roseolas had long since disappeared from her skin, there was no sign of a discharge, and the tumorous condition was gone as well. De Horne tracked her case further because of her history of the contagion and reported that the symptoms had not returned nor had she experienced long-term disabilities from the treatment.[39] Patients who received treatment from de Horne or other physicians like Gardane outside of the walls of Bicêtre had been the fortunate ones.

Efforts of men like Gardane and de Horne were significant in promoting a more humane regimen of treatment, but their work was limited. If venereal disease was destroying the "present race," it was also destroying the future population of France, and emergency measures were necessary. The Hospice de Vaugirard was one such measure, created to deal with the problem of newborns and infants who were infected with the venereal poison that was believed to be depopulating France. Fear of infection among wet nurses, infants, and their mothers was common. Gardane, for example, even asserted that wet nurses who carried the contagion could give it to their own children simply by sleeping with them or by sharing a spoon.[40] At Vaugirard, their treatment was strictly monitored with meticulous cleanliness and minimal doses of mercury, and infants carrying the disease were breast-fed solely by women who already carried the disease themselves. Vaugirard was not alone in awakening the French to the extent of the disease; an entire literature emerged condemning the wet-nursing industry and its ties to the spread of the venereal poison.[41]

The most significant French initiative concerning venereal disease, however, came in 1784 when Minister of the Interior Breteuil visited Bicêtre, whose distressing reputation had continued to grow. According to some reports, "fathers [even] took their daughters there in order that they would become 'disgusted by vice' and by the foulness of those who committed the vice."[42] The center of the debate had, in fact, become prostitution. What Breteuil found worse, however, was the stench of the closed corridors and humid pest-ridden rooms where straw mattresses and sheets were never changed and where the walls were black with filth and corroded by the presence of the ubiquitous quicksilver.[43] Finding the treatment of patients barbarous, Breteuil requested that they be transferred to another institution. The *lettres patentes* for the new institution were granted in 1785, setting aside a recently vacated building on the rue Saint-Jacques for "the poor of any age, of either sex, who have been attacked by venereal disease." This former convent of the Capuchins, which was finally occupied as the Hospice des Vénériens in 1792, was to provide a more humane treatment for carriers of the disease, whether they were prostitutes, miscreants, libertines, or innocents.[44]

For *most* victims of the venereal poison in Paris and particularly in the provinces, treatment had been arbitrary and experimental or entirely too expensive and therefore lacking. The new Hospice des Vénériens was intended to standardize treatment, to make it more available, and to become a model for other institutions. Even the location of the hospice was more suitable for medical care than Bicêtre had been. It was located south of the center of Paris in an area filled with low walls and gardens that did not impede the circulation of air or the view of the countryside farther to the south. Of the original twenty acres which had belonged to the former religious order, the government had retained about nine acres for the hospital. The rooms for treatment were not only larger than those at Bicêtre but they also had cross ventilation. Service areas were paved, promenades were planted with grass and shade trees, and the women's baths contained separate tubs. Perhaps even more important was the strict internal organization, which required careful record keeping, absolute separation of the sexes, and classification of the patients by age, condition, and complications.[45] The official assigned to oversee the operations, Michel Cullerier, had formerly been stationed at Bicêtre, that "tomb" of humanity which he had been powerless to change.

While mercury derivatives remained the proven remedy for venereal disease, Cullerier preferred to avoid the excessive use of the most stringent mineral treatments like mercuric chloride. Instead, he diluted his compounds and combined them with sudorifics. He also insisted that medication be given three times per day and that diets be improved to include a pound and a quarter of bread, a half pound of cooked meat, and a quarter liter of bouillon and milk each day, alternating the meat every other day with dried vegetables in winter and fresh greens and vegetables in summer. If the rations of solid food were decreased, then additional fluids, particularly bouillon, would be provided. He further recommended that the number of baths to reduce inflammation and rashes be increased. Mortality at the Hospice des Vénériens reflected his new regimen: only 2 percent.[46]

In the ledgers of the Hospice des Vénériens one finds Marie Dubuisson, age twenty. She came from the provinces but had been unable to find enough work as a laundress, so she had turned to prostitution during the three months before her incarceration. The treatment, using more diluted solutions in less quantity than would have been applied at Bicêtre, took 169 days or nearly six months.[47] For prostitutes like Dubuisson who had contracted the contagion, average treatment took nearly ten weeks; for nonprisoners and nonprostitutes, the treatment required less than half that time. Another victim, Julie Sabot, who had lived in Paris since the age of eight, was nineteen years old and allegedly working in the garment trade when she was admitted for venereal disease treatment. Showing serious skin eruptions, possibly venereal but certainly degenerative, she ultimately died. She was among the very few fatalities under Cullerier's care.[48] At the Hospice des Vénériens, one out of every forty-eight women who received treatment would not survive, rather than one out of seven as had been the case at Bicêtre.[49]

At the Hospice des Vénériens, Michel Cullerier had instituted his new order, consistent with the broader French revolutionary efforts to institute a regime of public health [*un contrôle sanitaire*]. This "Plan de constitution pour la médecine en France" spelled out an ideal *police de la médecine*, which would be organized by department so that epidemics and contagions could be handled with more expediency. The sweeping recommendations, most of which were finally incorporated into French law under the Directory and Napoleonic governments, included the supervision of all manner of liquid and solid consumables, surveillance of epidemics and contagious diseases, the care of those who had been rescued from asphyxiation drowning, the regulation of mineral waters, drugs, and medications, the suppression of charlatanism, the protection of public health by monitoring all establishments that affected workers and citizens (e.g., burial chambers, mines, marshes, sewers, canals, slaughterhouses, and butcher shops), as well as the general oversight of conditions in correctional houses, prisons, hospitals, and clinics.[50] In the case of monitoring venereal disease, which was cited among the epidemics of France, prostitution had become nearly the exclusive concern after issues of newborns and infants had been dealt with.

According to government officials, the spread of the contagion had to be curtailed, and France's population had to be restored. Police sweeps were authorized with impunity, not so much to sequester prostitutes over the long term as to subject them to *visites* so that treatment could be mandated and monitored if they were diseased.[51] An allegation or suspicion of soliciting, an inability to provide character witnesses, or the failure to have steady employment or a stable address added to the same police conclusion: the woman's entire body would be searched for any telltale signs of venereal disease. Prostitutes had been defined as "virtual vénériennes,"[52] and the *visite* had become absolute. By 1798 under the newly created Bureau Central of the Paris police, physicians established territories in the city, and extensive public records were kept on every gynecological examination, mandated or voluntary. Dispensaries were established, and between 1802 and 1805 the examination system was expanded, laying the basis for the nineteenth-century system of registered prostitution and venereal disease control.

While no statistical evidence exists to show whether or not the new methods of treatment and the policing of venereal disease proved effective in reducing the extent of the "epidemic," the numbers of victims seeking remedy and those unfortunates who were forced to undergo treatment increased dramatically. The number of admissions, for example, doubled at the Hospice des Vénériens between 1792 and 1810 while the death rate declined significantly.

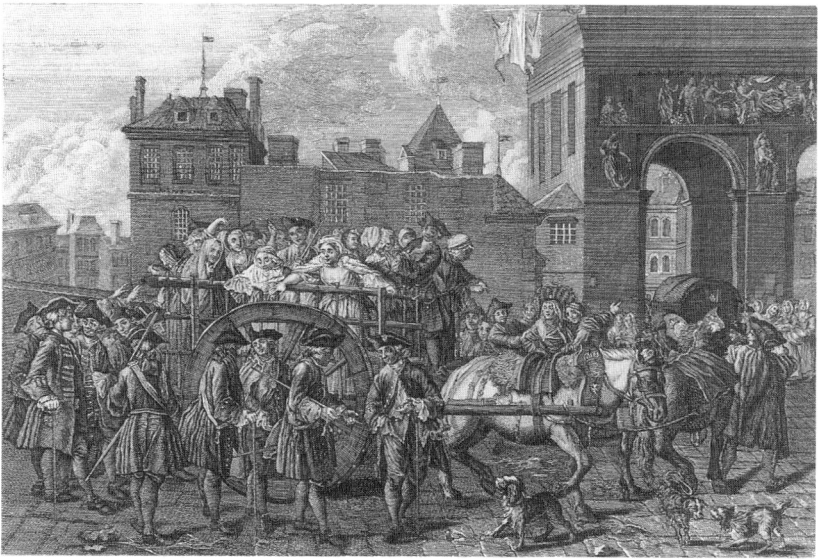

Fig. 2. Jean Benoit Winckler, "Le transport des filles de joye à l'hopital." Harvey Cushing/John Hay Whitney Medical Library, Yale University.

Even though unicists maintained control of authorized medical treatment in France and mercury remained "king," the "desolate picture," as one medical historian described it, of "women with the pox having series of abortions, decrepit children who survived looking like little old men, the eruptions which covered their bodies" became less the norm.[53] What replaced it was a more humane medical treatment, but that medical treatment was only created by expanding surveillance over individuals and their space, including, in the case of mandated *visites,* the very interiors of their bodies. In France, issues of social disease had ultimately become issues of social control.

NOTES

This research was made possible through the assistance of a research grant from Central Michigan University and a Travel to Collections grant from the National Endowment for the Humanities. I would also like to thank colleagues from Central Michigan University, the staff of the library of the Centers for Disease Control (Atlanta), and Craig Caldwell, M.D., for their assistance and suggestions on earlier drafts of this essay.

1. *Effets de la Tisane Caraïbe proposée la guérison des maladies vénériennes par le Nègre de Mondragon* (Paris, 1779), 79.

2. See Paul Delaunay, *Le monde médical parisien au dix-huitième siècle* (Paris, 1906), 234 ff.

3. Georges Morin, "Quelques bizarreries de la thérapeutique antisyphilitique au XVIIIe siècle," *Paris médicale,* no. 50 (1928): 508.

4. See, for example, Erica Marie Benabou, "'La maladie antisociale': le 'danger vénérien' à Paris au XVIIIe siècle," in *La France d'ancien régime: Études réunies en l'honneur de Pierre Goubert,* 2 vols. (Toulouse: Société de démographie historique, 1984), 1:47-54; Erica Marie Benabou, *La prostitution et la police des mœurs au XVIIIe siècle* (Paris: Librairie Académique Perrin, 1987); Jean Charles Sournia, "L'idée de police sanitaire pendant la Révolution," *Histoire des sciences médicales* 22 (1988): 269-75; Claude Quétel, *The History of Syphilis,* trans. Judith Braddock and Brian Pike (Baltimore: Johns Hopkins Univ. Press, 1990); and Georges Morin, "Quelques bizarreries," 507-11.

5. Voltaire, as cited by Alfred W. Crosby Jr., "The Early History of Syphilis: A Reappraisal," in *Social History of Western Civilization,* vol. 2, *Readings from the Seventeenth Century to the Present,* ed. Richard M. Golden (New York: St. Martin's, 1992), 1:222.

6. Bibliothèque nationale, Ms Fr.6062. S. Hardy, "Mes Loisirs ou journal des événements tels qu'ils parviennent à ma connaissance," 293.

7. Le Fébure de Saint-Ildephont, *Le médecin de soi-même ou méthode simple et aisée pour guérir les maladies vénériennes avec la recette d'un chocolat aphrodisiaque aussi utile qu'agréable par M. Le Fébure de Saint-Ildephont . . .* (Paris, 1775).

8. J.J. Gardane, *Manière sûre et facile de traiter les maladies vénériennes* (Paris, 1773), 1:17. A similar description is found in M. Vigarous, *Observations et remarques sur la complication des symptomes vénériens avec d'autres virus et sur les moyens de les guérir* (Montpellier, 1780), 8-9.

9. Jean Astruc, *Traité des maladies vénériennes traduit du Latin de M. Astruc* (Paris, 1777), 1:349.

10. Kenneth Clegel, "Changing concepts of the nosology of gonorrhea and syphilis," *Bulletin of the History of Medicine* 48 (1974): 574-75.

11. According to most historians of medicine, it was not until 1837 that American-born French doctor Philippe Ricord separated gonorrhea from syphilis as two distinct sexually transmitted diseases. This helped explain the phenomenon noted by some eighteenth-century surgeons: mercury treatments alone cured syphilis but had no effect on gonorrhea. The disease organisms of gonorrhea and syphilis, however, were not isolated until 1879 and 1905. Blood testing, which was begun in 1906, further aided in diagnosing the separate sexually transmitted diseases. See *Syphilis: A Synopsis* (Atlanta: Bureau of Disease Prevention and Environmental Control, 1968); and Vern L. Bullough, "Women, birth control, prostitution and the pox," *Transactions of the Conference Group for Social and Administrative History* 6 (1976): 20-28.

12. Erica Marie Benabou, *La prostitution et la police des mœurs*, 424-25; Jacques-Louis Ménétra, *Journal of My Life* (New York: Columbia Univ. Press, 1986).

13. Daniel Turner, *Dissertation sur les maladies vénériennes, ouvrage pratique, traduit de l'Anglois du Docteur Turner* (Paris, 1767), 2. See also Ludwig Fleck, *Genesis and Development of a Scientific Fact* (Chicago: Univ. of Chicago Press, 1979), 2; Theodore Rosebury, *Microbes and Morals: The Strange Story of Venereal Disease* (New York: Viking Press, 1971), 25 ff.; *Syphilis: A Synopsis*, chap. 1.

14. René Burgun and Paul Laugier, "Histoire des maladies vénériennes," *Histoire de la Medécine* 4 (1978): 303.

15. Antoine Deidier, *Dissertation médicinale sur les maladies vénéneriennes* (Paris, 1735).

16. *James's Medical Dictionary*, vol. 4, trans. Denis Diderot (Paris, 1747), quoted in Quétel, *History of Syphilis*, 78.

17. Ithier Menard, "Traité des maladies vénériennes," Bibliothèque de la Faculté de Médecine (Paris), Ms. 58, 18.

18. Benabou, *La prostitution et la police des mœurs*, 424.

19. Olwen H. Hufton, *The Poor in Eighteenth-Century France, 1750-1789* (New York: Oxford Univ. Press, 1974), 306.

20. A.N. F^{15}1816, "Réponses aux demandes faites par le Département des hôpitaux au sujet de la Salpêtrière, 19 mai 1790"; Louis Boucher, *La Salpêtrière: Son histoire de 1656 à 1790, ses origines et son fonctionnement au XVIIIe siècle* (Paris, 1883), 47-48.

21. Louis-Sébastien Mercier, as quoted in Christine Bertollier, "La population de l'Hospice des Vénériens entre 1792 et 1794, situation antérieur et evolution de l'hospitalisation," (master's thesis, University of Paris, 1973-74), 9.

22. A.N. F^{15}1816, "Bicêtre."

23. Michel Foucault, *Folie et déraison* (Paris, 1961), 105-6.

24. Michel Auguste Cullerier, *Notes historiques sur les hôpitaux établis à Paris pour traiter la maladie vénérienne* (Paris, Year IX [1801-1802]), 44-45.

25. Gardane, *Manière sûre et facile*, 1:33-38.

26. Pierre Lalouette, *Nouvelle méthode de traiter les maladies vénériennes par la fumigation avec les procès-verbaux des guérisons opérées par ce moyen* (Paris, 1776), 4-5, 10-11.

27. "Antisyphilitic," *Journal de Paris*, 21 June 1792. Purchase of the "suc végétal" could be made by contacting M. Naudier, Médecin, rue de Rohan, no. 64, Paris.

28. Laurence Brockliss, "Medicine," in *French Higher Education in the Seventeenth and Eighteenth Centuries: A Cultural History* (Oxford: Clarendon Press, 1987), 391-411; Laurence Brockliss, "L'enseignement médical et la Révolution française: essai de réévaluation," *Histoire de l'éducation*, no. 42 (May 1989): 79-100; Toby Gelfand, *Professionalizing Modern Medicine: Paris Surgeons and Medical Science and Institutions in the Eighteenth Century* (Westport, Conn: Greenwood Press, 1980); W.F. Bynum

and Roy Porter, eds. *Medical Fringe and Medical Orthodoxy, 1750-1850* (London: Croom Helm, 1987); and Paul Delaunay, *Le monde médical parisien.*
29. Brockliss, "L'enseignement médical," 90-91.
30. Delaunay, "Les cypridologistes," in *Le monde médical parisien*, 271.
31. Lalouette, *Nouvelle méthode*, and L. Elaut, "Les fumigations de mercure dans le traitement de la vérole: nouvelle méthode thérapeutique de Pierre Lalouette," *Histoire des Sciences médicales*, 11, no. 1-2 (1977): 80-88.
32. Delaunay, "Les cypridologistes," 252.
33. According to reports, the city of Brest, a seaport filled with sailors, consumed some 452 bottles of the ointment, providing an income of approximately 11,000 livres. See *Rapport sur l'analyse du Rob antisyphilitique du Sieur Laffecteur* (Paris, 1779); Laffecteur, *Recueil de recherches et d'observations, sur les différentes méthodes de traiter les maladies vénériennes, et particulièrement sur les effets du remède connu sous le nom de Rob anti-syphilitique* (Paris, 1797); and Henry Chaumartin, *Cythère XVIIIe siècle* (Paris, 1952), 30n. 23.
34. Delaunay, "Les cypridologistes," 279.
35. Royer's case was laid out in his work, *Nouvelles observations dans les hôpitaux militaires de la marine etc. pour constater la sûreté et l'effecacité des lavemens anti-vénériens* (London and Paris, 1771), 218 pp. Among the early assaults on baths was J.J. Gardane's *Mémoire sur l'insuffisance et le danger des lavemens anti-vénériens, pour faire suite aux recherches sur les différentes manières de traiter les maladies vénériennes* (London, 1770), 35 pp. The extensive debate on various mercuric and nonmercuric treatments can also be found in the writings of Turner and Jean Stanislas Mittié.
36. *Le Préservatif ou avis au public sur les dragées anti-vénériennes du Sr. Keyser* (n.p., 1756). See also Keyser's reply, *Lettre de M. Keyser à Mxxx, Docteur en Médecine servant de réponse à un faux article inseré dans le Journal Economique* (Paris, 1757).
37. Bibliothèque historique de la Ville de Paris (BhVP) Ms 941366, Stanislas Mittié, "Lettre adressée à la municipalité de Paris par M. Mittié, Docteur-Régent de la Faculté de Médecine."
38. De Horne, *Observations.* This two-volume catalogue was dedicated to Lieutenant-général de police Lenoir who authorized and supported his efforts to monitor drugs and venereal disease treatments. See also de Horne, *Instruction sommaire sur le traitement de la maladie vénérienne dans les compagnes* (Paris, 1797).
39. De Horne, *Observations*, 358, 405.
40. Gardane, *Manière sûre et facile*, 98-100.
41. See, for example, F. Doublet, *Symptômes et traitement de la maladie vénérienne dans les enfants nouveau-nés* (Paris, 1781).
42. BhVP, Ms 18400, pp. 15-61, cited in Benabou, *La prostitution et la police des mœurs*, 413n. 4 and Archives de l'Assistance publique (A.Asst. pub.), Ms D-256, "Recherches historiques sur l'Hôpital des Vénériens par M. Demay, jeune, chef du Bureau des hôpitaux, 2e division" (1830).
43. Em. Richard, *La méthode légère par extinction ne fut appliquée à Bicêtre qu'à partir de 1777*, cited in Delaunay, "Les cypridologistes," 238.
44. Michel Auguste Cullerier, *Notes historiques*, 41; and Berthollier, "La population de l'hospice des Vénériens," 44-45.
45. Cullerier, *Notes historiques*, 56-58.
46. Ibid., 65-66.
47. Archives de la Préfecture de Police (A.P.P.) A^92 (7 October 1793) and A.Asst.pub. 7.78 (7 October 1793).
48. A.P.P. A^93 (24 frimaire II) and A.Asst.pub. 7.78 (25 frimaire II).

49. Cullerier, *Notes historiques,* 66.
50. Sournia, "L'idée de police sanitaire," 272.
51. See Susan Conner, "Public Virtue and Public Women: Prostitution in Revolutionary Paris, 1793-1794," *Eighteenth-Century Studies* 28 (winter 1994-95): 221-40.
52. Benabou, "'La maladie antisociale,'" 53.
53. Quétel, *History of Syphilis,* 104.

Chapter 2

From Courtesan to Prostitute

*Mercenary Sex and Venereal Disease,
1730-1802*

Kathryn Norberg

Pox, the great [vérole, grosse]; . . . a virus which infects the body . . . rarely cured; . . . experience shows that not everyone who cohabits with an infected woman acquires the disease.

Courtesan; a debauched woman; much honored in Antiquity.
—*Encyclopédie*

IN DIDEROT'S *ENCYCLOPÉDIE*, THE WORDS *PROSTITUTE* AND *POX* REQUIRE NOT one but two separate entries. Under *pox*, the *Encyclopédie* discusses the virus and its symptoms, different cures, transmission to children, and effects on children. Virtually nothing is said about mercenary sex. "Public women" are discussed under a separate entry, that of "courtesan." Here the great *hetaerae* of Antiquity—Aspasia, Phryne, and Laïs—pass in review, but the common streetwalker (who certainly existed in the eighteenth century) is never mentioned. Her appearance is even more fleeting in the entry "prostitute." To prostitute, the *Encyclopédie* tells us, "is for a woman to give her body out of greed or libertinage" or "for a man of letters to write for money." Literary "prostitution" is then explored for several paragraphs; no more is said about the common, streetwalking whore. It is as if the prostitute—plebeian and diseased—did not exist.[1]

To a certain degree, she did not. Certainly, women sold their bodies nightly on the rue St. Honoré and in the Palais Royal as even the most casual reader of Rétif de la Bretonne or Mercier knows. But this woman was called a *fille du monde* or just a *fille*, and she was lovely and alluring, not diseased. Policemen, policymakers, and novelists could talk about prostitutes without mentioning that unfortunate consequence of venal love, the pox. The "venus of the crossroads" did not summon up images of sores and lesions.

This was certainly not the case in the nineteenth century. Syphilis and prostitution were inseparable. For Alexandre Parent-Duchâtelet and the other social hygienists of the July monarchy, "prostitute" was not an occupational category. It was an epidemiological group, what we would call a "risk group." As Jan Zita Grover has remarked, this notion of a risk group is far from innocent or "scientific." A risk group is a cultural concept that can (as it has in the AIDS epidemic) "isolate and condemn people."[2] Nineteenth-century hygienists subjected prostitutes to sequestration in official bordellos, to police surveillance, to arbitrary arrest, and to imprisonment in euphemistically named "hospitals" in the name of public health. Nineteenth-century moralists blamed "prostitutes" for everything from the fall of nations to the demise of the family, but mainly they blamed them for spreading "social diseases."[3] By 1848, France had an elaborate and expensive system of "sanitary regulation" designed to contain "social disease" by controlling the "social evil"—that is, prostitutes.[4]

The association of mercenary sex with venereal disease dates from the Empire and Restoration but has roots in the late eighteenth century. Between 1769 and 1802, important changes in attitudes toward mercenary sex and venereal disease occurred that drew together the whore and "her" disease, syphilis. Seemingly unrelated trends—the distress over depopulation and the hystericization of the female body (to use Michel Foucault's expression)—encouraged the marriage of the prostitute to venereal disease. This union was cemented in 1802 when the Parisian Dispensary was founded and police surveillance of prostitutes, complete with periodic health checks, was instituted. In slightly less than fifty years, the prostitute had become a health problem, a biological threat defined by syphilis.

However hard it is for us to believe, early-eighteenth-century men did not invariably link women of loose morals with syphilis or consider disease the most problematic aspect of venal love. Certainly, they knew that sleeping with a prostitute brought a risk of disease. Diderot is a case in point. In 1762, he recalled a summer thirty years before when he had barely escaped the deadly embraces of his neighbor in a Parisian rooming house. This alluring *fille de débauche* had casually offered Diderot her charms, but he resisted. "By the special Grace of Providence ... I escaped an accident at which the libertines laugh but which makes me shudder."[5] Physicians too knew that prostitutes brought special risks. La Mettrie used intercourse with prostitutes as a kind of empirical device to determine what kind of man is most likely to acquire syphilis and under what circumstances.[6] And French authorities had developed measures to deal with prostitutes' venereal disease. Since at least 1705, surgeons subjected arrested prostitutes to pelvic exams, often despite the women's fierce resistance. The infected were sent to a special hospital—la Salpêtrière—where treatment for venereal disease constituted part of the punitive regimen.[7]

Still royal officials, men of letters, and physicians did not regard prostitutes as the sole vector of the disease or its only victims. Prostitutes appear rarely in medical literature. Medical tracts from Turner to de Horne are happy to speculate on the origins of syphilis and attribute it to an exotic "other," to "dark skinned beauties of Zanguebar" to use Linguet's ironic but accurate description.[8] Otherwise, Enlightenment syphilogists had nothing to say about whores. They were more interested in offering cures that would attract a wealthy clientele. Astruc, for instance, says virtually nothing about whores and a great deal about respectable men and women.[9] Royal officials also tended to view syphilis as a scourge of the respectable and dishonorable alike. The principal Parisian hospital for the treatment of syphilis—the Bicêtre—was not destined for prostitutes but for anyone too poor to pay a private surgeon. When in 1775 the Parisian authorities offered to treat anyone suffering from syphilis for free, Bachaumont praised the initiative because it alleviated the suffering "of a most numerous and essential part of the nation."[10] If respectable workingmen caught the pox, so too did nobles and lords. As one poet explained:

> O Syphilis! O peste cruelle!
> Que ses ravages sont affreux!
> Que de cons désolés par elle
> Et que de fouteurs malheureux!
> C'est là le mal de l'opulence.
> Le mal français par excellence.
> Le mal commun dans tout pays,
> Le mal des prudes, des coquettes,
> Des duchesses et des soubrettes,
> Des portefaix et des marquis.[11]

For eighteenth-century men (to paraphrase Nougaret), syphilis was the disease that "all estates endure."[12]

Anybody, libertines and married women, working men and marquis, contracted syphilis, and the prostitute was not (yet) singled out as a biological threat. Prostitution was technically illegal (though widely tolerated), and whores were subject to unpredictable arrests and roundups.[13] But these measures were meant to secure the public peace, not protect public health. La Salpêtrière, where prostitutes were incarcerated and treated for syphilis, was more a prison than a hospital. It served as the major house of confinement for female criminals of all kinds, not just prostitutes, and it housed murderers, thieves, and banished women. Nor was la Salpêtrière regarded as the principal syphilis hospital of the capital. The Bicêtre hospice where both men and women received treatment had that honor.[14] Institutionally, prostitutes and the pox did not occupy the same space.

Nor did the fictional whore necessarily bear the marks of disease. The most famous prostitute in eighteenth-century literature is undoubtedly Manon Lescaut. The heroine of Abbé Prévost's 1731 best-seller, *L'Histoire du Chevalier des Grieux et de Manon Lescaut,* is typical of the literary whore. Manon is a curious creature, childlike and wily at the same time. She is "a study in opposites," to cite one literary critic, a charming creature who is sweet if inconstant, loving but also greedy.[15] She is paradoxical, and Prévost invests her with a mysterious, inscrutable quality. Whatever she is, Manon is certainly not diseased, and when she dies it is not of the pox but of love for her protector, the young des Grieux.[16] Manon's successors are just as robust. Rozette, heroine of Godard d'Aucour's *Thémidore,* is dangerous: she forces the hero to break with his family and defy aristocratic convention. But she does not infect him.[17] Similarly, Rosalie, Lucette, Mlle Cronel, and the other actresses, courtesans, and "girls" who enliven eighteenth-century fiction enjoy nothing if not good health.[18] Which is not to say that they are innocuous; on the contrary, they are scheming and devious. But they are beautiful and healthy, "right out of Boucher, Baudoin, or Fragonard," according to one critic.[19] When they attack the hero it is his heart, not his health, that suffers.

Even less likely to be diseased are the numerous refined and intellectual ladies of Antiquity and the Orient who play a little-appreciated role in eighteenth-century literature. As Pierre Fauchéry has remarked, the Enlightenment writers frequently cast their prostitutes as either sultanas or *hetaerae*.[20] Prévost, Benoit, Durand, Blain de Sainmore, and de Sacy to name but a few placed their novels in the harem or in ancient Greece.[21] The great courtesans of antiquity, Aspasia, Phryne, and Laïs, were particularly popular, and dozens of anonymous novels and stories sang their praises. Indeed, as late as 1772, Thomas undertook a spirited defense of the old-fashioned *hetaerae,* whose contribution to the arts and letters he deemed invaluable.[22] Nowhere in these texts does disease appear, and this is not just because syphilis was unknown in Antiquity. Smallpox, a common surrogate for syphilis, does not mark the bodies of these heroines, nor do they suffer a disfiguring and punishing death. On the contrary, most of the courtesans endure nothing worse than a broken heart, and they end their days in peaceful retirement enlivened by literature and art.

The pox does appear where one would least expect to find it: in the pornographic or libertine novel. In this genre, pox comes on the stage rather frequently and without masks or metaphoric veils.[23] The libertine whores—La Cauchoise, Eulalie, and la Duchapt—each have one bout with the "pox." Usually infection is the reward for an unpleasant encounter. La Cauchoise is given "the clap" by a *croc* (a client who refuses to pay for her services). She is not, however, dismayed. She calls for her surgeon, who assures her that her "retirement" will be brief and then has anal intercourse with her. She then exchanges *bons mots* with the man who infected her, getting the upper hand at least textually. To avenge herself on a cruel world, she gives the disease to a frisky cleric and then consoles herself in the arms of a young provincial who makes love to her despite her illness "because he would get it from me or someone else, what does it matter!"[24]

The prostitute may get sick, but she does not die of her pox. Recovery is ensured at the hands of either a doctor or surgeon whose treatment and mistreatment of the patient occupies a lot of textual space. Indeed, the pox often seems to be a pretext to bring a physician onstage who can then be mocked and derided. Sometimes, the surgeon ends up sleeping with his patient thereby catching the pox himself. Sometimes he insists on "knowing" the prostitute in unusual ways in order to avoid disease. Sometimes he is a base empiric; other times a learned professor. In any event, his remedies provide comic relief and a chance for the author to make fun of the medical profession. In Nougaret's *Lucette,* Lucette's illness precipitates a long scene in which four physicians quarrel over her nearly dead body. She is finally cured but only by a surgery student "who knew neither Galen nor Hippocrates by heart and who did not try to distinguish himself by big words." The triumph of "the messenger of the Gods" is complete, and Lucette comes out of her bout with the pox diminished but undaunted. Certainly, her charms do not escape untouched. Her complexion suffers. She is thin and "rattles around in her corset." She has lost her "freshness." She is, Nougaret tells us, "ugly enough to scare a person." Her cure, more than her disease, has cost her some of her charm, but not for long. She finds a wealthy bishop for a protector and returns to her old life "thanks to a little makeup, a whisper of lipstick and a deadly *mouche* well placed."[25]

Prostitutes might be "peppered," but their disease occasioned only momentary inconvenience, and their radiant looks hardly suffered. Eighteenth-century writers liked to think of their whores as beautiful creatures "made to be painted" [*faites à peindre*] even if they were also diseased women ready to be cured. Mademoiselle de la Chanterie, *L'Observateur anglais* reports, was "a chorus girl at the Opera, a rare beauty, an ingenue, a female angel." So lovely was la Chanterie that artists used her as a model. One painter borrowed her features for an altar picture of the Virgin, and the resemblance was striking. So striking, *L'Observateur anglais* reports, that a former lover remarked upon seeing the picture, "There is the Virgin who gave me the clap!"[26]

While the irony here is meant to provoke laughter, it reveals an essential truth: eighteenth-century whores were not diseased prostitutes but delicious courtesans closer in their looks to virgins than strumpets. The equation between mercenary sex and pox was not yet complete; graceful opera dancers, intelligent Aspasias, robust Rosalies, and healthy Manons graced French literature until the final third of the century.

Between 1767 and 1790, the diseased streetwalker emerged from the background to stand beside the elegant courtesan. She did not immediately eclipse her healthier and wealthier rival: as late as 1760 Turmeau de la Morandière had little to say about syphilis and less about streetwalkers in a long diatribe against courtesans.[27] But beginning in 1767, a set of proposals for the control of venereal disease through the regulation of prostitution appeared that focused on the common whore and "her" disease. These texts were not numerous—four at most—but they pointed to a new association between prostitutes and pox.

The earliest was Rétif de la Bretonne's *Le Pornographe ou les idées d'un honnête homme sur un projet de règlement pour les prostituées* published in Paris in 1767.[28] *Le Pornographe* was one of Rétif's first works and would remain one of his most infamous. The book is a curious mixture of epistolary novel, journalism, history, and political proposal. It liberally mixes fact and fiction, and the central part of the work—the proposal for the reorganization of prostitution—partakes as much of daydream as of social engineering. Nevertheless, here was a new portrait of the whore, a picture of a "prostitute," who is a streetwalker. *Le Pornographe* includes a painstaking analysis of the hierarchy of whoredom, and every class of prostitute from the highest—the *filles débauchées*—to the lowest—the *barboteuses*—pass through the text. But of the twelve "estates" of prostitutes described by Rétif, seven concern women who must sell their charms on the street. Rarely—if ever—had common hookers [*raccrocheuses*] received so much attention. Rétif does believe that courtesans are dangerous, but so too are the "dirty and diseased" streetwalkers with their "charming smile but infected breath" [180-81].

"The horrible malady which prostitution propagates," Rétif says, is the foremost of a "crowd of dangers that prostitution occasions" [41-42]. The streetwalker is not just dirty [*malpropre*]. She is also diseased [*malsaine*]: "poison circulates in (her) veins" and "she is dangerous because she infects the men she captures" [180-81]. The principal goal of Rétif's imaginary whorehouses, or Parthenions, is to extinguish disease. "Here is a nearly infallible means of eliminating the venereal leaven and of chasing that monster out of Europe" [157]. Rétif subjects every prostitute in his Parthenion to periodic pelvic examinations by specially trained matrons. Those found diseased will be strictly sequestered until cured.

Rétif's scheme with its closed houses of prostitution and health checks comes close to nineteenth-century regulation of prostitution, and no less an expert on social hygiene than its father, Parent-Duchâtelet, claimed Rétif as a forebearer.[29] But Rétif's proposal is fundamentally different from Parent-

Duchâtelet's in that it springs from different concerns, concerns unique to the late eighteenth century. For Rétif, syphilis is not a danger in and of itself; it is part of a larger peril, that of depopulation.[30] Syphilis is "contrary to population"; it infects "the descendants of humanity" and leads to "a deformed progeny."[31] Syphilis saps the vital energies of men and leads inexorably to "degeneration" and depopulation. Careful provision is made in Rétif's ideal whorehouse for the offspring of mercenary encounters. A special wing of the Parthenion is devoted to them, and Rétif himself devotes pages to how and when they will leave the house. The children are in fact key: if the extinguishing of syphilis is one of Rétif's goals, the cultivation of new subjects is even more important. At the Parthenion, "subjects otherwise lost to the world will be saved," and abortion will be punished by solitary confinement and a diet of bread and water. If nothing else, the prostitutes—"a crowd of beautiful girls"—will now be mobilized for the "use to which Nature destined them," that of procreation.

Rétif's obsession with depopulation summoned up a host of other anxieties. He bemoans the artificiality of manners, the spread of luxury, and the ill effects of urban life.[32] We need not dwell on these "perils to humanity" longer than to note that they, like syphilis, led directly to the prostitute. In eighteenth-century thinking, the whore was a creature of the city who wallowed in luxury and displayed a sweet but deceitful face. Venereal disease and prostitution were just one part of this larger degeneration of morals that produced depopulation.

A similar array of anxieties prompted an anonymous tract on syphilis, "Projet raisonné et moyens immanquables pour arrêter le progrès, empêcher la circulation et détruire jusqu'au principe des maux vénériens dans toute l'étendue du royaume," published in London in 1769. Like Rétif, the author is principally concerned with depopulation: "the corruption of the race," he claims, produces "that infinite number of weak, languishing, disfigured, disabled, and retarded individuals who are not capable of reproducing anything but their own deformations and imbecility" [5]. Syphilis is a part of this "decline": the "venereal germ" attacks both body and mind, leaving its victims unable to father healthy children. But syphilis is so closely related to the evils of urbanity as to be indistinguishable from the city itself. "When people remained in the provinces," the author observes, "no one knew about venereal disease." Paris, it appears, is the locus of infection, and the principal carrier is the Parisian whore. Innocent provincials curious to see the capital fall victim to the "nymphs" who "cover their poison with an alluring disguise." As soon as they return home, the provincials "make a present of what is called a gallantry to their wives or mistresses." The only solution, believes the author, is to cordon off Paris and subject all the prostitutes in the capital to periodic medical examinations [11]. The provinces will then be saved from Paris and the kingdom from the scourge of depopulation.

Fear of depopulation also inspired an anonymous pamphlet entitled "Code ou nouveau règlement sur les lieux de prostitution dans la ville de Paris" which was published in 1775. The author claims that Retif's *Pornographe* prompted him to write his text, and there is no reason to doubt him: the two books are almost identical in their recommendations. Like Rétif, the anonymous author condemned cities as sinks of iniquity and points to venereal disease as one cause of depopulation. To be sure, other "poisons" are also at work: luxury and too much delicacy have enervated the French, and the perversion practiced in bordellos has turned them away from procreative sex. Where the two authors differ is on how to deal with prostitution: the anonymous author would have it banned rather than regulated.

A strong case for regulation is made in the last and perhaps most persuasive of venereal disease tracts, *La santé de Mars,* published in Paris in 1790 by a Dr. Lecointe. Lecointe believes that the strength of nations is tied to the good health of armies. France, he argues, is vulnerable on this point. He deplores the filth in military hospitals and the need for better treatment on the battlefield. The ravages of syphilis are just as serious. He recounts an incident at a camp near Metz where one prostitute served over sixty cavaliers. "This brave trooper," he explains, "expired after sixty assaults, but it took only a week in the hospital for her to recover her health." Her "cavaliers" were less lucky: "Of the sixty who had commerce with her, fifty-eight acquired the pox." Lecointe asks, "How many brave soldiers are lost to this dreaded disease?" "Enervated," they cannot fight nor can they father the next generation of soldiers. Venereal disease weakens the system, and the joys of fatherhood pale by comparison to the venereal pleasures offered by prostitutes. "Paris contains forty thousand courtesans who do nothing but distract young men from their duties. What has happened to good families, to morals, to Nature?"

Again, depopulation is the result of this decay in morals. By removing attractive women from the pool of mothers and by distracting young men from their biological duty, prostitution deprives France of babies. Lecointe suggests setting up closed houses of prostitution in most garrison towns. Here strict hygiene would be observed, and all prostitutes would be periodically checked for disease. In these bordellos, soldiers could relieve their sexual tension without peril to their health or undue loss of reproductive fluids. Like Rétif, Lecointe is at pains to make allowances for the children that these institutions would produce. Indeed, he considers the offspring of his houses their greatest virtue. "Why," he asks, "should the strongest, most valiant soldiers not produce equally robust children?" Indeed, the male children could serve in the military thereby strengthening the army and the nation. Female children would be recycled back into the military bordello, so that they too could contribute to the "replenishing of the population."[33]

Reading these texts, one scholar has concluded that Frenchmen were seized in the late eighteenth century by a fear of syphilis of "panic" dimensions.[34] "Panic" is certainly too strong a word, and if there was a "panic" it concerned depopulation, not venereal disease. Still, the anxiety over depopulation had profound effects on perceptions of both syphilis and prostitution. The sources of depopulation—luxury, cities, and prostitution—tended to merge with venereal disease and make syphilis as problematic as falling population. At the same time, when linked to depopulation, syphilis ceased being a personal misfortune and became a social and political problem. Now more was at stake than the ill health of a few libertines; the fate of the kingdom was hung in the balance. Vigorous state intervention could now follow.

At the same time, the depopulationist panic colored views of those who contracted syphilis, including indirectly prostitutes. The worry over depopulation caused eighteenth-century physicians to invent a new category of syphilis sufferer—children.[35] These "innocent" victims benefited from the only real institutional "advance" of the period: the Vaugirard hospital for syphilitic infants created in 1780.[36] And one might expect these "unfortunate" children to have encouraged public toleration and acceptance of all syphilis sufferers whatever their age. But the opposite occurred. As AIDS activists have pointed out, the creation of an "innocent" category of victims only increases the turpitude of the "guilty."[37] Next to children, prostitutes looked more debauched and degenerate than ever before.

In fact, prostitutes were increasingly identified with syphilis, and syphilis was increasingly regarded as a visible sign of hidden moral corruption. This new attitude is particularly obvious in the salacious gazette or libel that flourished in the years before the Revolution. From the *Gazetteer cuirassé* and the *Chronique scandaleuse,* through the *Lettres d'un observateur anglais* and the *Gazette noire,* the telltale lesion unmasked the prodigality of the whore-loving aristocracy. Dukes and counts lavished fortunes on opera dancers who rewarded them with "a gallantry." Mlle Pélin "suffered from a supernatural *épanchement de lait* which she communicated to the Prince de Cont . . . who unknowingly passed it on to Madame the Duchess de B . . . who is capable they say of giving it to everyone."[38] "Mademoiselle Beaumesnil," one scandal sheet revealed, "having allowed a prince of the blood into her bed, has had to ask for six weeks off and will go to Bavaria where the great king Keyser will present her to his court."[39] The Duke of Berwick, another remarked, "infected with a terrible maladie, made a present of it to his flame (Mlle Dufresne)."[40] If the princes were polluted, so too were their princesses. Women of the highest birth slipped into Gourdan's famous bordello, it was rumored, and returned after an evening's dalliance corrupted and willing to infect others. "The public is warned," says the *Philosophe cynique,* "that an infection reigns among the girls of the Opéra and has now reached the ladies of the court who have communicated it to their lackeys."[41]

In these texts, syphilis reveals otherwise hidden decay, and the opera dancer, however aristocratic her ways, is just as diseased as a streetwalker. *L'Observateur anglais* does not hesitate to portray Madame Du Barry as a common prostitute who has "jumped from the bordello to the throne, from the arms of a lackey to those of the king."[42] The king's whore—and by extension the king himself—was no better than a servant, and the palace was just like a common bordello: sordid and diseased. The *Gazetteer cuirassé* took advantage of a courtesan's name—La Cour—to make the corruption of the court explicit: "Mlle La Cour," he tells us, "lost her palate [*palais*] to syphilis." This phenomenon, he goes on, is clearly explained by the following epigram:

> De Keyser craignons les secrets;
> De leur deplorables effets
> La Cour helas! est un exemple;
> Voulant purifier son temple.
> Elle a demoli son Palais.[43]

Syphilis acted as a metaphor for corruption, and the first years of the Revolution witnessed a correspondingly harsh attitude toward prostitution. When in 1791 Pierre Manuel published secret documents revealing that the Parisian police had tolerated—even encouraged—prostitution, a storm of outrage followed.[44] Officially, the new regime condemned prostitution and encouraged the Parisian police to lock up as many streetwalkers as possible.[45] The laws of 22 July 1791 and the municipal declaration of 4 October 1793 banned prostitution outright and authorized the arrest of any women found soliciting on the streets. Still, the repression was not directly linked to disease. "The regeneration of morals" was the stated goal of the campaign against prostitution, and prostitutes were condemned as "corruptors of morals and perturbers of public order."[46] The whore was not yet a medical problem to be dealt with by physicians.

Nor was she portrayed as such in Pancoucke's *Encyclopédie méthodique*, published in 1791. The entry on prostitution, written by former police functionary Peuchet, condemned prostitutes as "disorderly," "indecent," and detrimental to public morals. Like Manuel, Peuchet emphasized the corruption of the old regime police and bemoaned the "bad acquaintances, the poor habits and the counterfeiting of sentiments" that common prostitution encouraged.[47] But Peuchet departed from his predecessors and contemporaries in making one crucial distinction: he separated "private" prostitutes, or courtesans, from "public" prostitutes, or streetwalkers, and argued, like Parent-Duchâtelet a half century later, that only streetwalkers required the attention of the police. Courtesans, Peuchet observed, posed no threat to society and therefore should not be harassed by the police.[48] The common streetwalker, on the other hand, required close surveillance and monitoring. "Common prostitutes" were numerous, visible, and unsightly. Unlike their more elevated sisters, the courtesans, they caused "public scandal" and "disorders." As always the prostitute had to be monitored because she could occasion violence and crime. But Peuchet adds in passing a second "threat." "The hazards to one's health and the terrible consequences of the venereal disease that these prostitutes propagate ... makes this lowly form of prostitution additionally dangerous."[49] Gradually, the streetwalker was coming to dominate the discourse on prostitution, and she was perceived as an agent of disease as well as disorder.

During the Empire and Restoration, medical texts tightened the equation between prostitute and pox by describing the whore's body (syphilitic or not) as inherently diseased and abnormal. To a certain degree, the prostitute suffered the same fate as all women. Beginning with Bienville's famous *Fureurs utérines* published in 1771, medical treatises blamed the female reproductive organs for illness and physical debility. Because of their wandering and inflamed wombs, women suffered from vapors, hypochondria, various mental illnesses, lethargy, and mania. Women were sick by definition and therefore subject to medical surveillance. Because the seat of disease was women's reproductive organs, one wonders, like Yvonne Kneibler, if an extreme fear of female sexuality did not inspire this elaborate medical fantasy and shape attitudes toward prostitutes as well.[50]

In any case, during the Empire and Restoration the debauched woman, the prostitute, was allocated a special place among "diseased" females. Unlike eighteenth-century physicians who considered whores immune to hysteria, Restoration doctors attributed a particularly acute form of the disease to prostitutes. Writing in 1816, Louyer-Villermay asserted that "the abuse of venereal pleasures irritates the sensibilities and places public women in a moral and physical situation that makes them vulnerable to hysteria." "Excessive physical pleasure," he maintained, "far from dissipating hysteria, aggravates it."[51] According to Restoration doctors, prostitutes were "vengeful," "dominating," "whimsical," "changing," and of course "infertile." Even before she contracted syphilis, the public woman was sick, subject to fits, frenzy, even convulsions. Paradoxically, though a hysteric, a prostitute was also "unwomanly." "Prostitutes," Virey argued, "who have lost the appanage of their sex—modesty—are "hardly women at all."[52] Constantly exposed to sperm, prostitutes took on the qualities of men, acquiring "raucous voices," mustaches, and a tendency toward lesbianism.[53] Prostitutes were, in short, freaks, a foreign species best scrutinized by science, that is, by doctors.

The prostitute now belonged to the physicians, and public policy would henceforth treat her as a biological problem. In 1800, the Parisian police hired two physicians to examine prostitutes and inscribe their names in special registers.[54] Two years later the police established a "dispensary" in the rue Croixdes-Petits-Champs where prostitutes could be examined and receive medical help.[55] On 24 December 1810, Prefect Pasquier expanded the dispensary to include seven physicians and brought the institution under the direct supervision of the prefect. The same edict made registration and medical checks mandatory and set up a system of cards that replicated the dual registers already in use.[56] Similar institutions and policies were created in such provincial cities as Marseille and Lyon.[57] By 1812, the Napoleonic prefects had imposed compulsory registration and pelvic examinations on all prostitutes and had limited bordellos and streetwalking to small, officially designated red-light districts. The foundations of nineteenth-century regulation were in place: mercenary sex had become a medical problem and syphilis an object of state policy.[58]

Why was medical surveillance needed at this time? An increase in venereal disease would be an obvious explanation. The defenders of the new regulations did not overlook this argument: most claimed that prostitution and syphilis were on the rise. "The plague of prostitutes has multiplied," claimed one physician, who estimated the number of prostitutes to have grown from ten thousand in 1790 to thirty thousand in 1802. With more prostitutes came more syphilis. In Prairial XIII, one physician estimated "that one prostitute in nine was infected."[59] In 1812, the rate of infection had dropped to 1 in 24, only to rise with the occupation of Paris in 1814 to 1 in 17. Thereafter it declined until 1818 when Parent-Duchâtelet claims that 1 prostitute in 32 was contagious.[60] Even if these statistics are only approximate, they are surprising.[61] In an age that could neither cure nor prevent syphilis, one would expect virtually all prostitutes to be diseased. Anything less than a 100 percent rate of infection would seem surprising especially given the pitch and intensity of anti-prostitutional rhetoric during the Restoration and under the July monarchy.[62]

Statistics notwithstanding, nineteenth-century social hygienists, policemen, and novelists all assumed that every prostitute was diseased. In fiction, even the most elegant courtesan bore a secret infection. Her syphilis was like "an alien miasm, an evil gas that would burst into flame on contact with foreign heat."[63] "A corrosive poison runs through her veins," the hack novelist Cuisin warned.[64] "The disease," he elaborates, "descends on the courtesan from out of the heavens, like Divine justice," and in Cuisin's novel *Les femmes entretenues,* all of the heroines succumb to the "secret ailment." In several instances, the lord's executioner is appropriately a physician. Cuisin's Julie Sélicourt (otherwise known as the "yellow lady" because of her mania for the color) is literally tortured to death by a surgeon. Tied to an operating table, Sélicourt's "rhagades," "pustules," and "tumors" are exposed in the surgical amphitheater to a crowd of avid students: "The greatest silence reigned; the aids were at their posts penetrated with respect for the talents of the great surgeon who once again would display his dexterity; the scalpel, the lancet, and the knife were methodically spread out on the tray; she also saw spatulas, sponges, bandages, compresses, English tourniquets, silk thread, alkali and finally, worst of all, the burning stone for cauterizations."[65] With the instruments of her torture before her, Sélicourt begs forgiveness, but the great surgeon will not relent. She dies of a hemorrhage, imploring Divine mercy for a life of excess and debauchery.

The whore must now die of "her" disease; the equation between mercenary sex and syphilis appears to be complete.[66] Just how complete can be appreciated by looking at the treatment of prostitution in one of the successors to Diderot's *Encyclopédie,* Pancoucke's *Dictionnaire des sciences médicales.* Here in a medical compendium the prostitute is defined by a physician, the social hygienist Foederé. The prostitute is no longer the elegant courtesan of the past nor even a silly, "vaporous" hysteric of Restoration medicine. Now she is nothing less than "a threat to society" [*ennemie du corps social*]. She is the sole vector of syphilis, "a plague," a "disgusting object," "a corruption," according to Foederé. Forced by her metier to haunt the streets, she develops "a raucous, masculine" voice and is wholly degraded by "unwanted and vile caresses." She is bound to die of her pollution, for "virtually all prostitutes are completely devoured by syphilis, . . . their tissues and their humors are impregnated [with syphilis] which become sources of other maladies as well." So diseased are prostitutes that "most exercise their infamous metier for ten years or less and die in great numbers before the age of thirty of advanced syphilis."[67]

Only periodic pelvic examinations coupled with strict police measures can "stem the plague" that these "wretched creatures spread." Certainly, prostitution poses other dangers, especially to "wholesome" and honest women and girls who must be shielded from their contact and their bad example. But here again syphilis is the central problem, for honest women are most threatened by the infections that their unfaithful husbands bring from the bordello to the marriage bed.

Venereal disease is now *the* identifying characteristic of the prostitute.[68] The stage is set for nineteenth-century regulation and its obsessive linking of working-class disorder, female sexuality, and contamination. So lovely in the eighteenth century, the nineteenth-century *fille* is a repulsive figure who threatens to corrupt the very core of bourgeois society. Henceforth, the whore will be "the social evil."

Notes

1. *Compact edition of the Encyclopédie, ou Dictionnaire raisonné des sciences, des arts et des métiers par une société de gens de lettres* (New York: Reacex Microprint, 1969), 3:991. The *Encyclopédie* does cross-reference some things associated with mercenary love like "mauvaise lieu" or bordello. But the whore herself receives scant attention.

2. Jan Zita Grover, "AIDS: Keywords," in *AIDS: Cultural Analysis, Cultural Activism,* ed. Douglas Crimp (Cambridge: MIT Press, 1988), 27.

3. On the scapegoating of prostitutes in America see Alan Brandt, *No Magic Bullet* (New York: Oxford Univ. Press, 1985).

4. On nineteenth-century prostitution see Alain Corbin, *Les filles de noces* (Paris: Plon, 1978) and Jill Harsin, *Policing Prostitution* (Princeton: Princeton Univ. Press, 1985).

5. Patrick Wald Lasowski, *L'Ardeur et la galantrie* (Paris: Gallimard, 1986), 116-17.

6. Julien Offroy de La Mettrie, *Système de Monsieur Boerhaave sur les maladies vénériennes* (Paris, 1735), 51.

7. On treatment of venereal disease in prostitutes see Erica Marie Benabou, "'La maladie antisociale': le 'danger vénérien' à Paris au XVIIIe siècle," in *La France d'ancien régime: Etudes réunies en l'honneur de Pierre Goubert*, 2 vols. (Toulouse: Société de démographie historique, 1984), 1:47-54; Susan Conner, "Politics, Prostitution, and the Pox in Revolutionary Paris, 1789-1799," *Journal of Social History* 22 (1989): 713-34.

8. Simon Nicolas André Linguet, *La Cacomonade: Histoire politique et morale, traduite de l'allemand du Docteur Pangloss, par le docteur lui-meme depuis son retour de Constantinople* (Cologne, 1766), 21.

9. Jean Astruc, *A Treatise of the Venereal Diseases in Six Books Containing an Account of the Origins, Propagation, and Contagion of this Distemper*, trans. William Barrowby, M.D. (London, 1737), 2:78.

10. Louis Petit de Bachaumont, *Les mémoires secrets* 8 (1775): 91.

11. "O syphilis, o cruel plague! Your ravages are frightening. So many sad cunts and unhappy fuckers! You are the disease of opulence, the true French disease. The disease common to all the country, the disease of prudes, coquettes, duchesses and actresses, stevedores and marquises." *Les petites bougres au manège ou réponse de M*** en l'an second du rêve de la liberté* (Paris, 1793).

12. Pierre-Jean-Baptiste Nougaret, *Lucette ou le progrès du libertinage* (1780; reprint, Paris: Fayard, 1986), 360.

13. On prostitution in eighteenth-century Paris see Erica Marie Benabou, *La prostitution et la police des mœurs aux XVIIIe siècle* (Paris: Librairie Académique Perrin, 1987).

14. The Bicêtre like the Salpêtrière had, nevertheless, a variegated population. It housed not just the sick but also male "libertines" (young men whose families wanted them incarcerated) and pimps. See Louis Boucher, *La Salpêtrière: son histoire de 1656 à 1790, ses origines et son fonctionnement au XVIIIe siècle* (Paris, 1883); J. Bernier, *Hôpital de Bicêtre, 1763-1784* (unpublished memoire de l'École des Hautes Études, 1975).

15. On Manon see Philippe Laroch, *Petits-maîtres et roués: Evolution de la notion de libertinage dans le roman français du XVIIIe siècle* (Québec: Les Presses de l'université de Laval, 1969), 70-73. Also important for any consideration of the libertine novel is Jacques Rustin, *Le vice à la mode: Étude sur le roman français de la première partie du XVIIIe siècle* (Paris: Ophrys, 1979).

16. Generally, in eighteenth-century fiction, the pox does not figure as the just reward of a corrupt character, a frequent occurrence in nineteenth-century fiction. One clear exception exists in eighteenth-century fiction: Madame de Merteuil in Pierre Choderlos de Laclos's *Liaisons dangereuses* who is disfigured by smallpox, a clear reference to syphilis. Coming as it does on the eve of the Revolution, *Les Liaisons* manifested a new attitude toward the disease and provided readers with an ongoing critique of libertinage. Merteuil certainly gets what she deserves, the disease "at which libertines laugh," to quote Diderot, but Laclos certain does intend for the reader to laugh.

17. Godard d'Aucour, *Thémidore ou mon histoire* (Paris, 1745; reprint, Paris: Robert Laffont, 1993).

18. Charles Palissot de Montenoy, "Les Courtisanes ou l'école des mœurs," in *Oeuvres complètes de M. Palissot* (Paris: Bastier, 1779), 3:133-73; Chevrier, *Le colporteur* (Paris, 1774); Coustillier, *Lettres à Fillon* (Cologne, 1750); Pierre Alexandre Gaillard de la Bataille, *Histoire de la vie et des mœurs de Mademoiselle Cronel dite Frétillon, écrite par elle meme, actrice de la Comédie de Rouen* (Paris, 1739).

19. Raymond Trousson, ed., introduction to *Romans libertins du XVIIIe siècle* (Paris: Robert Laffont, 1993), 271.

20. Pierre Fauchéry, *La destinée féminine dans le roman européen du dix-huitième siècle* (Paris: Armand Colin, 1972), 439.

21. Abbé Prévost, *Histoire d'une femme grecque* (Paris, 1733); Mlle Bedacier de Durand, *Les belles grecques ou l'histoire des plus fameuses courtisanes de la Grèce* (Paris, 1755); Blain de Sainmore, *Lettre de Sapho à Phaon* (Paris, 1766); Claude de Sacy, *Les Amours de Sapho et Phaon* (Paris, 1775); Jean Castre d'Auvigny, *Histoire et les amours de Sapho de Mytilene* (Paris, 1724); Madame Benoit, *Erreurs d'un jolie femme ou l'aspasie française* (Paris: chez la veuve Duchesne, 1781).

22. Antoine Leonard Thomas, *Essai sur le caractère, les mœurs, et l'esprit des femmes dans différents siécles* (Paris: Moutard, 1772).

23. Eighteenth-century authors were not opposed to piquant euphemisms. The most general term for syphilis and gonorrhea was "une galanterie" (Nougaret, *Lucette*, 359).

24. *La Cauchoise ou mémoires d'une courtisane célèbre* (1784; reprint, ed. Michel Camus, Paris: Fayard, 1985), 456-62.

25. Nougaret, *Lucette*, 370, 409.

26. *L'observateur anglais* (London: John Adamson, 1779), 2:102-3.

27. Turmeau de la Morandière, *Représentations à Monsieur le lieutenant général de police de Paris sur les courtisannes à la mode et les demoiselles de bon ton* (Paris: Imprimerie d'une Société de gens ruinés par les Femmes, 1760). Turmeau devotes only two pages (155-56) to venereal disease in his two-hundred-page tract. He believes that the primary danger posed by courtesans are the excessive spending they provoke and the luxury they cultivate.

28. Rétif de la Bretonne, *Le Pornographe ou les idées d'un honnête homme sur un projet de règlement pour les prostituées propre à prévenir les malheurs qu'occasionne le publicisme des femmes* (Paris: Au Palais Royal, 1767; reprint, Paris: Editions d'aujourdhui, 1983).

29. Alexandre Jean Baptiste Parent-Duchâtelet, *De la prostitution dans la ville de Paris* (Paris: Chez Baillière, 1837), 1:38-39.

30. Which is not to say that traces of the old depopulationist argument don't crop up in *De la prostitution*. They certainly do, but they are not the principal reason for his advocacy of regulationism.

31. Rétif, *Le Pornographe*, 171.

32. For a summary of the late-eighteenth-century critique of the city see Henri Coulet, ed., *La ville au XVIIIe siècle: Colloque d'Aix-en-Provence, 29 avril-1 mai 1973* (Aix-en-Provence: Centre Aixois d'Études et de Recherches sur le XVIIIe siècle, 1975).

33. Jourdain Lecointe, docteur en medicine, *La santé de Mars ou moyens de conserver la santé des trouppes en temps de paix; d'en fortifier la vigueur et le courage en temps de guerre; d'assurer la salubrité des hopitaux militaires; et de produire un surcroit de population suffisant pour tenir complets tous les régimens du royaume* (Paris: Chez Briand, 1790), 101, 219-20, 231.

34. Here I take issue with Erica Marie Benabou. While I heartily agree with her picture of the horror inspired by the syphilis hospitals like Bicêtre, I don't think that there was much fear of the disease itself. Certainly, what anxiety there was never reached the proportions found at the height of the post—World War I scare (Benabou, *La prostitution et la police des mœurs*, 429; Claude Quétel, *Le Mal de Naples: Histoire de la syphilis* (Paris: Seghers, 1986).

35. E. Jeanselme, *Histoire de la syphilis* (Paris: Doin et Cie, 1931), 217-18.

36. On the Vaugirard hospice see Quétel, *Le Mal de Naples*, 133-34; Jeanselme, *Histoire de la syphilis,* 258-65, 365-71.

37. Douglas Crimp, "Thinking about Magic Johnson," paper read at the UCLA Center for the Study of Women, Los Angeles, March 1991.

38. *La gazetteer cuirassé* (1771), ed. Jean Hervez (Paris: Bibliothèque des curieux, 1912), 289, 287.

39. *La chronique aretine ou recherches pour servir à l'histoire des mœurs aux XVIIIe siècle* (1789), ed. Jean Hervez (Paris: Bibliothèque des Curieux,1912), 183-84.

40. *Gazetteer cuirassé,* 309.

41. Ibid., 1.

42. *L'Observateur anglais,* 2:100.

43. "Let us fear Keyser's secrets and their deplorable results; The court alas! is an example; Hoping to purify its temple it demolished its palace" (*Gazetteer cuirassé,* 307).

44. For an example of this outrage see *La chronique scandaleuse* (1791), introduction by Octave Uzanne (Paris: A Quantin, 1879), 219-50. *La Chronique* reproduces many of the documents discovered by Pierre Manuel and subsequently published under the title *La police de Paris dévoilée* (Paris: L'an II). The insights of Pamela Cheek on this and other "unveilings" of police records are pertinent: Cheek, "Prostitutes and Political Institutions," *Eighteenth-Century Studies* 28 (1994-95): 207-14.

45. Susan Conner, "Public Virtue and Public Women: Prostitution in Revolutionary Paris, 1793-1794," *Eighteenth-Century Studies* 28 (winter 1994-95): 221-40; also see her "Politics, Prostitution, and the Pox in Revolutionary Paris, 1789-1799," *Journal of Social History* 22 (1989): 713-34.

46. This legislation is reprinted in Parent-Duchâtelet, *De la prostitution,* 2:55.

47. Jacques Peuchet, "Jurisprudence; police," *Encyclopédie méthodique* (Paris: Pancoucke, 1791), 112:678-94.

48. Ibid., 678. See also the entry by Peuchet under "Courtisanne," ibid., 608-13.

49. Ibid., 679.

50. Yvonne Kneibler, "Les médecins et la 'Nature Feminine' au temps du Code civil," *Annales* (1976): 824-45.

51. M. Louyer-Villermay, *Traité des maladies nerveuses ou vapeurs et particulièrement de l'hysterie et de l'hypocondrie* (Paris: Chez Mequignon, 1816), 37.

52. J.J. Virey, *De la femme sous ses rapports physiologiques* (Paris: Chez Crochard, 1825), 99, 100, 215, and 216.

53. Kneibler, "Les médecins," 835. The reader will recognize in this discourse the same themes that appear repeatedly in Parent-Duchâtelet and subsequently other nineteenth-century social hygienists. On Parent-Duchâtelet see Alain Corbin's introduction to Alexandre Parent-Duchâtelet, *La prostitution au XIXe siècle* (Paris: Seuil, 1981), 9-55.

54. Archives de la police, AD 230.

55. Parent-Duchâtelet, *De la prostitution,* 2:63.

56. Bibliothèque historique de la ville de Paris, "Dispensaire de salubrité: Compte général de surveillance administrative et sanitaire pour l'exercise de 1816," cote provisoire 4476.

57. On Marseille and Lyon see Docteur Hippolyte Mireur, *La prostitution à Marseille* (Paris: Chez Dentu, 1882); Docteur Potton, *La prostitution et le syphilis dans les grandes villes, dans la ville de Lyon en particulier* (Paris: J-B Baillière, 1842).

58. Although there was much talk under the Republic and the Empire about containing syphilis, particularly in the army, not much was actually done. Financial constraints inevitably prevented local authorities from establishing new institutions. However, the prefects appointed by Napoleon probably made the regulation of prostitution possible. The prefects were much more powerful than their predecessors and able to undertake and enact such policies.

59. Bibliothèque historique de la ville de Paris, cote provisoire 4476; F.F.A. Béraud, *Les filles publiques de Paris et la police que les régit* (Brussels: Meline, Cans, 1859), 1:86.

60. Parent-Duchâtelet, *De la prostitution*, 2:128.

61. Indeed, the earlier figures are highly dubious. They are based on a population of only 250 prostitutes, all of whom reported voluntarily to the Dispensary, suggesting that they suspected they had venereal disease (Bibliothèque historique de la ville de Paris, cote provisoire, 4476). It is important to note that Parent-Duchâtelet gives a much higher rate of venereal disease for the *insoumises*, the women who would not submit voluntarily to the dispensary regime. His wholehearted advocacy of regulation makes these statistics also dubious (Parent-Duchâtelet, *De la prostitution*, 2:142).

62. When I have shared these statistics with my colleagues at the UCLA School of Public Health, they are disbelieving. Based on their experience with AIDS, they cannot believe that the rate of syphilis did not approach 100 percent in a population with no effective means of prevention.

63. Pierre-François Cuisin, *Les nymphes du Palais Royal* (Paris: Chez Roux, 1815), 16.

64. Cuisin, *La galanterie sous la sauvegarde des lois* (Paris: Plancher, 1815), 142.

65. Cuisin, *Les femmes entretenues dévoilées dans leurs fourberies galantes* (Paris: Cordier, 1820; reprint, Bruxelles: J-J Gay, 1883), 2:179.

66. Which is not to say that there are not "positive" depictions of prostitutes. The period is in fact particularly rich in such portraits, the most famous being Eugène Sue's Fleur de Marie. But the regulationist mentality did not exclude positive valuations of prostitution. On the contrary, Parent-Duchâtelet himself regarded whores as a "necessary" evil much preferable to a host of others.

67. *Dictionnaire des sciences médicales* (Paris: Pancoucke, 1820), 45:491.

68. Susan Sontag has remarked that some diseases confer "identities" on their victims. Tuberculosis made those who contracted it "sensitive" or "artistic." AIDS makes its victims "perverts." Syphilis appears to have given prostitution its distinctive characteristics in the nineteenth century (Susan Sontag, *AIDS and Its Metaphors* (New York: Farrar, Straus and Giroux, 1989).

Chapter 3

"Laying Aside Any Private Advantage"

John Marten and Venereal Disease

Roy Porter

IT HAS BEEN MAINTAINED THAT ENGLAND UNDERWENT A CONSUMER REVOLUtion in the eighteenth century, resulting in the first consumer society. Even historians who balk at these bold claims can have no quarrel with the notion that England was becoming intensely commercialized, with London its driving force.[1] One element of this transformation was what would today be called a "media revolution"—a startling growth in the output of newspapers, magazines, primers, educational works, advice manuals, and light reading. Not least, "Grub Street" sprang up, the term denoting the actual quarter of the metropolis where journalists operated but also, symbolically, the new trade of hack was born.[2] Drowning in a sea of ink, critics complained that the whole world had turned scribbler: authorship seemed to be the universal means of authentication.[3]

And medicine too was seen to be falling under what high-minded physicians condemned as the pestilential influence of commerce—though, of course, numerous medical entrepreneurs cheerfully availed themselves of new opportunities of making profits out of pain. Supplanting the traditional image of medicine as a rigid tripartite hierarchy, medical historians now tend to speak of the eighteenth-century "medical marketplace," in which healing was practiced more as a trade than as a profession.[4] Largely as a consequence, the boundaries between medical fringe and medical orthodoxy, between regular doctors and so-called quacks, grew enigmatic and furiously contested.[5] Medical publications increased by leaps and bounds with the compiling of potboiling domestic medicine and kitchen physic texts.[6]

In view of the circumstances just mentioned, it is no wonder that a bunch of practitioners emerged specializing in venereal complaints[7] and promoting their practice by ventures into print. Such publications could take diverse forms, ranging from the blaring handbill that trumpeted the charlatan[8] to long-winded learned treatises, festooned with Latinate erudition. Print had become the medium through which to stake claims to fame.

The main features of the venereal disease business in Georgian Britain have been expertly analyzed by Bynum.[9] Over a hundred separate works dealing with the topic were published during the century, and sexually transmitted diseases formed the site of massive controversies between "generalists" and "specialists," between physicians and surgeons, and between regulars and empirics. Venereal diseases constituted a highly lucrative field but one in which, in view of its sensitive nature—it was often called "the secret disease"—it was particularly essential, yet especially difficult, for medical practitioners to establish their bona fides and so convince the doubting world that they were not simply exploiting what James Boswell called "Signor Gonorrhoea" and similar shameful conditions in the manner of arrant quacks. Rival practitioners did not merely denigrate opponents to demonstrate their own superior credentials and skills. They battled over the very concept and essence of venereal infection—not least whether it was one disease or many. Conflict raged as to who was entitled to advance the best authenticated notion of the disorder—the most "scientific," true to experience, philosophical, or simply appealing. The venereal wars involved the very framing of the disease.[10]

One of the most prominent of those specializing in venereal medicine was the surgeon John Marten (d. 1737). Little is known about his early life and career. He claimed to have studied under the surgeon Joseph Green and to have been judged qualified by the Surgeons' Company. He also tells us that he attended the sick and wounded in an Irish hospital. He had a brother, James, who was an apothecary in Thumen Street, while he himself kept an apothecary's shop in Barnaby Street, though practicing from a house in Hatton Garden. He informed readers that he had a flourishing practice and had married a rich woman.[11] Presumably to publicize his practice, Marten became a miscellaneous medical writer, cashing in on the burning medical topics and diseases of the day. His *Attila of the Gout* (1713) addressed one great scourge of high society—a topic to which he returned in *The Dishonour of the Gout* (1737). Such works enjoyed a brief blaze but left no lasting impression.

Yet Marten had the distinction of writing two of the more conspicuous medico-sexual works to appear in early eighteenth-century England. His *Treatise of all the Degrees and Symptoms of the Venereal Disease in Both Sexes*, published in 1704 by S. Crouch and running through several subsequent editions, fully justifies its somewhat boasting title. By its sixth edition it had swollen to over four hundred small-print pages that imparted a mass of medical detail with a certain garrulous eloquence. The sixth edition of that work will be the primary focus of the following discussion, but mention should also be made of his later *Gonosologium Novum, or A New System of All the Secret Infirmities and Diseases*, also published by Crouch, the British Library copy of which is bound up with the sixth edition of the *Treatise* (1708).[12] Drawing very heavily upon—plagiarizing might be the better term—Nicolas Venette's *Le Tableau de l'Amour Conjugal*,[13] this was a manual of sexual information, delineating the anatomy and physiology of the genitals, depicting the sexual act, and explaining generation.[14] Marten's *Gonosologium Novum* thus mapped the terrain of sexual pathology, within which the *Treatise of all the Degrees and Symptoms of the Venereal Disease in Both Sexes* focused on a specific topic, venereal disease, which was barely touched on in the other work.

As its table of contents makes clear, Marten's *Treatise* is divided into four bulging chapters. The first discusses "The Nature, Causes, and Signs of the *Venereal Disease;* the various ways of Infecting, with the Difference and Degrees thereof; the Certainty of knowing whether infected or not, and how to prevent, or hinder Infection." Having thus expounded the nature of venereal infections, he proceeded in his second chapter to explore remedies. To catch the sufferer's eye, Marten made a point of stressing "The easiness of Curing the *Venereal Disease,* and the Reasons why so many daily miss of Cure." To further ingratiate himself with readers, he added "some Directions, whereby the Patients themselves may know when, and when not, they are in safe and skilful Hands for Cure."[15]

Having emphasized the rapidity and reliability with which venereal infections might be cured by proper practitioners like himself, Marten advanced to the polemical core of his work, an assault on quacks and their "cobweb Assurances" [xxxi]. This third chapter was thus devoted to the "Mischiefs caus'd by Ignorant Pretenders"—with some account of rescues he had performed upon those whose health, imperiled by the pox or a clap, had been further wrecked by charlatans. The final chapter continued the tirade against fakes and frauds by drawing the reader's attention to "Old *Gleets,*" that is to say, chronic gonorrhea, typified by whitish urethral discharges, strictures, and burning pissing-pains. Customarily produced through deleterious management by "*Imposters, Cheats, Fortune-tellers, Mountebanks, Doctresses, &c.*" [xxxvi], gleets were harmful in their own right, and they also led to barrenness, thereby frustrating the ends of sexual intercourse. They were widely believed to be irreversible, but, Marten noted, that was merely because "mercenary Miscreants" [xxix] lacked the skill to heal them; in the hands of a "regular honest surgeon," they could be cured.[16]

It would be tedious to try to hack through the thickets of Marten's texts, but it is worth exploring his strategies for establishing his credentials to pronounce on venereal complaints. It was, first, no small claim of his to possess more solid knowledge than other writers: he liked to portray himself as the most learned of writers on such topics. The point was forcefully made in the preface to the sixth edition of the *Treatise*, as he bragged over the swelling size of his *opus*. The first three editions, each running to a thousand copies, had enjoyed, he noted, such brisk demand that no opportunity presented itself between editions to insert revisions. But by the fourth edition, overwhelming desire to be "useful to the Publick" left him with no alternative but to add further information and case histories, "*whereby it became swell'd to more than treble the number of Sheets contain'd in the three former Editions, and the price consequently rais'd from* One Shilling *(which was what they were sold at) to* Two Shillings and Sixpence" [i].

And when a fifth revision was required, the same applied again, and he "*found more and more occasion of amending it, and upon several accounts, saw it also necessary to add some material Matters, that had since occurr'd in my Practice, insomuch, that the Half-Crown Book was throughout interspers'd with many advantageous Things, not taken notice of in the others, and became swell'd to much more than double the number of Sheets contain'd in that* Fourth *Impression*" [ii]. And, once more, when that edition had sold out, he had "*found reason at the same time, (from longer Practice and Experience in the Cure of that* Disease*) to make many further, but notable* Additions *thro' the whole, which tho' to the amount of a fourth part more than the* Fifth *Edition contain'd, yet by its being printed in a lesser Letter, neither the bulk or the price is advanc'd, but continu'd as before, at* Four Shillings, *(tho' according to rate a six Shilling Book, the charge being considerably more) and is the very Book I here present the Reader withal*" [ii].

Size was not everything—Marten also insisted upon the quality of his pen. He made a great parade of his book learning, quoting over a hundred earlier medical authors, Greek, Islamic, and Renaissance alike, and giving numerous pharmacological recipes. He cited such philosophers as Lucretius and "that great man, St Austin," and, not least, sprinkled his text with snatches of verse, Latin proverbs and tags ("mens sana in corpore sano," "habent sua fata Libelli," etc.), to create a show of erudition.[17] And complementing such bookish learning he also stressed the cardinal value of "matters of fact."[18]

Blending scholarship and experience, Marten aimed to display a deeper theoretical grasp of the character of venereal disease than that possessed by sufferers themselves, by rank-and-file practitioners, and, above all, by those disreputable quacks "*who have no other Foundation, than Ignorance and Impudence, to bubble so many Thousands out of their Money and Lives*" [*Treatise*, xxxiii]. To convince his readers, he set about proving that venereal infections were far from simple; indeed, they required a sophisticated grasp of the body system and its susceptibility.

For one thing, venereal disease was far more widespread than met the inexpert eye. A variety of symptoms and debilities, seemingly unconnected with venereal origins, would be discerned by the sharp-eyed inquirer to entail a syphilitic component of some sort, originating perhaps many years previously or even hereditary in nature. Astute diagnostic skills would confirm the truth that "the *Pox* is a Monarch, all other Diseases are its Subjects."[19]

Thus, venereal infections were an iceberg of which only the tip surfaced to public view. Equally, Marten claimed that a subtle theoretical grasp and an experienced diagnostic eye were needed because the disorder constituted "a moveable Disease" [*Treatise*, 94]. Though originating in the genitals, it readily migrated to other locations and organs where inept practitioners would fail to suspect its venereal source. Such disorders and afflictions thus had venereal roots, for "after a long Travel," Marten informed his readers, the pox "fixes at last upon some one Symptom, as a *Hectick, Ulcer* of the *Kidneys* or *Bladder, Consumption* of *the Lungs, Megrim, Node, Tophe, Dropsie, Night-Pains,* &c." [*Treatise,* 225]. Not least, venereal infections were protean in character: claps would turn into poxes, and syphilis into gonorrhea; indeed, infinite individual infections were possible, dependent on different personal constitutions and local circumstances.[20]

Marten thus aimed to convince readers of the sophistication of his comprehension of the disease. Unlike the simpleminded, he was alert to its individual and changeable character. Disorders presented differently in every person, and even then they would be continually migrating, changing location and disposition. Diagnosis was an art requiring special expertise.[21]

A subtle theory was also needed, argued Marten, to master the pattern and pathways of its transmission. A shallow view was abroad—perhaps encouraged by those for whom such doctrines were comforting—that the pox could be caught only from genital sexual intercourse involving penetration and emission. Marten demurred: venereal infections could be acquired through a multitude of more or less sexual acts. In the *Treatise* he cited the case of a gentleman who consulted him with a *"Clap."* Though this had been acquired after picking up a woman at a playhouse, the party nevertheless protested that he had not actually copulated with the woman but had merely been "accommodat'd" by her hand (which he clearly expected to secure safe sex). Marten, however, entertained no doubt that, if the woman were herself infected, it was "possible to get the Infection that way, and that by Friction or rubbing the *Yard* with a warm Hand, just wet with a virulent *Venereal* Matter, the *Pocky* contagious Miasms may enter into the Pores of the erected heated *Yard,* and prove infectious."[22]

The more insidious character of venereal infections proposed by Marten had major implications for therapeutics. Because venereal disorders were not "specific," conforming to a single, direct cause-and-effect model, there could be no "specific" medication. For that reason, the quack faith in a panacea, arcanum, or catholicon was foolish and hazardous.[23] Marten was equally concerned with another consequence of ineffectual, indeed harmful, therapies. Misunderstanding venereal complaints, the ignorant practitioner would tout "cures" that would do no more than palliate or suppress symptoms—that is, stopping the "runnings" commonly associated with gonorrhea or clearing up syphilitic rashes. Such "cures" created dangerous illusions. "The same Mischiefs also often happen," Marten explained. "No Method is more irrational than as the Custom is (for the sake of a quick Cure) to use after five or six Purges, *Astringents* inwardly, or *Restringent*, or Stiptick *Injections*, which stops the *Running*, till the *Blood* is spoil'd and the *Pox* confirm'd."[24] The medicines commonly used failed to cure the disease. They merely suppressed its manifestations, drove the morbific matter inwards, intensified its poisonous qualities, and in the end rendered it chronic and far more perilous.

In short, venereal maladies were intricate and intractable, and it was essential to possess a shrewd grasp of constitutional disorders and therapeutic strategies. By adopting this stance Marten was signaling his adherence to orthodox physiological disease-theory and so confirming he was a regular practitioner, upholding mainstream medical philosophy. As will be noted later, he was also leaving open the possibility of exploiting his concept of venereal disease for panic-making and empire building.

To cap this theoretical adroitness, Marten laid claim to superior bedside experience, much of his book being given over to case histories displaying his practical skills while also giving readers the opportunity both to identify with sufferers (in "before and after" accounts) and to learn how to be a model patient. Recording as they do the give-and-take between himself and patients seeking his aid, there is a typical structure to the narrative of such cases.[25] The sick person solicits help and unfolds his tale of woe. It often transpires that, at some earlier stage, perhaps because of cheapness, embarrassment, or the itch for secrecy, the sufferer had consulted an inept practitioner or quack, who predictably had made bad worse. Once approached, Marten then diagnoses the true nature of the complaint and works a cure, at which point the satisfied patient expresses eternal gratitude and rewards Marten handsomely.

> One poor Fellow in particular, came lately to implore my assistance, that had been in his [a quack's] Hands for a mild *Clap*, many Months, till all his Mony was gone, and render'd worse instead of better, which the *impostor* perceiving, would do no more for him, unless he would bring him more Money, and then he should have a Diet-Drink, which he told him would Cure him: He carried all the Mony he could get, by borrowing a little of one, and a little of another, (being in a Condition not able to follow his Employ to get any) to purchase this Drink, and then bid to come such a Day and he should have it, which

he did, and then was put off till another Day, with the pretence of forgetting it; at another time not leisure to make it, and so drill'd him on, from time to time, for several Weeks, till his Distemper had so advanc'd, that had he not met with my Book and come under my Care, (and who I undertook more out of Charity than any thing else) he might have died in Ditch, (for the care his Doctor took) but, under God I cur'd him, and is now in his Business, as Well, Hearty, and Strong, as ever he was in his Life. [*Treatise*, 261]

This was a narrative style Marten frequently deployed, doubtless because he assumed it would chime with the circumstances of many of his potential patients:

T'other Day there comes a young Fellow to me with a Clap, *for Cure of which he said he had apply'd to the Foreign* Quack *at the Hand and* Urinal *in* Holborn, *who, after managing him according to his skill; and before the Malignity was expel'd, gave him a pint Bottle of Turpentine-drink and a Powder, for which he took ten Shillings, and by which he told him his Running would be stopt, which indeed was so to a tittle, for it was immediately dislodg'd and thrown down upon one of his* Testicles, *to the creating a very big inflam'd and painful humoral Tumour, which if had not been forthwith remedied, or had been under his Outlandish Direction, would have prov'd sufficiently mischievous and dangerous.* [*Gonosologium Novum*, A6]

Though most of the patients thus recorded were male, a few were of the opposite sex (all of whom Marten chivalrously stated had been infected by their husbands). "A Gentlewoman, some time since, came to me by direction of a Friend of hers that I formerly Cur'd," one such tale commenced. This unfortunate lady

had a Venereal Running, *which she got from her Husband, and had been for Cure in the Hands of one of the* Quacks *aforemention'd, who telling her 'twas only the* Whites, *gave her Restringents which stopt it, and told her she was well, she believ'd the same, and paid him three Pounds for doing it; but a while after she fell into Pains, and Breakings out almost all over her Body, and at length complain'd of a Soreness in her Throat and Palate, which, upon inspection, I found to be Ulcerated, both Tonsils and Palate; I put her into a proper method and Cur'd her, which otherwise would have been her Ruin.* [*Gonosologium Novum*, A6]

These narratives incorporate numerous hints, asides, circumstantial details, and other devices designed to display Marten's integrity and competence, while instructing the sufferer in proper medical etiquette: strict obedience, prompt and handsome payment. Above all, it was Marten's literary technique to lard his tales with letters and other documentation purportedly from the hand of the sufferer, praising his nonpareil skills. They might, for example, corroborate his reputation as a celebrated author. *"A Gentleman who was afflicted with Incontinency of Urine, tho' but by Drops or Dribbling, and which was generally foul, and came away with some sharpness, and sometimes had stoppage of Urine, sent me the following Letter from the* Queen's-Arms *Tavern near where I liv'd then,"* Marten informed his readers.

Worthy Sir

THE useful Learning, great Integrity, and universal Compassion to Mankind, you have shown the World in your two Treatises, the one of the *Venereal Disease*, the other in the Translation of Dr. *Greenfield de Cantharidibus,* with large Additions, give me full assurance of speedy help by your Assistance, desir'd by one unknown to your Person, but an Admirer of your Virtues, and

Humble Servant,

X Z, &c.

Be pleas'd Sir, to favour me with your Company at the *Queen's-Arms Tavern* in *Aldersgate-Street.*[26]

Other encomiastic letters did not dwell particularly on Marten's expertise but displayed those attitudes of supplication, expectation, and gratitude he evidently wished to inculcate in would-be patients.

The testimonial was a key weapon in Marten's rhetorical armory. "I have many scores of Letters by me that I can produce," he boasted, *"only concealing the Writers Names, &c. from among the number of which take these that follow (as a Specimen) and be referr'd to more in the Book, from page* 156 *to* 218, *as also from page* 275 *to* 284; *which Letters here, as also those inserted in the Book"* [*Treatise*, iv]. Yet he clearly felt somewhat uneasy about such material, since recourse to testimonials was widely denigrated as the trick of the quack, and it was standardly assumed that such material was fabricated. Marten acknowledged there would be reader resistance to accepting the genuineness of the article, feeling obliged to protest that his testimonial letters *are exactly (as I have observed therein) agreeable to the Originals, as the Printer and his Men can justifie, and as all Persons (unless such that resolve they will not be convinc'd by the plainest Matter of Fact) may be satisfy'd by reading page 218; and I do assure them, that the same (and many hundreds more not taken notice of here) are real and genuine, and were not sent by my Desire or Knowledge, (as some would basely insinuate) for that I knew nothing of, or concerning them, till they came to my hands, which assurance, as I hereby solemnly declare to be Truth, will I think be sufficient to justifie the most scrupulous Person that is.* [*Treatise*, iv]

In the eighteenth-century medical marketplace, establishing public authority was obviously not a simple matter. The author who, like Marten, sought to recruit to his cause the *vox populi*, or at least the patient's voice, could not easily absolve himself from the charge of medical demagoguery or, worse still, the forging of fictions.[27]

In the *Treatise*, as has been seen, Marten deployed the voice of learning and also the voice of the patient, first supplicating and later grateful. A third voice is also prominent—that of salutary warning. Marten presented himself as the guardian of the public good, fired by moral zeal and benevolence to bestow good counsel upon an abused world—an honest man who, at enormous personal cost, was prepared to tell the naked truth against conniving knaves and fools. The nation, according to Marten, was suffering ghastly sexual miseries: impotence, infertility, venereal infections. Such troubles were the outcome of ignorance or misinformation from ignorant quacks, most of whom, after all, were but *"obscure Mechanicks, as* Weavers, Taylors, Nailers, Coblers, Barbers, *or some Broken Tradesmen, that know nothing of the matter, or the Business they undertake, any farther than to get the Money, which they take care to chouse the Patient of, and which is yet much worse, cheat them of their Cure, and too often deprive them of their Lives"* [*Treatise*, 126].

As this and earlier quotations make clear, Marten cast himself as crusading against the quackish infidel. Despite being predatory, greedy, and unprincipled, such rogues had nevertheless become entrenched, possessing a seductive appeal for those suffering from mysterious disorders:

There are a great many People, who under such misfortunes . . . out of a modest reservedness, instead of applying to the Physicians, they in other Cases make use of because they would not that any who know them, shou'd know their Secret Infirmities, *do choose to run to This and That* QUACK *for Cure, and the more obscure he lives, the better as they think it suits their Purpose, and who, upon their assuring them of Cure, they presently trust, till at length they find their Mistake, by their Ignorance and Unsuccessfulness, there being so many* Quacks, Mountebanks, Fortune-tellers, *&c. in the Town, and all pretend to great Matters, that it is a great Chance but they fall into the Hands of one or the other.* [*Gonosologium Novum*, A5]

Marten hence professed himself duty-bound to act as a quack-finder general, identifying those villains and warning the public of their evil ways: *"tis necessary therefore to point out who are* Quacks, *at least those that profess by their Bills distributed about the Town, and pasted up at every pissing Place, the Cure of Venereal and other Diseases, which as they know nothing of, so the People by knowing them, may avoid and shun them*" [*Gonosologium Novum*, A5].

Occasionally quacks were lethal, but their ministrations typically resulted in something far more insidious: they wrecked their clients' health and created chronic maladies that in effect delivered them into their clutches as permanent patients: *"It is by them that many poor Wretches are deluded and bubled out of their Mony and Lives; and if they escape Death, are frequently brought into some languishing condition . . . which by their Villainous management are too often render'd past the Power of Art to rectify*" [*Gonosologium Novum*, A5]. Marten thereby insinuated to his readers that those who found themselves racked by chronic ill health were probably the victims of some form of iatrogenic (i.e., *quack-originated*) disorder. Poor health was a symptom of having frequented quacks.

Marten's blitz on the quacks need not be chronicled in detail. It consists of predictable denunciations of ignorance, self-promotion, duplicity, swindling, and indifference to others' welfare. The point that needs to be addressed here is that Marten himself was roundly and soundly attacked for being the spitting image of what he denounced: a quack. In two pamphlets, *Quackery Unmasked* (1709) and *Venus's Botcher* (1711), John Spinke judged Marten a classic case of the pot calling the kettle black. Marten's *Treatise*, Spinke charged, was nothing other than "one large quack bill."[28]

Marten might be regarded as having invited such retribution, since his writings abounded in the faults he found in his foes. He accused quacks of ad hominem sniping, yet he did just that himself in jingling verses:

> For *Quacks* by Shoals, with Boldness in this Place,
> As *T——g, W——ll, K——us* Doctor *C——e,*
> *S——k, C——m,* and *N——y,* and th' rest o'th' *Quacking* Crew;
> Practice for Gain the People to undo.[29]

It was in the nature of quackery to puff up one's abilities and magnanimity, and every quack, Marten revealed, stuck up bills in "Pissing-Places," boasting his profound Skill in the Art of Physick, and his Charitable readiness to assist the languishing Poor, and the like; and among the many thousands of great Cures in every Distemper that he tells you he has perform'd, acquaints you at last, what Success he has had in the *Pox,* how he has Cur'd Thousands thereof, making the Conditions of them, which he tells you he has Cured, so lamentably bad, (altogether Incredible but with the Vulgar) that none but himself was able to Cure them, and that if he had not undertook them, they could never have been Cur'd, &c. [*Treatise,* 254-55]

Blowing one's own trumpet was thus a mark of quackery. Yet what else was Marten doing in page after page of his own work? *"But taking no more notice of Letters here, and laying aside any private Advantage,"* he confided at one point to the reader, *"I may fairly, and I think without Ostentation, assert, That the Benefits which have accru'd to many hundreds by means of this* Treatise, *are so extraordinary, that otherwise they might have been led on in Ignorance, not discerning whether they were in the* right *or* wrong *Method of Cure, 'till the succeeding ill Symptoms and Effects had too plainly made manifest, they were rendred incurable"* [*Treatise,* xv].

Likewise, Marten denounced nostrum mongering as a mark of quackery. Yet he also promoted his own arcanum, the "tinctura gloriosa" or his "grand preservative" (price 7s. 6d.), which he promised would keep buyers pox-free even if they were to have sex with infected companions.[30] Marten also laid himself open to the other charge repeatedly leveled against contemporary medical popularizers: that of being a closet pornographer, one of the growing tribe of Grub-Street hacks shamelessly pandering to the market for titillation by exploiting filth under the guise of medical necessity and the public interest.[31]

Marten was as lurid and sensational (yet also coy) as any. In his discussion of the diverse modes of contracting venereal infections, he noted that these were not exclusively heterosexual, gratuitously elaborating the point while denying he was so doing. One way of catching "the *Venereal* Infection," he observed, was by "one Man's conversing with, or having the Carnal use of another Man's Body, *viz.* B———ry, an abominable, beastly, sodomitical and shameful Action; an Action, as its not fit to be named" [*Treatise,* 68]—though of course Marten both named it if, through studied ellipsis, he didn't quite do so. Indeed, he had no compunction about describing in copious detail those sexual acts not "fit to be named": "And which is still worse, this Distemper is also gotten after another manner of Conversation, *viz.* by a Man's putting his erected *Penis,* into another Persons (Man or Woman's) Mouth, using Friction *&c.* between the Lips; a way so very Beastly and so much to be abhorr'd, as to cause at the mentioning, or but thinking of it, the utmost detestation and loathing" [*Treatise*, 68]. So shocking to him were these practices that Marten could not resist a pious ejaculation, apparently over his Bible:

> O monstrous! thought I, that Men otherwise, sensible Men, should so vilely debase themselves, and become so degenerate; should provoke God so highly, contemn the Laws of Man so openly, wrong their own Bodies so fearfully; and which is worse (without sincere Repentance) ruin their own Soul eternally. A Sin so heinous and aggravating, that God particularly expresses his Anger against those that commit it, as being hardned and given up by him to uncleanness, speaking of such in Rom. l. ver. 4. *Wherefore God also gave them up to Uncleanness, through the Lusts of their own Hearts, to dishonour their own Bodies between themselves.* [*Treatise*, 69]

Despite being sure he would be "blam'd" and "censur'd" for his apparent immodesty (or, rather, courage) in writing on forbidden topics, Marten defended himself on the grounds that *"there is nothing herein but what is discours'd in a Physical way, and in the modestest Terms Anatomy would allow"* [*Gonosologium Novum*, A4]. And, as so often, he recruited the authority of the learned: "*Venette* tells us," he maintained, launching into a double denial of responsibility, *"if modestly speaking of affairs of the Secret Parts be blamable, either St. Austin, St. Gregory of Nice, nor Tertullian should be perus'd, who all speak of Conjugal Affairs in such terms, as he durst not Translate. And by the same rule, one would suppress the Book of Secrets of Women, by Albertus Magnus wherein he sets forth a great many things to provoke to Love. And in fine, the Books of Physicians and Anatomists ought not to be seen, if the Complaints above recited were just and reasonable"* [*Gonosologium Novum*, A4v].

Beyond a certain point it is futile to pry into an author's intentions, scruples, or disavowals, for the paradoxes may principally be structural to the discourses, inseparable from the very project of writing on such topics as venereal disease in which the equivocal status of the subject may require utterance (to protect innocence against filth) while that act in itself may be accused of contributing to obscenity. Talking the taboo thus appears inherently paradoxical. Yet it would not be hard to accuse Marten of hypocrisy in exploiting public susceptibilities and capitalizing on the role of anxiety maker.[32]

We will never know whether Marten was callously exploiting the susceptibilities of alarmed readers, but it may be suggestive that he chose to devote some pages to the "Hypochondriack Distemper," a malady which he noted

> changes it self, *Proteus*-like, into any shape, representing some-

times in the space of a few Hours, almost every Disease incident to Mankind, bringing the Patients under such dismal apprehensions, and rendring them so unaccountably Whimsical, that it is really the hardest Task imaginable to perswade them to the contrary, notwithstanding the Reasons given them to be back'd with never so plain and undeniable Arguments. This, I say, is the nature of the Hypochondriack Disease, which yet has a much worse effect upon those People that have once had the *Venereal* Distemper, or that have but once gone the way to get it, tho' at the same Time they have really had the good hap to escape it: I say, upon those has this Disease had such an effect, that several have came to me and would not be satisfied 'till I had given them something for that purpose; and scarcely then would they be easie. [*Treatise*, 41]

It would not be impertinent to infer that Marten was opportunistically stating that sufferers from the "Hypochondriack Distemper" (i.e., those we would today call hypochondriacs) were sure to experience venereal complaints through a spectrum of symptoms; hence in such patients, almost *any* symptom might be venereal in origin, and it would be proper for the practitioner (i.e., Marten) to treat it with placebos.[33]

It would be pointless, however, to conclude by putting Marten in the dock, or on the couch. The point of this study has been to suggest that his books suitably demonstrate that, paralleling the "protean" nature of the venereal complaint as constructed in his own writings, the relations between medical practitioners and the public in the era of medical Grub Street were no less protean and equally perilous.

Notes

1. Neil McKendrick, John Brewer, and J.H. Plumb, *The Birth of a Consumer Society: The Commercialization of Eighteenth-Century England* (London: Europa, 1982); see also the introduction to John Brewer and Roy Porter, eds., *Consumption and the World of Goods* (London: Routledge, 1993).

2. Pat Rogers, *Grub Street: Studies in a Subculture* (London: Methuen, 1972); S. Parks, *John Dunton and the English Book Trade: A Study of His Career with a Checklist of His Publications* (New York: Garland, 1976); Gilbert D. McEwen, *The Oracle of the Coffee-House: John Dunton's "Athenian Mercury"* (San Marino, Calif.: Huntington Library, 1972); R. Straus, *The Unspeakable Dr. Curll* (New York: Kelley, 1970).

3. Much has been written of late on authors and authority. One germane article is Harold J. Cook, "Good Advice and Little Medicine: The Professional Authority of Early Modern English Physicians," *Journal of British Studies* 33 (1994): 1-31.

4. Dorothy Porter and Roy Porter, *Patient's Progress: Doctors and Doctoring in Eighteenth-Century England* (Cambridge: Polity Press, 1989); Roy Porter and Dorothy Porter, *In Sickness and in Health: The British Experience, 1650-1850* (London: Fourth

Estate, 1988); Roy Porter, *Disease, Medicine, and Society in England, 1550-1860* (London: Macmillan/Economic History Society, 1987); Mary E. Fissell, *Patients, Power, and the Poor in Eighteenth-Century Bristol* (Cambridge: Cambridge Univ. Press, 1991); I.S.L. Loudon, *Medical Care and the General Practitioner, 1750-1850* (Oxford: Clarendon Press, 1986).

    5. Roy Porter, *Health for Sale: Quackery in England, 1660-1850* (Manchester: Manchester Univ. Press, 1989); W.F. Bynum and R. Porter, eds., *Medical Fringe and Medical Orthodoxy, 1750-1850* (London: Croom Helm, 1987); R. Cooter, ed., *Studies in the History of Alternative Medicine* (London: Macmillan, 1988).

    6. Paul Slack, "Mirrors of Health and Treasures of Poor Men: Uses of the Vernacular Medical Literature of Tudor England," in C. Webster, ed., *Health, Medicine, and Mortality in the Sixteenth Century* (Cambridge: Cambridge Univ. Press, 1979), 237-74; Roy Porter, ed., *The Popularization of Medicine, 1650-1850* (London: Routledge, 1992), and especially the articles therein by Mary E. Fissell: "Readers, Texts and Contexts: Vernacular Medical Works in Early Modern England," 72-91, and by Andrew Wear: "The Popularization of Medicine in Early Modern England," 17-41; C. Lawrence, "William Buchan: Medicine Laid Open," *Medical History* 19 (1975): 20-35; Charles Rosenberg, "Medical Text and Medical Context: Explaining William Buchan's *Domestic Medicine*," *Bulletin of the History of Medicine* 57 (1983): 22-24; Lamar Riley Murphy, *Enter the Physician: The Transformation of Domestic Medicine, 1760-1860* (Tuscaloosa: Univ. of Alabama Press, 1991).

    7. For venereal disease itself, see Claude Quétel, *The History of Syphilis*, trans. Judith Braddock and Brian Pike (Oxford: Basil Blackwell, 1990); Theodore Rosebury, *Microbes and Morals: The Strange Story of Venereal Disease* (New York: Viking Press, 1971); Allan M. Brandt, "Sexually Transmitted Diseases," in W.F. Bynum and Roy Porter, eds., *Companion Encyclopedia of the History of Medicine* (London: Routledge, 1993), 561-83.

    8. For analysis of such bills, see Roy Porter, *Health for Sale*, chaps. 4 and 7.

    9. W.F. Bynum, "Treating the Wages of Sin: Venereal Disease and Specialism in Eighteenth-Century Britain," in *Medical Fringe and Medical Orthodoxy*, 5-28. The next two paragraphs summarize Bynum's argument.

    10. Much has been written about the construction of disease. See Charles E. Rosenberg and Janet Golden, eds., *Framing Disease: Studies in Cultural History* (New Brunswick, N.J.; Rutgers Univ. Press, 1992).

    11. John Marten, *A Treatise of all the Symptoms of the Venereal Disease, in both Sexes*, 6th ed. (London: Crouch, 1708), preface. For information on Marten, see Philip Pinkus, *Grub Street Stripped Bare* (London: Constable, 1980).

    12. John Marten, *Gonosologium Novum, or A New System of All the Secret Infirmities and Diseases, Natural, Accidental, and Venereal in Men and Women* (London, 1709). Subsequent quotes from this work will be cited in the text.

    13. For the English impact of Venette's work, see Roy Porter, "Spreading Carnal Knowledge or Selling Dirt Cheap? Nicolas Venette's *Tableau de l'Amour Conjugal* in Eighteenth-Century England," *Journal of European Studies* 14 (1984): 233-55; Roy Porter, "Love, Sex and Medicine: Nicolas Venette and his *Tableau de l'amour conjugal*," in *Erotica and the Enlightenment*, ed. Peter Wagner (Frankfurt: Lang, 1990), 90-122; Lesley Hall and Roy Porter, *The Facts of Life: The History of Sexuality and Knowledge from the Seventeenth Century* (New Haven, Conn.: Yale Univ. Press, 1994).

    14. For contemporary theories, see P. Darmon, *Le Mythe de la Procréation à l'Age Baroque* (Paris: J.J. Pauvert, 1977); F.J. Cole, *Early Theories of Sexual Generation* (Oxford: Clarendon Press, 1930).

15. Elsewhere referred to as "the many unhappy, ah! too deservedly unhappy Votaries of *Venus*, or rather of Hell and Ruin": Marten, *Treatise*, 6th ed., 206.

16. "Old Gleets, whether *Venereal* or *Seminal*, the former being generally procur'd by ill Management, and by most (tho' too often mistakenly) deem'd incurable; Wherein the Nature, Seat, and Difference of *Gleets* are demonstrated, and their true way of Cure, both from Reason and Experience ascertain'd. In order to which, the Parts ministring to Generation in both Sexes, their Situation, Action, Use, Abuse, &c. are necessarily consider'd, and why *Gleets* hinder Procreation, causing (as sometimes they do) impotency, &c. in *Men*, and Sterility &c, in *Women*; with several remarkable Cases of that kind added": Marten, *Treatise*, 6th ed., table of contents.

17. Bernard Mandeville commented on such devices in *A Treatise of the Hypochondriack and Hysterick Diseases* (2d ed., London: Tonson, 1730; reprint, Hildesheim: Georg Olms, 1981), a fascinating account, *inter alia*, of the devices used by physicians to create authority. See discussion in Roy Porter, "'Expressing Yourself Ill': The Language of Sickness in Georgian England," in *Language, Self, and Society: The Social History of Language*, ed. P. Burke and R. Porter (Cambridge: Polity Press, 1991), 276-99.

18. Marten, *Treatise*, 39; for the preoccupation of the new science with such "matters of fact," see S. Shapin and S. Schaffer, *Leviathan and the Air-Pump: Hobbes, Boyle, and the Experimental Life* (Princeton: Princeton Univ. Press, 1985).

19. Marten, *Treatise*, 94. It was another century before modern notions of tertiary syphilis were developed. It is not here being claimed that Marten was a precursor of nineteenth-century views.

20. Ibid., 105. Marten was here adhering to orthodoxy on venereal complaints, as expressed later, notably, by John Hunter: P.J. Weimerskirch and G.W. Richter, "Hunter and Venereal Disease," *Lancet* 1 (1979): 503-4; D.J.M. Wright, "John Hunter and Venereal Disease," *Annals of the Royal College of Surgeons of England* 63 (1981): 198-202.

21. For the medicine of internal flows and migration, see Malcolm Nicolson, "The Metastatic Theory of Pathogenesis and the Professional Interests of the Eighteenth-Century Physician," *Medical History* 32 (1988): 277-300; Malcolm Nicolson, "The Art of Diagnosis: Medicine and the Five Senses," in *Companion Encyclopedia of the History of Medicine*, 797-821; Barbara Duden, *The Woman beneath the Skin: A Doctor's Patients in Eighteenth-Century Germany*, trans. Thomas Dunlap (Cambridge: Harvard Univ. Press, 1991). It is, of course, a remnant of humoralism: see V. Nutton, "Humoralism," in *Companion Encyclopedia of the History of Medicine*, 281-91.

22. Marten, *Treatise*, 34. Marten concludes: "I cured him." See also 31 and 50. For Marten, the pox is typically communicated by direct sexual contact; a clap was transmitted by various forms of sexual excess.

23. Marten, *Treatise*, xxxi: "*We have seen that This and That Medicine, under the specious Title of* Panacæa, Arcanum Catholicon, *&c. have been so in Vogue as to have a Run for a while as universal Medicines, to Cure all Diseases, in all Persons, as your* Aurum Potabile *of* Silius, *your* Goddard's Drops, Lockyer's *Pills,* Daffy's *Elixir, and the like which after all, by failing in three Cases perhaps in four, have at last dwindled and come to be rejected, as much or more than before they were admir'd.*" Marten denounces quack "panaceas" at great length: 315 ff.

24. Marten, *Treatise*, 105. Such premature "cures" made matters worse: "For if a *Gonorrhoea* be consider'd as an *Ulcer*, as most certainly it is, those that suddenly dry it up with *Astringents* before the malignity be destroy'd, do most certainly (unless the Infection be very small indeed) throw their Patients into an early or late *Pox* which their whole Posterity may prove too sensible of; and I even found that when the *Ve-*

nereal Taint is once extinguish'd, and the Humours that flow to the Part diverted, the *Running* will gradually and most certainly abate of it self, and with a very little help" (105-6).

25. Case studies and the art of medical narrative have been widely analyzed in recent years. See Mary E. Fissell, "The Disappearance of the Patient's Narrative and the Invention of Hospital Medicine," in *British Medicine in an Age of Reform*, ed. Roger French and A. Wear (London: Routledge, 1992), 92-109; Kathryn Montgomery Hunter, *Doctors' Stories: The Narrative Structure of Medical Knowledge* (Princeton: Princeton Univ. Press, 1991); Arthur Kleinman, *Illness Narratives: Suffering, Healing, and the Human Condition* (New York: Basic Books, 1988); H. Brody, *Stories of Sickness* (New Haven, Conn.: Yale Univ. Press, 1987), and also Brody's *The Healer's Power* (New Haven: Yale Univ. Press, 1992); Suzanne Poirier et al., "Charting the Chart—An Exercise in Interpretation(s)," *Literature and Medicine* 11 (1992): 1-22; William Frank Monroe, Warren Lee Holleman, and Marsha Cline Holleman, "'Is There a Person in This Case?'" *Literature and Medicine* 11 (1992): 45-63.

26. Marten, *Treatise*, xii. He reports a happy ending: *"I went to this Gentleman, who told me his Case as above describ'd; I put him into a proper Course, by which he soon recover'd. He came and thank'd and gratify'd me; and acknowledg'd he could not but admire at the efficacy of what I gave him, and with what Ease and Expedition he was cur'd of that which had baffled the Efforts of many others before"* (xiii).

27. For testimonials see Roy Porter, "'I Think Ye Both Quacks': The Controversy Between Dr. Theodor Myersbach and Dr. John Coakley Lettsom," in *Medical Fringe and Medical Orthodoxy*, 56-78; and Porter, *Health for Sale*, chap. 7.

28. John Spinke, *Quackery Unmasked* (London: D. Brown, 1709); John Spinke, *Venus's Botcher* (London: D. Brown, 1711). The quotation is in *Quackery Unmasked*, 77. Spinke accuses Marten's "poxy book" of using the "Rhethorick of a scandalously ignorant Quack" (2). It may be noted that Marten followed the practice of many quack authors in giving his address in his books: "From my House in *Hatton-Garden*, on the Left-Hand beyond the Chappel, turning in from *Holborn, John Marten*, Surgeon, being writ over the Door."

29. Marten, *Treatise*, xxx. For identifications, consult C.J.S. Thompson, *The Quacks of Old London* (London: Brentano's, 1928). John Case is one of a small number that Marten actually names (208).

30. Marten, *Treatise*, 312. Spinke, *Quackery Unmasked*, 13, not unreasonably suggested this was a scandalous incitement to vice. Marten stated (65) that he could not, of course, disclose the contents of his preservative "lest it should encourage any to commit that Sin, which the more to be lamented, is too predominant already."

31. An indictment was brought at Queen's Bench in 1709 against Marten for his *Gonosologium Novum*. "'Being evil disposed and wicked', Marten, the alleged accusation, 'intending to corrupt the subjects of the Lady the Queen and seduced by cupidity, published and sold a scandalous book entitled Gonosologium novum, or a new system of all the secret infirmities and diseases natural accidental and venereal in men and women . . . written by way of appendix to the 6th edition of his book of the venereal diseases lately published and done with the same letter on the same paper, that those who please may bind it up with that.'" Noted in David Foxon, *Libertine Literature in England, 1660-1745: With an Appendix on the Publication of John Cleland's "Memoirs of a Woman of Pleasure," Commonly Known as "Fanny Hill"* (New York: University Books, 1965), 31. The charge against him was dismissed.

32. Alex Comfort, *The Anxiety Makers: Some Curious Preoccupations of the Medical Profession* (London: Nelson, 1967).

33. The best contemporary discussion of hypochondria is in Bernard Mandeville's *A Treatise of the Hypochondriack and Hysterick Diseases,* 2d ed. (London: Tonson, 1730; reprint, Hildesheim: Georg Olms, 1981). See also S. Baur, *Hypochondria: Woeful Imaginings* (Princeton: Princeton Univ. Press, 1988).

Chapter 4

Exposing the Secret Disease

Recognizing and Treating Syphilis in Daniel Turner's London

Philip K. Wilson

Contemporary sources suggest one particular socially constructed view of venereal disease that existed during this period: its secret nature. A 1730 London advertisement promoted both a lotion and an elixir for the "Secret Disease," local parlance for venereal disease.[1] Sufferers and healers generally claimed syphilis was contracted through coupling the secret parts. If contracted through secret dalliances, the inflicted kept their predicament secret from their spouses, at least initially. In fear of his reputation, one victim paid a quack twenty-five guineas for his treatment, ten for "its cure" and fifteen for "Secrecy."[2] Some obtained their treatments through secret shop entrances, often during the night, and medicines were sent through "utmost Privacy" to other individuals, many of whom used "Feigned Names."[3] Some patients even wore masks to keep their identity secret when personally calling upon practitioners.[4] And numerous advertised medicines claimed their panacean powers were derived from secret ingredients. Given this context, it is not surprising that venereal disease had become known as the "secret disease."

What did practitioners and patients recognize as the "secret disease" during this period? This article begins to answer this question along with others: How many venereal diseases were there? Was the presentation of the disease related to selecting who should treat the disease? Were these diseases curable? If so, what was used in the treatment? Were treatments directed only to alleviate external manifestations, thereby keeping the disease a secret? What distinguished orthodox treatment from quack remedies?

As I am primarily interested in the surgical and medical career of one contemporary London practitioner, Daniel Turner, my emphasis lies upon his

Exposing the Secret Disease

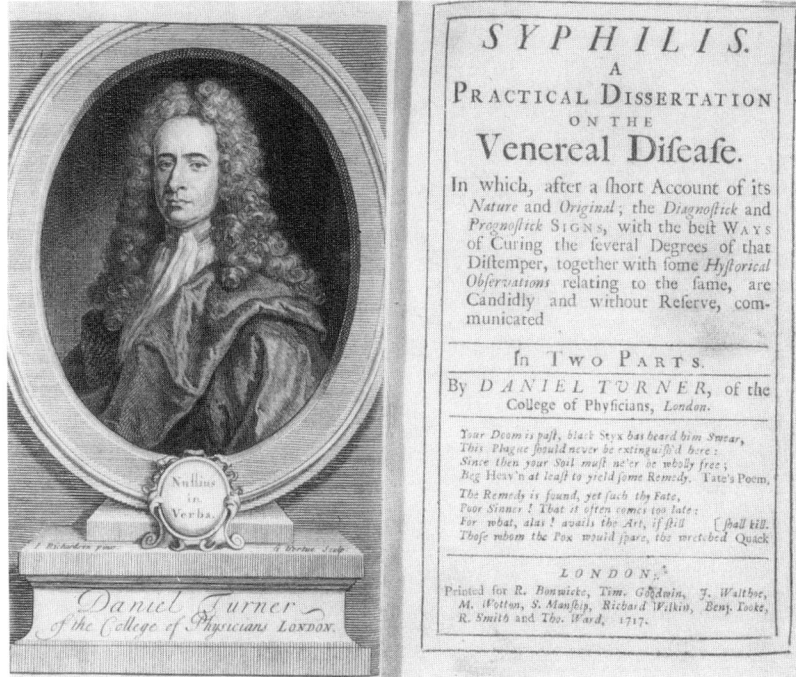

Fig. 3. Daniel Turner, engraved by G. Verture after J. Richardson, c. 1712-14. the title page of Turner's first treatise on venereal disease (1717). Wellcome Institute Library, London.

writings, the patients he treated, the treatments he administered, and the criticisms against these treatments. I selected Turner's writings over those of his contemporaries as he was London's most outspoken author on venereal disease for over twenty years (see fig. 3). But to better contextualize my account, I discuss Turner's writings in relation to those of his explicit allies and opponents. Among these were his compatriots John Marten, William Cockburn, Thomas Dover, Joshua Ward, and John Douglas, as well as contemporary French authorities on this disease, including François Chicoyneau and Pierre Desault.

Conceived in the year of London's Great Fire of 1666, Daniel Turner, the son of a tallow-chandler, was born into the London so eloquently described by his contemporary, Daniel Defoe. Turner apprenticed seven years under a surgeon of London's Barber-Surgeons' Company and commenced his own city practice in 1691. After twenty years of practice, he relinquished his position within this company and was admitted, after examination, as a licentiate into London's College of Physicians—a position which officially allowed him to practice physic (i.e., medicine), but not surgery, in the capital city.

He later obtained a medical degree, not through a university education as most of his colleagues had done, but through bartering twenty-five books to the College of the Academy at Yale in the colony of New Haven. This was to be the first medical degree offered by any American colonial school.[5] Little, however, is known of Turner's medical practice if, indeed, he practiced much medicine at all. Rather, he claimed his new medical career allowed him more leisure to devote his time to writing than did his toilsome surgical practice. Many of the thirty-four texts and treatises Turner published before his death in 1741 discussed one of his incessant career concerns: the treatment and control of venereal disease.

Some practitioners distinguished syphilis from skin diseases more upon a patient's moral fiber than upon any outward manifestation. One 1721 account claimed that if a patient presented with "Ulcers or running Sores, red, yellow, blue, or dark Spots, Pimples, or Blotches on the Face, Arms, Legs, or any other Part of the Body" and was deemed to be of "sober discreet" character, he was diagnosed with scurvy. But if he was "inclined to wantonness by reason of his Youth, or sly Countenance," then he was diagnosed with "the Pox."[6]

Most authors, however, directed readers to watch for the pathognomonical signs of infection, yet cautioned them that these signs might not appear all at once or even at all on everyone who became infected. Contemporary accounts typically discussed recognizable sequences or patterns of signs appearing at different stages or degrees of infection. Turner distinguished venereal disease as being either recent or confirmed [*Syphilis*, 1717, 17]. He identified a recent or first infection by a "dripping" of purulent matter from the urethra, often accompanied by a genital chancre which, he claimed, produced much "Pain and Smart" when making water. This infection, which Turner preferred to call *stillicidium purulentum*, was known among contemporaries as the dropper, the burning, gonorrhea, gleets, or more colloquially the clap. If this infection was not "dried up" and if its "venom" was not "evacuated," Turner argued, "a Pox may [then] happen to commence" [*Syphilis*, 1717, 24-25]. Turner described the pox (i.e., syphilis, lues, the great pox, or the French disease) as the confirmed or second stage of venereal disease. More specifically, it was the "usual Consequence" of an untreated, "ill-treated," or "empirically flubber'd over" clap [*Syphilis*, 1717, 81].

The idea that different venereal diseases were malignant or corruptible into other forms was consistently expressed among most contemporaries. This finding supports the notion that the "metastatic translation" of diseases was, as Malcolm Nicolson has convincingly argued, "virtually [a] constant feature" of eighteenth-century disease theory.[7] Extending this argument, I find that patients and practitioners apparently shared the belief that venereal diseases spread through the body in some "malignant," "corruptible," or "sequential" fashion.

Recognizing this shared belief helps explain why those who were suspicious of having "been clap'd" sought immediate curative remedies. This action was uncommon among Londoners who often suffered disorders, particularly surgical disorders like ulcers, tumors, and hernias for many months, even years, before seeking care [*Syphilis,* 1727, 218]. What, then, prompted those who believed themselves venereally infected to seek immediate care?

For many, perhaps most, it was fear. Fear of developing a more painful state of venereal disease. Fear of being "found out" by their spouse. Fear that the "telling" signs of the disease would "risque their Characters in the [business] World" [*Syphilis,* 1727, 218]. This fear, Turner argued, particularly existed "among the Tradesmen or Citizens" who worried that without rapid treatment syphilitic throat infections would cost them the "proper Tone of their Voice" and consequently "their Reputation" [*Syphilis,* 1727, 217-18]. "Syphilophobes" loomed large in the anecdotal literature. Scores of English vernacular publications from the first half of the eighteenth century indicate that fear drove people to obtain any medicine advertised as an immediate cure.

Selling a curative product largely depended on effective advertising, and London was filled with advertisements for "curing" venereal disease. The public was made aware of potential cures through the handbills persistently passed their way and posted on signboards throughout the city, through the practitioners hawking their cures on the streets, through booksellers or coffeehouses, and through the many pages of advertisement in the rapidly expanding periodical press. Those thinking themselves venereally inflicted could shop for remedies as a consumer shopping for goods.

Case study evidence indicates that many venereal sufferers first turned to the local, self-acclaimed healers whose advertisements had appeared most convincing. Other sufferers, particularly middle-class men who had not initially sought out street practitioners, often called upon the advice of "gentlemen" in coffeehouses or barbershops, those "dens of male comradeship."[8] Here, not only could they confirm their suspicions with the experience or knowledge of their comrades but they could also select from a variety of remedies sold within. Although the ingredients of the remedies most barbershops offered were secret, the name brands were often the same as the products advertised on "quackbills" posted around the city. Thus, the same product appears to have been distributed to different classes of patients through different venues and, at times, for different prices. This commercial exchange suggests an intra-London drug trade had already been well formed.

Most of the contemporary literature, together with most surviving case history evidence, suggests to me that caring for syphilis patients was recognized as an aspect of the surgeon's calling. That is, surgeons were both publicly and occupationally recognized as caretakers of syphilis, at least of the stubborn, resilient, recurrent, or previously mismanaged cases of syphilis. I offer several reasons as to why this form of the disease remained part of general surgical practice.

English surgeons were traditionally provided practical written instructions in treating syphilis at least as far back as the late sixteenth century.[9] At this time, and in the early eighteenth century, orthodox surgeons were primarily treating externally manifest disorders whereas internal disorders were handled by physicians. Syphilis was recognized and diagnosed primarily upon its external appearance; therefore, its care, as many surgeons argued, fell to the surgical trade. Turner, for one, claimed that "if we consider many of the [Signs] and Symptoms" of syphilis, undertaking its "Cure" was by "right" the surgeon's province, for the cure often required much "manual Operation." Treating syphilis implied having to apply caustics to "lay open the Venereal Abscesses, to rub down the Verrucae, to extirpate Carbuncles; ... to lay bear rotten Bones, or [to apply] Cauteries ... [upon bones] for Desquamation." After providing this scenario, Turner concluded, "it must be granted, that the Surgeon is the most proper Person to be consulted" for treating syphilis [*Syphilis*, 1717, preface].

Surgeons were also the primary caretakers of syphilis on the Continent. By the early eighteenth century, the syphilis treatises of François Chicoyneau, Jean Louis Petit, Augustine Belloste, Vincent Brest, and Pierre Desault had been translated into the vernacular and were sold in London bookstalls. The manual treatments these authors recommended were explicitly cited by many later English surgical authors, indicating the adoption of some foreign methods in treating this disease. The French writings appear to have held particular influence with English surgeons; what better way than to emulate French treatments for what the English so readily referred to as the "French disease" or "French pox"?[10]

Surgeons also appear to have been accustomed to manually administering long, labor-intensive treatments. A contemporary case book from St. Thomas's Hospital, for example, indicates that surgeons William Cheselden, Josiah Paul, and James Ferne routinely attended many "foule" (i.e., venereally diseased) patients throughout their standard twenty-one-day or thirty-one-day courses of treatments.[11] London surgeon John Douglas recorded that patients outside the hospital often received a surgeon's care for one or two months.[12]

From what we know about contemporary medical practice, many London physicians, particularly those of the College, were less likely to embark upon such time-consuming, labor-intensive types of treatment.[13] They typically treated, or at least are described as having treated, upper-class patients, whereas surgeons appear to have treated any who sought their care and were brought to their surgery. Of course, not all individuals who sought help from a surgeon were persuaded to undergo the extensive treatments he recommended. Surgeons who succeeded in these negotiations, which often involved setting the patients up in the surgeon's own home or in a nearby rented accommodation, were able to contract a set length of service for set fees. And since thousands of people appear to have been afflicted with some venereal disorder, securing syphilis treatment as part of their trade offered surgeons a way to gain a constant, predictable business.

Most important, the willingness of syphilitics to seek a surgeon's care suggests that surgeons were able, or at least were thought to be able, to cure this disease. Evidence abounds that syphilis was curable.[14] For example, Samuel Palmer, admitting surgeon to the Lock Hospital in Southwark and a correspondent of Turner's, reported that between January 1719/20 and January 1720/21, 108 of the 115 syphilitics he admitted to the Lock were later "cured and discharged."[15] At St. Thomas's Hospital, nearly all of the thirty-four "foule" patients treated between 1 May and 1 September 1726 were discharged as "cur'd." John Douglas, surgeon to Westminster Infirmary, claimed to have never sent one of his "several hundreds" of venereally diseased patients away "uncured."[16] Edward Dunn and William Cockburn attest to similar curability in their public (i.e., nonhospital) practices. Before explaining how they achieved these cures, I first examine what contemporary surgeons considered "cured." Specifically, I compare Turner's descriptions of cure in a series of thirty syphilis patients' case histories with his depictions of the cures that "quacks" claimed to have achieved.

Twenty-six of the thirty patients Turner described in his 1727 *Syphilis: A Practical Dissertation of Venereal Disease* were "cured" through his treatment. Turner used the term *cure* when any one of the following therapeutic objectives had been reached. Cure involved "eas[ing] the Smart" of making water, "lessening the Running" of the clap, "mending the colour" of the urine, and "drying up" scabs and pustules. In addition, he sought to "resolve" the buboes, "mundify" the "chankerous" ulcers, "reduce" nodus protuberances, restore the ability to swallow with ease, preserve the voice, and "relieve" the "Great [nocturnal] Pain" in the head and legs.

To achieve these cures, Turner's patients often underwent months of therapy. For example, salivating a patient, a common therapy more fully described below, required that a patient be "laid down" (i.e., confined to bed) for a month. "Strictly conform[ing] to the Rules prescribed" (i.e., keeping to one's "Chamber the whole time"), Turner argued, greatly "contribute[d] to the success of these Cures." Yet, he claimed that "'tis seldom" surgeons "have such Opportunity" of this "Convenience" [*Syphilis*, 1717, 147]. Despite the public belief that incompletely treating the clap often led to a confirmed pox, Turner acknowledged that surgeons often compromised ideal treatments according to the patient's demands [*Syphilis*, 1717, 32].

Distinct from our present-day understanding of "cure," cure in the early eighteenth century appears to have been the general state of a patient's health at the time he was "dismis'd" from private care or "discharg'd" from the hospital. Few contemporaries reported what we would call patient follow-up. Turner did, however, provide glimpses into the futures of five venereally diseased patients he claimed to have cured. One gentleman was described as "fat and lusty" a year later, and the cure of another "stood firm" some two years after treatment [*Syphilis*, 1727, 271 and 300]. Another gentleman married a year after his treatment, but, whether through his previous infirmity or his advanced age, this patient complained to Turner that "his [marital] Abilities" were "not answerable to his Inclinations" [*Syphilis*, 1727, 208]. Another patient, being "well tired with Venus's wars . . . enter'd those of Mars" in which he was "not long after . . . kill'd in an Engagement" [*Syphilis*, 1727, 275].

All of the above-mentioned criteria for cure were, for Turner, aimed at removing the "venereal venom" that was lurking within. This point distinguishes Turner's meaning of cure from the "Aim" of "London Quacks." The latter, he argued, only sought to stop the urethral running and heal the outward sores, disregarding any possible consequence of a confirmed case of the pox [*Syphilis*, 1717, 36]. London physician Edmund Packe claimed it was a problem to judge cure only by absence of visible signs. "Nothing is more common," he claimed, "and indeed unavoidable, than a Return of Distempers (with their Symptoms) . . . one Day after . . . [many practitioners] believe they are cur'd."[17] To overcome this calamity, surgeon John Douglas urged orthodox practitioners to pursue their course of treatment until "the symptoms have all disappeared, and some little time after" [Douglas, pt. 2, 37].

No single universally accepted treatment existed to cure syphilis. Rather, exponents of a variety of therapies appeared in the contemporary surgico-medical literature. However, many of these remedies as well as those in quack handbills contained some form of mercury. Prince's Powder, for instance, a red precipitate of mercury, was one of the most common "Chemical Quack Remedies" and was also prescribed in Quincy's *Pharmacopoeia*.[18] Mercury was among the most common ingredients present in the remedies distributed gratis to charity patients, sold to commoners in local shops, and offered to the aristocracy, the nobility, and the royal household.

Like most London practitioners of the 1710s treating venereal disease, Turner was a mercurialist. He claimed mercury was the "specifik" or "antidote" for syphilis [*Syphilis*, 147 and 154]. During this time, various forms of mercury were available for use by surgeons, physicians, and quacks. White sublimate, calomel, red, white, yellow, and green precipitates (i.e., oxides of mercury), natural and artificial cinnabar (mercury and sulfur), as well as crude mercury or quicksilver could be obtained from apothecaries.[19] Mercurial products were administered internally by mouth or externally by frictions, fumigations, salivations, clysters, or impregnated plasters applied on the limbs, worn as girdles or as socks.

Numerous disputes ensued over selecting the precise form of treatment. Turner distinguished himself from some mercurialists by restricting his use to particular forms of external and internal administration. Topically applied mercurials, he claimed, digested, deterged, and cicatrized external syphilis ulcerations. For "mild" forms of the pox, Turner frequently prescribed the use of calomel (i.e., mercurous chloride) to be "given inwardly."[20] Indeed, he became incensed over many contemporaries' use of crude mercury as a panacea to treat all forms of venereal disease. Crude mercury, he argued, was quacked from London streets and distributed by "Plowmen, Farmers, [and] Swineheard" who were "destroying" local inhabitants as "people do with Buckets of Water, to quench the Fire of another Nature" [*Syphilis*, 151]. Turner claimed firsthand knowledge of its effects, having used it on patients early in his surgical career [*Syphilis*, 100-107]. But the hazardous consequences he observed in his and other surgeons' patients had prompted him to abandon its use, and he urged fellow London surgeons to stop using it, too.[21] Specifically, Turner urged practitioners to reduce the amount of external mercury they applied and to quit administering crude mercury orally.

Turner did not completely reject the use of crude mercury, only its oral administration. Indeed, he quite favored its use when applied "in the way of Unction," rubbing it into the body. In the 1710s and 1720s, mercurial unctions were commonly used to bring forth internal venereal poisons through the excessive production of spital or saliva, a process labeled salivation or ptyalismus. Turner advocated salivations for both the mild and the "stubborn or rebellious" pox.

In 1736, Turner claimed that "several hundred Persons" were salivated "yearly, in the Cities and suburbs of London and Westminster."[22] Earlier in the century, salivation had become the standard for treating "foule" patients admitted to St. Bartholomew's and St. Thomas's Hospitals, London's "sacred sanctuaries for the sick."[23] One hospital pupil at St. Thomas's specified that these methods "may safely be us'd according to Turner."[24]

When a patient would not salivate, Turner recommended the use of a cinnabar fumigation [*Syphilis*, 84 and 217]. Cinnabar was a mixture of mercury and sulfur. If the patient's whole body was to be fumigated, he or she was placed upon a seat that was "perforated" somewhat "like the close Stool." A blanket was wrapped around the patient, entirely "enclosing" his body and head, and was secured to a hook in the ceiling [*Syphilis*, 1727, 173]. Cinnabar was "sprinkled on" a hot iron placed below the seat, and the fumes ascended through the chair, guided by an inverted funnel so that they would flow "all round the Diseased Parts" [*Syphilis*, 1717, 51] (see fig. 4). If fumigating was to be used primarily for treating stubborn syphilitic ulcers in the nose, mouth, and throat, as Turner recommended, the blanket-enclosed patient was directed to hold the cinnabar in an earthen platter on his knees and to inhale the fumes repeatedly. Turner generally "smoked" or fumigated these patients in the "Night and Morning ... for about a week" [*Syphilis*, 1717, 62-63]. As in salivating, Turner urged practitioners to keep patients "confined" to their house "During the Course" of treatment. Fumigation, however, more readily allowed patients whose "Business would not permit" the confinement that salivations required to go "about their Affairs as usual, only wearing a bit of Flannel under their chin, as a Muffler, to keep their Throat warm" [*Syphilis*, 1717, 173].

Turner regarded it as quackery for a surgical or medical author to "conceal ... from the Reader" anything he knew that might be of help to patients [*Syphilis*, 1717, preface]. In particular, Turner despised any author promoting secret remedies. It was this fault, Turner claimed, that lay at the heart of a work entitled *The Symptoms, Nature, Cause and Cure of a Gonorrhoea* (1713). He rebuked the author of this work, his contemporary and fellow licentiate of the College of Physicians, William Cockburn, for keeping the remedy he promoted a secret.[25]

In contrast to Cockburn's quackery, Dr. Thomas Dover openly disclosed his venereal disease remedy: orally administered quicksilver. Although Turner was a mercurialist, he was opposed to this form of mercurial administration. He also expressed outrage at Dover for promoting this remedy as a "panpharmicon" or panacea. Indeed, Dover recommended using large doses (i.e., several pounds) of mercury as a cure not only for venereal disease but also for hysteria, intestinal infestation and obstruction, scrofula, infertility, asthma, elephantiasis, and scorbutic ulcers.

A publishing war ensued over this "crude-mercury mania," chiefly between Turner and Dover, but backed by respective allies as well.[26] Dover defended his claims of quicksilver on grounds of both theory and practice. According to Dover, injuries resulting from any medicinal agent were due to the agent's shape or form. Hazardous agents, he argued, were always marked with "spiculae, points, and edges." Thus, quicksilver, which always retained its "globular form," was perfectly harmless. Dover added further support of mercury's efficacy by publishing eight signed testimonials.

Dover's detractors, including Turner, provided much first- and second-hand case evidence that the large quantities of mercury Dover used had produced hazardous effects. They scorned him for returning to the practice of the "Ancients," i.e., seventeenth-century practitioners who administered mercury in the much more unregulated fashion. Turner claimed he "might forgive [Dover's] Quackery if he would [only] quack safely."[27] As in many contemporary medical disputes, no quick resolution over Dover's medicine was reached.[28] Neither the College of Physicians nor the Society of Apothecaries made an official pronouncement regarding Dover's treatments. Rather, each side continued to gain adherents by publicly denigrating their opponent.[29]

Exposing the Secret Disease

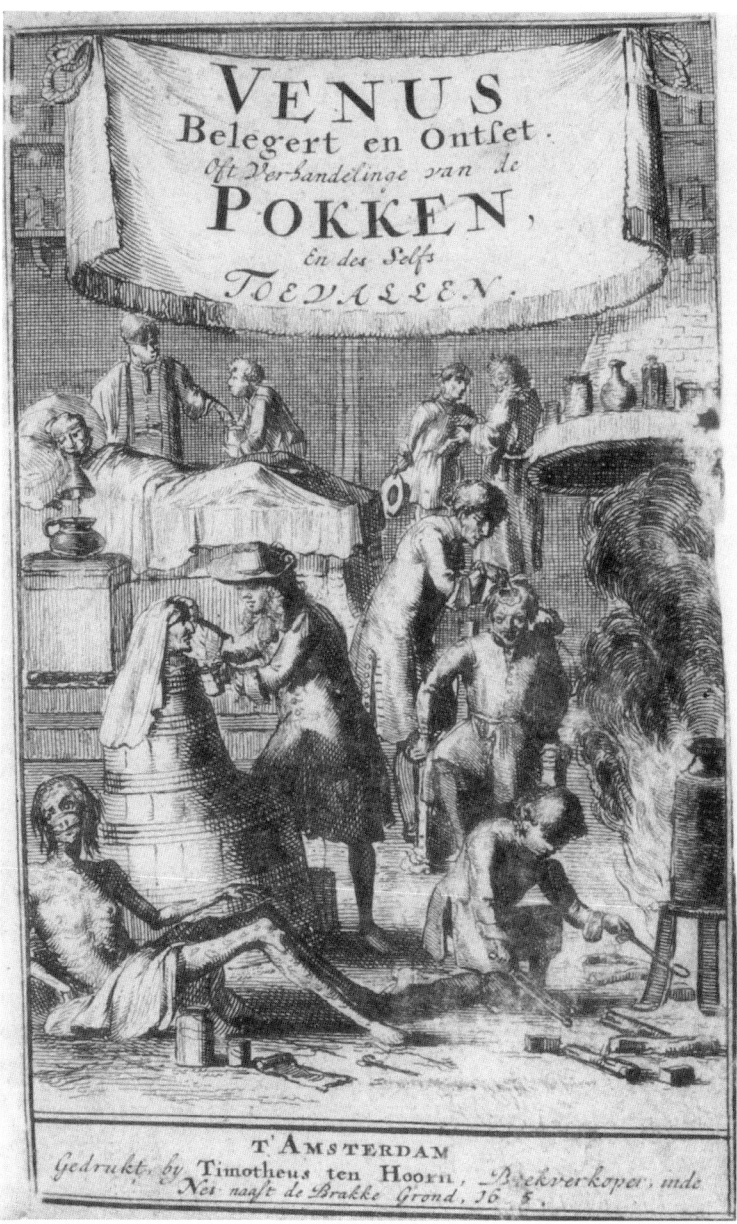

Fig. 4. The scenario of various syphilis treatments, including fumigation and salivation. Frontpiece to Steven Blankaart, *Venus Belegert en Ontset* (1685). Wellcome Institute Library, London.

To resolve the contemporary dilemmas over selecting the most efficacious and least harmful form of therapy, Turner proposed that a more open and accurate method of reporting case evidence was needed. His efforts to compile case studies as evidence are best exemplified by his tirade against Joshua Ward. Trained as a drysalter with no qualification in physic, surgery, or pharmacy, Ward developed a reputation as a dispenser of his emetic "Pill & Drop," a medicine Marjorie Nicolson rightly claimed was "one of the most notorious medicines of the XVIII Century."[30]

Principally, Ward advertised his "Pill & Drop" as effective in treating numerous disorders, not the least of which was venereal disease. He claimed that some twenty thousand individuals had benefited from this remedy during Ward's first nine months in London. But opposition to Ward's remedy, as well as to his possible popish intentions, quickly followed. He was first attacked in the *Daily Courant* on 28 November 1734. *The Daily Journal*, *The Advertiser*, and *Gentleman's Magazine* soon joined the campaign against Ward. His most relentless foe was the *Grub Street Journal*.[31]

Turner became one of Ward's "most active critics."[32] To demonstrate how Ward's claims ran contrary to what he represented as orthodox practice, Turner gathered much case evidence demonstrating the "mischief" that he attributed to Ward's medicine. One "poor Fellow," for instance, who had been Turner's patient "for a Venereal Head-ach," produced "between sixty and seventy Stools" and was in "the most imminent Danger of his Life" after taking only "One single Pill." Turner reprinted twelve similar incidents that had previously appeared in the *Grub Street Journal* and *Gentleman's Magazine* for the "Satisfaction of all those in whose Hands" these periodicals had "not fallen."[33] He was soon joined by many allies seeking to depose Ward by exposing the identity of the "Pill & Drop." By gathering testimonials as evidence of the previously untold miseries resulting from Ward's remedies, they hoped to convince the public to quit using his medicines.

Turner appealed to the public to "send an Account of what they know . . . from taking of these Medicines" (fig. 5). He requested reports of both the "Good and Bad Consequences," claiming that only in such gathering of information can "equal Justice . . . be done." He specified that contributors provide "Facts" that they had "truly" observed, together with the "Patient's Names and Places of Residence." Turner specifically urged parish clerks to "lay the strictest Injunction" upon parishioners to "make a true Report" of the incidents "immediately ensuing" upon taking Ward's medicine. This information was to be left in a letter addressed to Turner at John Clarke's Bookshop under the Royal Exchange. Turner swore to keep the informer's name confidential, if so desired.[34] Thus, the public would compile the data of which Turner viewed himself the ultimate arbiter.

Whatever responses Turner may have received remain unknown. But

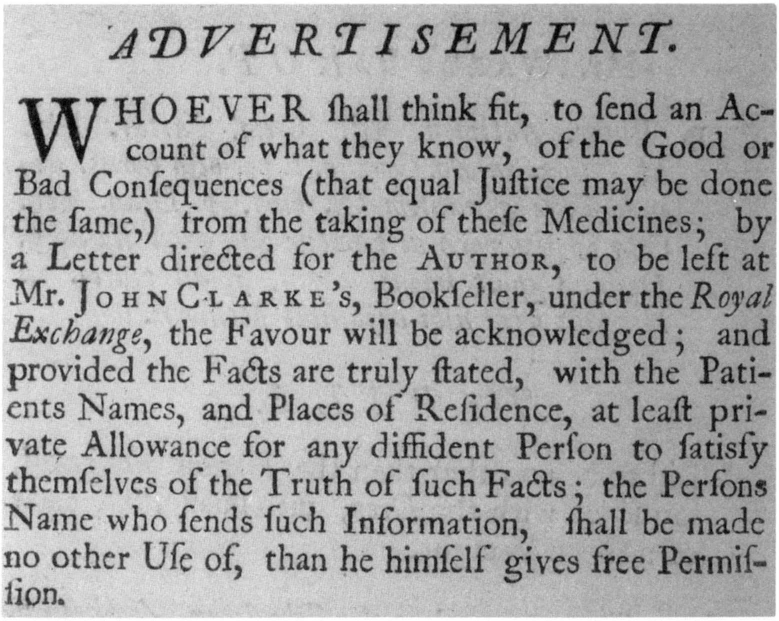

> ## ADVERTISEMENT.
>
> WHOEVER shall think fit, to send an Account of what they know, of the Good or Bad Consequences (that equal Justice may be done the same,) from the taking of these Medicines; by a Letter directed for the AUTHOR, to be left at Mr. JOHN CLARKE's, Bookseller, under the *Royal Exchange*, the Favour will be acknowledged; and provided the Facts are truly stated, with the Patients Names, and Places of Residence, at least private Allowance for any diffident Person to satisfy themselves of the Truth of such Facts; the Persons Name who sends such Information, shall be made no other Use of, than he himself gives free Permission.

Fig. 5. Daniel Turner's public appeal for firsthand testimonials regarding the efficacy of Joshua Ward's "Pill & Drop." From Daniel Turner, *The Drop and Pill of Mr Ward Consider'd* (1735). Wellcome Institute Library, London.

the publicity of the campaign against Ward's remedies appears to have actually supported his business. Ward established three privately run infirmaries in London for whose patients, primarily charity patients, he took direct charge. This business captured the attention of some of Turner's professional colleagues. Dr. Edmund Packe, for example, supported Ward's claims for his "Pill & Drop" after seeing firsthand how Ward was treating his patients. He wrote an invective against Turner's "injurious Treatment of Mr Ward" and encouraged Collegiate physicians to follow the "God-like" example he claimed Ward exemplified by dispensing such "extraordinary" medicines to the poor.[35] This dispute over Ward's claims illustrates the diversity and discordance over ideas about medicines and medical practice during this period.

Just as Turner regarded purging as necessary for treating the clap, he argued it was also needed to cure the pox. Not all contemporaries, however, agreed with this view. François Chicoyneau, a physician in Montpellier, claimed to have cured many syphilitics without ever administering a purge. More adamantly, he denounced salivations as an "ineffectual & pernicious" form of treatment. Instead, he recommended that only small doses of "Quicksilver Ointment" be applied by "friction." These frictions had gained some acclaim on the Continent where, as later in England, they became advertised as the "Montpellier Method."[36] Turner completely disagreed with Chicoyneau's argument. In remarking upon each of Chicoyneau's points, Turner claimed experience had taught him to the contrary. Salivation had, he argued, annually cured "Hundreds" of London patients, many of whom had "fruitlessly" undergone previous treatments only with frictions [*Syphilis*, 1727, 352].

Another French physician, Pierre Desault of Bordeaux, claimed that the "whole Secret" of curing syphilis derived from "keeping the Patient's Body open by Clysters" [*Syphilis,* pt. 2, 164]. Thereby, in modifying the "Montpellier Method," Desault recommended that syphilitics be treated primarily by purging, in addition to using only mild frictions. More emphatically, like Chicoyneau, Desault disdained salivation. Consistent with his earlier dispute, Turner opposed Desault's method and claimed never to have "seen or known" anyone with an inveterate pox to be cured without submitting to salivation.[37]

Desault met Turner's objections through correspondence, but their differences were aired to a wider audience through the intervention of London surgeon John Douglas. Douglas claimed to have treated "several hundreds" of venereal patients by friction and gentle purgation without ever sending "one away uncured."[38] In 1739, Douglas published an "Answer" to Turner's "bitter Invectives, false Insinuations and Gross Misrepresentations" of Desault's method of cure. Can "T——r and company" not see, he argued, the difference between "spitting four, five, or six pints a-day, for a month, sometimes two [while suffering with] all of the parts of the mouth inflamed, ulcerated, tumified, and excessive[ly] painful, the face puffed up, the voice suppressed and inarticulate, and [with] such a difficulty in swallowing that it is seldom possible to get [even] the smallest quantity of liquids down, . . . *and* taking two or three gentle purges a week, and eating heartily all the while?" [Douglas, 27]. Douglas identified four surgeons and six physicians in London who also favored frictions without salivation, and he claimed he was working to have all the local hospitals "fitted up" to use purges and only mild frictions.[39] He also insinuated that Turner retained the practice of salivation primarily because it was more "profitable" than short-term frictions.[40]

Comparing Douglas's writing from 1737 to 1739 with that of Turner's over the preceding twenty years offers important insight into the change of accepted orthodox syphilis treatment. By the late 1730s, Douglas was promoting the use of only small amounts of mercury through frictions, certainly not enough to bring on the salivation that he despised. Working back through the literature, I find that support for frictions as opposed to salivation began gaining strength in the early 1730s. It was also at this time that guaiac, Dover's mercurial remedy, and eventually Ward's "Pill & Drop" began to gain public and professional support as well.[41] Thus, it appears there was a general, though gradual, movement toward finding alternatives to salivation as a method for treating syphilitics. Why was this so, and what does this say about Turner?

Neither the College of Physicians nor the Barber-Surgeons' Company formally urged practitioners to quit salivating patients in favor of other methods. Indeed, a constituency of both physicians and surgeons may be found among the supporters of each alternative therapy as well as among the old guard of "sworn salivators." Thus, promoting an alternative to salivation was not, at this time, so clearly divided along surgeon/physician lines as some historical accounts have suggested.[42] Instead, subscribing to salivation as a public practitioner in the late 1730s appears to have been passé. Although salivating hospital patients does not appear to have declined, salivations by public (i.e., nonhospital) surgeons under whom patients had more say over their treatment distinctly lost the level of support it boasted of ten years earlier. Instead, several new alternatives were available whereby patients had more time to go about their day-to-day business, without having to be "laid down" for a month. Only brief contact with practitioners was required, regardless of whether the practitioners were qualified or quack.

Quackery was not exclusively a term used to describe the practice of unqualified mountebanks. Advocating particular remedies was enough for some members of the orthodoxy to identify any supporter of these remedies as a quack. Indeed, in 1739, many qualified London practitioners no longer considered salivation as an orthodox form of treating syphilis. What then of Turner? If Douglas be our guide, and he is the only contemporary guide we have to this issue, he insinuates that by his "bigotry" to "antiquity," by his adherence to "old" outmoded "notions" and practices rather than adopting the less hazardous "modern" forms of treatment, and by retaining "old forms" of treatment merely "because they are profitable," Turner was nothing better than a quack. "Rail T[urner] rail! Your Craft's in danger, if the truth prevail" [Douglas, pt. 3, 153]. Having led London's crusade against quackery from as early as 1695 through 1739, Turner's practice was ultimately designated as quackery by a similarly aged, similarly trained surgical colleague. What an ironic turn for Turner, the physician probably most keenly attuned to abolishing quackery in all London. Turner's situation, at least from Douglas's view, exemplifies W.F. Bynum's dictum that "quack is as quack does" [Bynum, "Treating the Wages of Sin," 12].

Notes

1. *The Practical Scheme of the Secret Disease* (London, 1730). R.P.T. Davenport-Hines labeled the chapter of his historical investigation into venereal disease as "The Secret Disease" in *Sex, Death, and Punishment* (London: Collins, 1990), 16-54, and James Cleugh depicted syphilis in the title of his *Secret Enemy* (London: Thames and Hudson, 1954).

2. Daniel Turner, *The Modern Quack, or The Physical Imposter Detected* (1718), as cited by W.F. Bynum, "Treating the Wages of Sin: Venereal Disease and Specialism in Eighteenth-Century Britain," in *Medical Fringe and Medical Orthodoxy, 1750-1850*, ed. W.F. Bynum and Roy Porter (London: Croom Helm, 1987), 20.

3. *Practical Scheme*, 5.

4. D. Turner, *Syphilis: A Practical Dissertation on Venereal Disease* (London, 1717), 319. Unless otherwise noted, subsequent references to *Syphilis* are taken from the fourth edition, 1732.

5. Philip K. Wilson, "Reading a Man through His Gifts: Daniel Turner's 1722 Book Donation to Yale College," *Yale University Library Gazette* 69 (1995): 129-48.

6. *Medicina Flagellata, or The Doctor Scarify'd* (London, 1721), 18.

7. Malcolm Nicolson, "The Metastatic Theory of Pathogenesis and the Professional Interests of the Eighteenth-Century Physician," *Medical History* 32 (1988): 281.

8. Davenport-Hines, *Sex, Death, and Punishment*, 41.

9. William Clowes, *A Briefe and Necessarie Treatise, Touching the Cure of the Disease called Morbus Gallicus* (London: Flesher, 1587).

10. Jeremy Black noted the English gentry's preference for French surgeons in treating venereal disease in *The British and the Grand Tour* (London: Croom Helm, 1985), 111.

11. Charles Oxley Notebook, case notes of surgical patients admitted to St Thomas's Hospital, 1725-26," MS. S2.a.6., final section "Observationes and Ptyalismum pertinented." Medical Library, St. Thomas's campus, United Medical and Dental Schools of Guy's and St. Thomas's Hospitals. I discuss these treatments in "'Sacred Sanctuaries for the Sick': Surgery at St Thomas's Hospital (1725-26)," *London Journal* 17 (1992): 53-54.

12. John Douglas, *A Treatise on the Venereal Disease* (London: printed for the author, 1739), pt. 3, 27.

13. It is frequently speculated that many London physicians spent their days in coffeehouses writing prescriptions, some never actually seeing most of their "patients." Yet, physicians of the early eighteenth century appear to have been more sympathetic to venereally diseased patients than European physicians whom Ulrich von Hutten said typically "fled from the presence of syphilitics" two centuries earlier. Hutten, *De Morbo Gallico* (1519), as cited by Davenport-Hines, *Sex, Punishment, and Death*, 24.

14. James J. Walsh provides an interesting psychological explanation in *Cures: The Story of Cures That Fail* (New York: Appleton, 1923), vii-ix, 1-12.

15. Daniel Turner, *Remarks upon Dr. Willoughby's Translation of Monsieur Chicoyneau's Method of Cure* (London, 1727), appended to *Syphilis*, 1727, 377-78. Similar reports for 1731-37 appear in Turner's *Syphilis*, pt. 2, 233.

16. Douglas, *Treatise on Venereal Disease*, pt. 3, 53.

17. Edmund Packe, *An Answer to Dr. Turner's Letter to Dr. Jurin* (London: J. Roberts, 1735), 20.

18. Turner noted the quack's common distribution of the Prince's Powder in *Syphilis*, 1717, 66. This same remedy was recommended in Quincy's *Pharmacopoeia Officinalis & Extemporanea, or A Complete English Dispensatory*, 2d ed. (London, 1719), 663, as cited in Leonard Goldwater's *Mercury: A History of Quicksilver* (Baltimore: York Press, 1972), 239.

19. Quincy's *Pharmacopoeia*, 1719, listed sixteen forms of mercurials including crude quicksilver, Arcanum Joviale, Mercurius Sublimatus, Calomel, Mercurius

Resuscitatus, Mercurius Praecipitatus ruber, albus, and viridus, the Prince's Powder, Panacea Mercurii rubra and alba, Turpethum Minerale, Arcanum Corollinum, Aethiops Mineral, and Cinnabar Nativum and Factitium. John Marten's *Treatise of Venereal Disease*, 663, includes even more preparations of mercury.

20. D. Turner, *Syphilis*, 1717, 106. George Urdang constructed a historical survey of the preparations and uses of calomel in "The Early Chemical and Pharmaceutical History of Calomel," *Chymia: Annual Studies in the History of Chemistry* 1 (1948): 93-108.

21. Among the harmful consequences of crude mercury treatment Turner described were hemorrhages from the "Lungs by the Mouth, and from the Brain by the Nose," blood vessels of the adnata (or albuginea) of the eye "burst[ing] open," and the loss of vast quantities of blood in the stool. See Daniel Turner, *A Discourse on Quicksilver*, in his book *The Ancient Physician's Legacy impartially Survey'd* (London: J. Clarke, 1733), "By Way of Postscript," 131-80. John Marten, among many others, also noted that "Ill prepared" and "untimely Administration" of mercury often led to "Tremors, Spasms, Pains, Weaknesses, Lamenesses, Impediment of Speech, loss of hearing, Tasting, Smelling, [and] decay of Sight." See Marten's *Treatise of Venereal Disease*, 651.

22. T.D. [i.e., Turner, Daniel], translation of Aloysius Luisini's *Aphrodisiacus, Containing a Summary of the Ancient Writers on the Venereal Disease . . . with a Large Preface by Daniel Turner* (London: J. Clarke, 1736): xxxv.

23. Turner's phrase for the two hospitals as used in his *Apologia Chyurgica: A Vindication of the Noble Art of Surgery* (London: J. Whitlock, 1695), 115.

24. "Observationes and Ptyalismum pertinented," in the "Charles Oxley Notebook."

25. Daniel Turner, *A Discourse Concerning Gleets* (London: J. Clarke, 1732), 417.

26. Graham Everett's term for this "furore," as used in *Doctors and Doctors: Some Curious Chapters in Medical History and Quackery* (London: Swan, Sonnenschein, Lowrey & Co., 1888), 104, 106.

27. D. Turner, *Ancient Physician's Legacy . . . Survey'd*, 59.

28. Dover's work continued through at least eight editions, the last printed in 1771. And after both Dover and Turner were dead, respected authorities like George Cheyne continued to laud mercury as the "only true Panacea, and Universal Antidote." See Cheyne's *The Natural Method of Cureing the Diseases of the Body and the Disorders of the Mind* (London: G. Strahan and J. and P. Knapton, 1742), 119. David Hartley discussed similar outcomes of disputes in his "Honour and Property: The Structure of Professional Disputes in Eighteenth-Century English Medicine," in *The Medical Enlightenment of the Eighteenth Century*, ed. Andrew Cunningham and R.K. French (Cambridge: Cambridge Univ. Press, 1990), 138-64.

29. Turner entered into a similar dispute against the French physician Augustine Belloste's panacean claims for his mercury pill. See Daniel Turner, as cited by [T. Dover], *Encomium Argenti Vivi: A Treatise upon the Use and Properties of Quicksilver* (London: for Stephen Austin, sold by J. Roberts, [1733]), 61-64.

30. Marjorie H. Nicolson, "Ward's 'Pill and Drop' and Men of Letters," *Journal of the History of Ideas* 29 (1968): 177. For other accounts of Ward, his reputation, and his medicines see H. Selfe Bennett, "Joshua Ward, 1685-1761," *Proceedings of the Royal Society of Medicine. Section of the History of Medicine* 9 (1916): 100-112, and W.A. Campbell, "Portrait of a Quack: Joshua Ward (1685-1761)," *University of Newcastle Medical Gazette* (June 1964): 118-22.

31. The campaign lasted several years, and according to a historian of periodi-

cal publication, Ward's "Pill and Drop" was given more space in the *Grub Street Journal* than any other subject in the paper's history. James T. Hillhouse, *The Grub Street Journal* (Durham, N.C.: Duke Univ. Press, 1928; reprint, New York: Benjamin Blom, 1967), 272.

32. Eric Jameson, *The Natural History of Quackery* (London: Michael Joseph, 1971), 45.

33. Daniel Turner, *The Drop and Pill of Mr. Ward Consider'd* (London: J. Clarke, 1735), 15, 29-32.

34. Ibid., 38.

35. Edmund Packe, *An Answer to Dr. Turner's Letter to Dr. Jurin* (London: J. Roberts, 1735), 34.

36. For a description of this method, see François Chicoyneau, *The Practice of Salivating shewn to be of no Use or Efficacy in the Cure of the Venereal Disease*, trans. C. Willoughby (London: J. Roberts, 1723), and R. Brown, *A Letter from a Physician in London . . . giving an Account of the Montpelier Practice* (London: J. Roberts, 1730).

37. Turner published correspondence from Desault's countryman, Monsieur Perochon of Bordeaux, in favor of salivation in which Perochon claimed Desault's method was "entirely exploded" such that he knew no one still following this practice in Bordeaux. D. Turner, *Syphilis*, pt. 2, 245-46. It is noteworthy that this is the only contemporary Frenchman whose writing or practice Turner explicitly favored. More often, Turner reflects the national tradition of remaining what Jeremy Black describes as "Natural and Necessary Enemies" against France. See Black's *Natural and Necessary Enemies: Anglo-French Relations in the Eighteenth Century* (London: Duckworth, 1986).

38. Douglas, *Treatise on Venereal Disease*, pt. 3, 53. He claimed that although they were "well cured" without the "least visible sign of the distemper remaining," "two or three . . . still pretended to have pains here and there" due to the "fear of paying" for their treatment.

39. Ibid., 154-55. "What say ye to this?" he added, "Is not the milch cow [his depreciating terms for Turner] in danger of going dry?" Douglas identified physicians Mead, West, Douglas, Sanders, Nisbett, Owen, and Wodrow in support of friction as well as surgeons Paisely, Deverell, Glen, and Horton.

40. Ibid., 153. Jean Astruc, France's most authoritative venereologist, also argued that "all Degrees" of venereal disease could be removed by "mercurial Remedies without [bringing the patient to] salivation." J. Astruc, *A Treatise of the Venereal Diseases* as cited by D. Turner in *Aphrodisiacus*, xxx-xxxi. Astruc held little regard for Turner's writing style, claiming it was "not so methodically delivered . . . nor placed in . . . order as might have . . . afforded a fuller Insight into the Nature of this Distemper," as cited by Turner, *Syphilis*, pt. 2, viii. Turner, too, disapproved of Astruc's writing agenda to compile an encyclopedic account of "useless Divisions" and "unnecessary Distinctions" that were "superfluous and foreign" to practical means of cure (Turner, *Syphilis*, pt. 2, 53-61).

41. Guaiac, also known as *Lignum vitae*, the "pock wood," and the "Indian cure" or "Indian Decoction," was a wood introduced into Spain and Portugal from the New World in the early sixteenth century. By 1728, the "guaiacum vogue" was "once again revived." Robert S. Munger, "Guaiacum, the Holy Wood from the New World," *Journal of the History of Medicine* 4 (1949): 218.

42. C. Willoughby anticipated that opposition to salivation would generate a similar response from both physicians and surgeons as the response had been to proposals for safer and gentler methods of treating smallpox. See the introduction of his translation of François Chicoyneau's *The Practice of Salivating*, iii.

Chapter 5

John Burrows and the Vegetable Wars

MARIE E. MCALLISTER

ALL AGES HAVE THEIR DESPERATE ILLS, DISEASES WHOSE ONLY KNOWN CURE IS AS terrible as the sickness itself. The frightened patient prepares to enter into a dreadful course of treatment, in which physical suffering will be compounded by months of confinement and lingering aftereffects, with no certainty that the cure will be complete. The disease itself, although common enough to be the subject of both pity and jokes, carries severe social consequences. The workman may lose his job, the prostitute her last means of support, the eminent citizen his public character, the married couple their happiness: "How often has the Peace and Union of Families been disturbed by the ignominious Traces of Debauchery, which a young Bride has discovered on her Bridegroom!"[1]

Small wonder that such patients turn eagerly to alternative medicine. Small wonder either that some fall prey to quacks and hucksters for whom the pain of others means easy profit. In the eighteenth century, when the problem was venereal disease the profits could be immense. The inventor of Godbold's "Vegetable Balsam," a former gingerbread baker, was said to have made ten thousand pounds a year from his syrup, while Isaac Swainson (an active participant in the vegetable wars of my title) earned enough from his remedy to purchase a fine Twickenham estate and create an extensive botanical garden on its grounds.[2] In France, Laffecteur's antisyphilitic nectar, guaranteed mercury-free, was such a success that its inventor became official supplier to the French navy—obviously a lucrative commission.[3] In England, the potential revenues from antivenereal medicines were so great that competitors stole each other's trade names and spent their proceeds on pamphlets accusing one another of medical malpractice.

How, two hundred years later, can the researcher evaluate the eighteenth century's alternative medicine and sort profit seekers from serious prac-

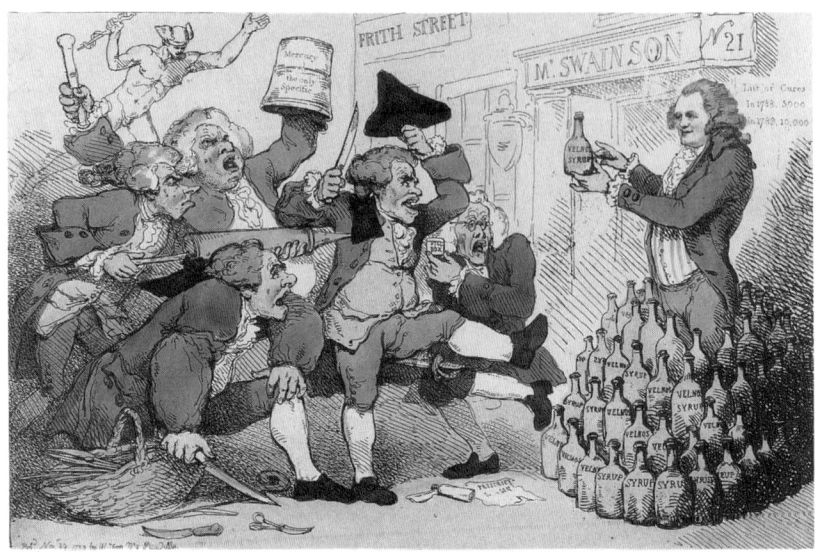

Fig. 6. Thomas Rowlandson (1789), "Mercury and his Advocates defeated, or Vegetable Intrenchment." Harvey Cushing/John Hay Whitney Medical Library, Yale University.

titioners? Some venereal disease medicines seem from the perspective of our own time to have been utterly fraudulent, the work of charlatans interested only in lining their own pockets. Others, however, make sober scientific claims or are supported by reputable eighteenth-century physicians. Patients, even if they could distinguish, might be tempted to try both. Mercury, the treatment program supported by the eighteenth-century medical establishment, proved ineffective or physically intolerable for many venereal disease patients. These sufferers could try a host of alternative treatments, some of which made the same claims alternative medicines make today: they relied on natural ingredients; they sought to heal the whole person; they were based on a science untainted by contemporary prejudices. Such remedies also offered the possibility of health to patients whom the medical establishment had already failed—and of course today mercury therapy is no longer given. Once the science has changed, is the alternative medicine necessarily more dubious than its mainstream counterpart?[4]

This article considers one branch of eighteenth-century alternative medicine, plant-based nonmercurial remedies purported to cure venereal disease. I am quite unable to say whether such remedies did anyone any good. Perhaps they staved off mercury doctors long enough for nature to heal some problems mistakenly diagnosed as venereal. What interests me more than the efficacy of such drugs is the picture of eighteenth-century life gained by examining the culture that produced them. By surveying the ideas behind plant medicines and by looking particularly at the career and writings of one advocate of nonmercurial remedies, we glimpse the spectrum of eighteenth-century medicine and learn something about how the trade of alternative medicine was practiced. This essay, then, tells the story of a reputable physician turned patent medicine salesman, of the vegetable wars in which he engaged, and of the rhetoric he used to persuade scientists and lay readers to consider his "New Vegetable Remedy." Dr. John Burrows's personal and professional lives remain for the most part a mystery, but what we can learn of his scientific and commercial practice opens an interesting window into the world of nonmercury veneral disease healers.

Mercury treatments constituted the preeminent "cure" for venereal disease in the eighteenth century, but mercury's side effects—and its limited efficacy—had aroused opposition for centuries. By the time my subject, John Burrows, began advertising his vegetable syrup in 1772, nonmercurial alternatives had a long pedigree and the support of certain schools of scientific thought. More supportive still were the patients for whom mercury had proved useless or physically intolerable. Vegetable-based remedies promised good health coupled with secrecy. They could be taken without the supervision of a physician (a possibility touted by apothecaries and frowned on by doctors), and any side effects could be concealed, unlike the excess salivation associated with mercury treatments.

Several different theories provided support for nonmercurial treatments. The first derived from the Renaissance belief that unbalanced humors cause illness: by inducing vomiting and diarrhea, or salivation and sweating, morbid humors would be expelled and the body cleansed of disease. Thus, when Dr. Burrows argues for the superiority of his vegetable syrup as compared with mercury, he stresses the ability of the syrup to spread into and cleanse even the tiniest channels of the body: "The Vegetable Remedy does not act by Dint of Weight; it is not by forcing the Obstacles that it tends to destroy them . . . it mixes with the Humours, with them it conveys itself into the obstructed Vessels, reanimates their languid Motion, and disposes them efficaciously to operate upon the dense Matter which causes the Obstructions. It envelopes [sic] the Venereal *Miasmata*, alters their Nature, allays their Acrimony, and as it were *neutralizes* them."[5]

Vegetarianism as a moral and a therapeutic movement provided additional support for plant-based medical regimens. Virginia Smith has provided the most extensive analysis of eighteenth-century beliefs associated with vegetable diets, including "cooling" therapies such as bathing in cold water and eating raw fruits and vegetables. Smith neatly summarizes the old theoretical split dividing "post-Paracelsian 'heroic' chemotherapy" from "the humoralist/ mechanist paradigm of bodily harmony, the cool *vis medicatrix naturae*." On one side of this divide stood the mercury practitioners, fighting disease by increasingly technical chemical means. On the other stood practitioners of traditional and folk medicine, social reformers for whom vegetable diets symbolized moral purity, charlatans interested only in vending their own nostrums, and the occasional physician suspicious of mercury's purported benefits.[6]

Specific plant-based remedies had pedigrees almost as long as the theories on which they were based. The oldest well-known vegetable remedy for venereal disease was guaiacum, or "the bark," the wood of a New World tree (probably *Guaiacum officinale*), which appears to have had good short-term effects in some venereal cases. Owsei Temkin offers the most complete history of this remedy, which he traces back at least as far as 1518, when it was being imported from the West Indies. The humanist Ulrich von Hutten tried guaiacum then with temporary success, and a poem he wrote in its praise helped spread the bark's reputation—even after his death a few years later from syphilis. The famed Swiss physician and alchemist Paracelsus was more skeptical, attacking the treatment in 1529 as ineffective and entirely motivated by profit. Such skepticism had its roots in the mineral/vegetable split discussed above: Paracelsus rejected humoral theory and advocated the use of chemical specifics including mercury. But while Paracelsus's view eventually dominated, guaiacum held its own for several centuries. It, sarsaparilla, Peruvian bark (quinine), and other "sudorific woods" remained important medicinal ingredients throughout the eighteenth century.[7]

Theories about the origins of syphilis helped perpetuate the use of guaiacum and other woods. Many eighteenth-century British histories of syphilis have the disease originating in France or brought to France from Naples. Others argued that it had been brought back from the New World by Spanish explorers, and since guaiacum was a product of the Americas, it could thus be claimed as a specific for the American disease.[8] In another version of the same story, John Burrows argues that vegetable remedies must have value because venereal disease is supposedly endemial (endemic) in Africa toward "the coast of Guinea. This, I apprehend, implies, that these People had some kind of Remedy for this Distemper before the Properties of Mercury were discovered." Since European explorers found the inhabitants of Guinea "entirely unskilled in the Art of extracting Metals from the Bowels of the Earth," whatever medicine kept the disease endemic rather than epidemic must have been plant-based, not mineral.[9]

In addition to guaiacum, patients could avail themselves of a number of other plant-based remedies. The physician Buchan, writing in 1796, mentions guaiacum, sarsaparilla, mezereon (a European shrub with an acrid medicinal bark), opium, and Peruvian bark; a mercury supporter himself, he values each largely as it helps patients tolerate mercury. The recipes for most proprietary medicines were kept secret, but critics frequently guessed at the ingredients. Buchan, for instance, believed mezereon to be the active ingredient in Velnos's Syrup, "Dr. Kennedy's Decoction," and the "Lisbon Diet Drink"—the last of which he felt certain also secretly contained mercury.[10] Indeed, scandals involving the inclusion of mercury in supposedly vegetable cures emerged throughout the period. Isaac Swainson, for one, spent years trying to refute the claim that his vegetable syrup had been tested and found to contain mercury. His defense involved tarring his competitors as well as arguing for his own product: at the same time as he threatened, and published letters of retraction from, those who had impugned his formula, he accused all competitors (John Burrows included) of secretly dealing in mercury with utter disregard for their customers' health.[11]

Among the best-known English nonmercury remedies was Velnos's Vegetable Syrup, alternately referred to as Velno's, Velnos', de Velnos', and De Velnos's syrup. The variant titles may represent typographical preference or, as I shall discuss below, outright piracies of the name. Fortunately for the student of venereal disease, the various proprietors of this medicine or medicines were a literary lot, obligingly quick to defend their product in print and proclaim their exclusive right to the recipe. I have thus been able to reconstruct a significant portion of the syrup's rather scandalous history. It should be noted, though, that variations on de Velnos's concoction represent only a small proportion of the nonmercury medications available. Untitled proprietary medicines were widely advertised: "Dr. Henry begs leave to acquaint his friends and the public, that he continues dispensing at his home . . . his vegetable drops and balsam . . . for curing venereal disease, rheumatism and scurvy." Other such remedies had recognizable trade names, like the "real and only genuine Growland's Vegetable Lotion" of which Robert Dickinson advertised himself the "sole proprietor and preparer."[12]

The vegetable remedy or remedies that for simplicity's sake I will call Velnos's has by far the most vexing history of the nonmercury medicines I have reviewed. At least six different names come up in conjunction with the medicine; at least three writers claimed to be sole proprietor of the genuine article. Best of all, the man who took out a patent on the medicine is not among the last three. The origins of the syrup are murky, but the concoction was probably invented by Vergery de Velnos, either working with or succeeded by one Dr. Mercier.[13] About these original figures I have thus far discovered next to nothing. Thereafter, a number of treatises by different authors appear in defense of the syrup, each trumpeting its virtues and lambasting the effects of mercury. At one stage John Burrows patented the medicine; he was subsequently attacked by two different proprietors who claimed exclusive rights to the formula. The extensive pamphlet war that ensued seems to have had little long-term effect; before the century's end, variants on Velnos's Syrup were being widely marketed, and the cure was so popular that "Velno's Vegetable Syrup" takes pride of place in a 1792 Gillray cartoon of the Prince Regent.[14]

Many participants in the vegetable wars concerned themselves with attacking mercury as well as each other. The title of a work by Henry Saffory, who claimed to own rights to the medicine in 1773, is typical: *The inefficacy of all mercurial preparations in the cure of venereal and scorbutic disorders, proved from reason and experience. To which are added, a dissertation on M. de Velnos's vegetable syrup, which radically cures every species of the above disorders; and an accurate analysis of that medicine.* Saffory's title employs the language of enlightenment science in both his attack on mercury—"reason and experience"— and his defense of the accurately analyzed syrup. More dramatic is a title chosen by Isaac Swainson, who put himself forward as "sole proprietor of the genuine medicine" in the 1780s and 1790s: *Mercury Stark Naked. A Series of Letters, Addressed to Dr. Beddoes; Stripping that Poisonous Mineral of its Medical Pretensions; and Showing, That it Perpetuates, Increases, and Multiplies all Diseases for which it is Administered* (1797). Swainson, the man who supposedly bought a Twickenham estate with his profits from Velnos's Syrup, was among the most prolific writers on nonmercury medicines. Previous to *Mercury Stark Naked* he had published multiple editions of five works designed to encourage readers to apply to "Mr. Swainson in Frith Street" for their medicinal needs. *Directions for the Use of Velnos' Vegetable Syrup*, which first appeared in 1786, advertises that Swainson is "only successor to Mr. de Velnos and Dr. Mercier" and forcefully discourages clients from seeking out his competitors: the subtitle promises *a summary view of the artifices, by which Impostors have attempted to substitute ineffectual or poisonous preparations for the genuine syrup.*

The medicine men listed thus far—de Velnos, Mercier, Saffory, and Swainson—create a tangled history in themselves. How did de Velnos's medicine reach England? What was Mercier's role? From whom did Swainson purchase his rights? But more exciting complications remain. In February 1772, a full year before any of his competitors' treatises, Dr. John Burrows applied for and received a patent for "a medicine, called Velno's Vegetable Syrup."[15] He also published his treatise on venereal disease, *A Dissertation on the Nature and Effects of a New Vegetable Remedy*, which went through multiple editions over the next decade.

The vegetable wars began at once. Saffory's 1773 attack on mercury also attacked Burrows. Burrows replied with *Remarks on Certain Passages Contained in a Scurrilous Pamphlet, Published by Henry Saffory.* Saffory seems to have retreated, but the date of Burrows's patent next comes into question: by the third edition of his *Dissertation*, Burrows is claiming that the patent was received back in 1765. To complicate matters still more, in the mid-1780s

Isaac Swainson begins cautioning his readers against "spurious" versions of Velnos's Syrup, and in 1786 he lists Burrows prominently among those "impostors" whose "poisonous preparations" are being passed off as the genuine article. Burrows seems to have died before the vegetable wars reached their peak in 1792; at that point Swainson accused Burrows outright of obtaining his patent under false pretenses, passing off an inferior recipe as the genuine syrup, and essentially stealing the de Velnos name.[16]

Although Burrows responded to Saffory's 1773 attack, he appears to have held himself aloof thereafter. Perhaps Burrows did so to distinguish himself, as an M.D., from the medically unqualified Swainson.[17] Or perhaps his silence represented prudence consequent upon guilt. His publications carefully refer to a "New Vegetable Remedy," not "Velnos's Syrup," although his patent would seem to grant him clear title to the de Velnos name. Either he found the name not worth using, or he came under external pressure not to make free with the name of a preexisting remedy.

Swainson's indignation, which he expressed at great length in publication after publication, stems from several sources. He resents the competition—or, to put it more positively, he fears that patients will be harmed by inferior imitations of Velnos's Syrup. By 1792 he also worries that his recipe may be made public. The Royal College of Physicians, we discover, has asked to examine his medicine, perhaps suspecting again that it contains mercury. Indeed, the College is about to insert Burrows's recipe (apparently filed with the patent) into its Pharmacopoeia as the recipe for Velnos's Vegetable Syrup, an action that would put Swainson out of business. The unhappy proprietor must therefore prove that his "genuine" remedy differs from Burrows's, and he must insist on his right to preserve the secret formula for the true Velnos's Vegetable Syrup.[18] Perhaps by this point Swainson was regretting the hysterical tone of his 1791 attack on John Hunter's *Treatise on the Venereal Disease:* Hunter was an esteemed surgeon writing for other medical men, and the Royal College cannot have been much amused by Swainson's information that Hunter "was brought up, and, I am credibly informed, actually worked, as a common carpenter."[19]

Since the origin of Velnos's Syrup remains unclear, it is hard to weigh the merits of each participant's case. In the interpretation most favorable to Burrows, for example, Swainson's protests mean simply that the "sole proprietor" of Velnos's syrup was annoyed to find Burrows not only selling a competing product but also in possession of a royal patent. An interpretation less favorable to Burrows has him concocting some product similar to the existing Velnos's Syrup, then rushing to patent his formula under an already advertised, but not protected, name.

Swainson mentions three other doctors—Hodson, Baylis, and Moulsdale—in his attack on Burrows. Although he singles Burrows out for particular condemnation, he accuses all four of vending "pernicious preparations under similar names."[20] Hodson indeed authored two pamphlets on venereal disease while Baylis published a "practical botanic physic," but I have thus far been unable to trace any imitation Velnos's Syrup they may have sold. Others, however, clearly made use of the name. Two 1800 advertisements by James Pidding suggest its staying power: "A Few Testimonials of the Efficacy of de Velno's Vegetable Pills" and "Proofs of the Efficacy of de Velno's Vegetable Pills" are both listed in the *Eighteenth-Century Short Title Catalogue*, bound into copies of the *Critical Review*, *Gentleman's Magazine*, and the *Monthly Review* from that year. Pidding names himself the sole proprietor of de Velno's pills. Swainson must have been apoplectic.

So how does a medical doctor like John Burrows become involved in the sale of patent medicines and in the pamphlet wars accompanying that rich market? Biographical information that might help us understand Burrows's career trajectory is hard to come by.[21] Betty Rizzo has traced a significant portion of Burrows's professional life, which appears in its early days to have been reasonably successful, but Burrows's own publications remain the chief source of information on his metamorphosis from reputable doctor to more marginal figure.

Burrows is first traced as the personal doctor of the duchess of Bridgewater and her new husband, Sir Richard Lyttelton; he traveled with them as attendant physician after their marriage in 1745. Lyttelton proved a good patron, and when in 1763 Lyttelton was named captain general and governor of Minorca, "John Burrows, Esq." became secretary to the governor.[22] Four years later Burrows published his first work, a pamphlet on the treatment of cancers. Over the next two decades he repeatedly reissued this and his 1772 treatise on venereal disease.

Changes in approach between the first cancer treatise and Burrows's subsequent publications suggest that at some point between 1767 and 1772 his fortunes began to slide; Lyttelton's death in 1770 may have precipitated the change.[23] By this time Burrows had a wife and at least one child, a daughter, to support. He presumably lived for some years as a physician, then in 1775 engaged to travel to Cartagena with John Sherratt, who had just been appointed consul there. It is not clear whether he was hired as an attending physician or as an administrator with previous experience in a Spanish-speaking territory. Whatever the job, Burrows would probably have taken it: he appears to have been in terrible financial trouble at this point. According to Sherratt's later comments, Burrows had been arrested many times for large debts, and he had had two executions (the rough equivalent of modern bank auctions) in his house. Sherratt helped Burrows save some household possessions by shipping them to Cartagena along with his own.[24]

Burrows's ill luck appears to have followed him. Relations between the two men quickly soured, culminating when Sherratt physically attacked Burrows in a public tavern. After two months' imprisonment in the Spanish castle, Sherratt returned to England unemployed. Burrows, who had never been paid, was left to raise the money for his own return. If we are to believe the evidence of the fourth edition of his venereal disease pamphlet, Burrows spent the years 1775 to 1779 in Spain; that edition includes a testimonial from a Spanish nobleman praising Burrows's skill in physic.[25] Thereafter, Burrows surfaces only as the author of subsequent editions of his treatises on cancer and venereal diseases. He died sometime between 1784 and 1790.

Was Burrows, then, a reputable medical man, as his association with Lyttelton, Sherratt, and the Spanish court might suggest, or was he a quack, peddling a nostrum whose very name was stolen from a competitor? Was he simply a once-reputable M.D. fallen on hard times? A definitive answer seems impossible, but certainly Burrows's integrity grew more and more shaky over the course of his career. The case of his cancer pamphlets says a great deal about Burrows the venereal doctor. In 1767 Burrows published a short volume, *A New Practical Essay on Cancers,* anatomizing the kinds and causes of cancer and explaining those remedies he has found most effective in his own practice. An eighteenth-century reader might have picked up the essay with some suspicion, for cancer was every bit as much as venereal disease the province of the quack. Its contents, however, would have been reassuring. Burrows begins by laying out the history of the disease and its treatments. He examines formerly accepted treatments, questioning the merits of some. In careful scientific language he then divides cancers into four groups based on their causes: from venereal infections, from a scorbutic or scrofulous humor, from complications arising from such humors, and from external injuries. He treats the first with mercurials, the second with antimony, the third with a combination of medicines, and the last with the milk of goats fed on hemlock. He also uses external "antischirrous and anticancerous medicines" designed to ease pain, induce cleansing suppuration, and "relax the fibers" of the afflicted part. However doubtful these cures may now seem, an eighteenth-century reader in search of relief would likely have felt reassured by Burrows's historical knowledge, his scientific attempt at classification, and his willingness to match the treatment to the particular disease.

The "new edition" of *Cancers* that Burrows published in 1783, however, would have left its readers more doubtful. Largely a resetting of the original, the 1783 edition contains one highly disturbing change. The classifications Burrows offered in 1767 remain, but where in 1767 he accepted the use of mercury, antimony, and hemlock, by 1783 the only acceptable medicine, no matter what the case, is "my anticancerous elixir." No details about the contents of this elixir are offered, but it is proclaimed "the most safe, efficacious, and only certain method of cure" for all cancers. The elixir's source is equally questionable: "In my progress through the Levant, I met with an Armenian physician, who practiced there on cancers with astonishing success. On my hinting to him the superior efficacy of his medicine to any I had ever known . . . he generously imparted to me the valuable discovery."[26] The new edition's introduction also mounts a defensive-sounding attack on those who would discourage trained physicians from seeking out new cures. Perhaps Burrows was aware that he had crossed a line his fellow M.D.s still maintained.

Burrows's "anticancerous elixir" may well be a medicine different from the antivenereal "Vegetable Remedy." He makes no mention of the cancer elixir being plant-based nor does he go into the same laudatory details as in his vegetable treatise, and no patent is mentioned. Whatever its composition, however, the elixir's value can be questioned for reasons other than its supposed universal efficacy and its exotic origins. Numerous details from the 1783 treatise suggest that Burrows's medical practice was by then less than above-board. Unlike the original, the new edition trumpets the doctor's address on the title page and ends with a long compendium of testimonials. The testimonials themselves inspire doubt: reading Burrows on cancer of the breast—in which any swelling or inflammation related to breast-feeding seems to be classed with tumors of the breast—certainly raises the credit of those eighteenth-century doctors who claimed that most patients "cured" by proprietary medicines had been misdiagnosed all along.

Let us turn now to Burrows's "New Vegetable Remedy," which presents ethical problems of its own. The title of Burrows's publication already makes stronger claims than an impartial physician might have wanted: *A Dissertation on the Nature and Effects of a New Vegetable Remedy, an Acknowledged Specific in all Venereal Scorbutic & Scrofulous Cases.*[27] Like the cancer pamphlet, the *Dissertation* begins with a short treatise on its subject. Here Burrows reviews the history of venereal disease treatment, reminds readers of the problems associated with mercury regimens, and calls for further research, citing authorities—Boerhaave, Sydenham, and Fernel—who support the possibility of vegetable medicine. Burrows's language is scientific and rational, as when he explains that the current blanket acceptance of mercury has suppressed the search for other mineral cures, let alone possible plant- or animal-based remedies [12, 20]. Avoiding the melodramatic presentation of later writers (*Mercury Stark Naked*), he admits that mercury is not intrinsically bad, simply dangerous because of variations in physician skill, patient constitution, and medicine preparation; he even chastises the eminent Fernel for "over-strain[ing]" his attack on mercury [4, 16]. He then offers scientific explanations for the efficacy of plant-based medicines and describes the beneficial effects of the New Vegetable Remedy. (Briefly, plant medicines are soluble and can thus circulate throughout the body, pushing the disease out of channels mercury cannot reach and invigorating the entire physique.)

Yet however scientific the presentation and however correct his catalog of mercury's faults, Burrows's findings remain problematic. We might begin with the description of his medicine: "This Remedy... derives its Antivenereal Virtue from a certain Number of Plants, whose Efficacy in destroying the Venereal Virus, which they possess in an eminent Degree, was never so much as suspected" [25]. No mezereon, no China root, no guaiacum, no opium; whatever ingredients the syrup contains have never before been tried in connection with venereal disease. Then, too, whatever the particular symptoms—gonorrhea, syphilitic ulcers, swollen testicles, skin eruptions, nodes on the bones, and worse—the Vegetable Syrup, like the anticancerous elixir, can be counted on to do the trick. The patient can even administer his own remedy, although the doctor's supervision is advised. This last item, of course, brings out the remedy's selling point: it can be taken in complete secrecy, and leaves no aftereffects to shock a new spouse or deprive the patient of general society [37, 44].

Despite the occasionally technical approach of its initial section, Burrows's *Dissertation* is clearly directed toward potential purchasers rather than the scientific community. One interesting offshoot of this choice is Burrows's complete avoidance of moral comment. Where contemporaries interested in prevention and treatment address the spread of venereal disease through sexual contact, Burrows carefully avoids offending potential buyers by reproving them or warning them against sexual contact. Two hundred years earlier William Clowes had cautioned in his 1579 *Morbus Gallicus* that the existence of a book on cures must not be taken as encouragement to sinners who wished to continue their dissolute ways. In the eighteenth century William Buchan, Burrows's highly respected contemporary, goes substantially further, insisting that a man must inform his partner if he has been "off his guard at one time or another" and stressing the cruelty of communicating the disease to an "innocent" party: wives whose husbands "want honesty or resolution to tell them of their danger," children nursed by a carrier, nurses infected by their charges and unable to afford the treatment that would save their own families in turn.[28] Where a mainstream physician like Buchan stresses prevention and honesty or discusses the regulation of prostitution, Burrows remains silent, seeking to attract business, not forestall it. Like his less medically qualified fellows in the patent medicine business, Burrows writes for his audience rather than the greater good of medicine.

The most interesting part of the *Dissertation* may be the section of case studies and testimonial letters appended to the treatise itself. For the most part the format of these sketches is standard; testimonials attached to any similar treatise from the period contain the same litany of earlier failed treatments, new hope, and miraculously speedy cure. Yet despite their apparently formulaic aspect, the testimonials repay study. They represent storytelling at its simplest; they also reveal society in all its complexities.

To establish his veracity in these testimonial case studies, Burrows employs all the rhetorical techniques most commonly used by medicine peddlers. The precise symptoms of each sufferer are cataloged, sometimes in gruesome detail. Also recorded is the time elapsed before the remedy cleared up each symptom in turn: pain gone in days, throat ulcers healed two weeks later, tumors in the groin "radically cured" after a two-month course of Vegetable Syrup, and so forth. W.F. Bynum and Peter Wagner have discussed treatises in which an analysis of venereal disease becomes an excuse for including sexually explicit material, but Burrows's examples avoid mention of how the disease was contracted, and all references to anatomy serve only to show the miraculous healing powers of the syrup.[29] Of the twenty-five cases in the third edition, nineteen are carefully dated, and the dates themselves cover a span of seven years, presumably to reassure potential buyers of the medicine's illustrious history and continuing support. Most important of all, Burrows includes the names of, and other identifying details about, many of his satisfied patients. Eleven of Burrows's patients are named, with two more identified by initials or a last name. In those cases where no name is given, some other identifying detail appears in all but three instances: the name of a patient's employer, his doctor, or the merchant, clergyman, or other reputable person who will happily testify to the cure. Three of the cases take the form of letters from contented patients, while several of the case studies are also signed or witnessed.

Naturally, the question of authenticity arises at once. Were these real patients and witnesses? Or were they paid supporters, even inventive fictions? I have made no attempt at a complete answer, but a little digging uncovers a response largely favorable to Burrows. Easiest to trace from this list are professionals such as the doctors who have put themselves on record, according to Burrows, as having witnessed the fine effects of the Vegetable Remedy. One surgeon and one physician among those cited can be identified with reasonable certainty based on the locations of their practices (although Burrows spells the surgeon's name wrong and fails to identify which Dr. Morris he means of the two who were "physician to the army and the Westminster Infirmary").[30] Since both Ainsley/Ainslee and Morris (a or b) could have been traced with some ease by potential patients, they must be presumed to have supported Burrows's remedy, whether from belief or self-interest. Five other doctors mentioned by name are less easy to trace today, but since the locations of four are given, they too would probably have been detectable as fictions had Burrows simply invented his witnesses. This possibility can thus be ruled out.

Burrows could, of course, have used the doctors' names without permission, as did many of his contemporaries.[31] Certainly he makes free with whatever eminent names can be connected with the patient: Dr. Hinchliff, who was indeed "Lord Bishop of Peterborough and Master of Trinity College Cambridge" and who will supposedly testify to the cure of farmer James Cole;

Sir Richard Spry, who was indeed "Commodore" and whose servant Burrows cures of a persistent clap. With many of the witnesses and patients identifiable, though, it seems most likely that Burrows had permission to include the names he gives. Any would-be patient could have asked for the china painter Charles Weyman at the Bow manufactory in Middlesex County, or checked with the coachmaker Henry Saltkill "at Walham Green in the parish of Fulham" to see if John Astle still worked there and whether his symptoms had recurred. Almost certainly, either Burrows's medicine had its admirers or he paid off a fair number of people—and neither his probable financial condition nor the eminence of a few of his witnesses makes the latter likely.

But Burrows's sources are not all unimpeachable. The witnesses to four of his cases are booksellers or merchant firms. Booksellers are easy to trace, and it is quite clear that Burrows did not invent Mr. Berrow in Worcester or Fletcher and Hodson in Cambridge. But booksellers, of course, were interested parties, since many sold patent medicines for venereal and other diseases. Fletcher and Hodson, moreover, were the Cambridge booksellers for Burrows's first edition, a conflict of interest that casts some doubt on their ability to serve as impartial witnesses to the cure of Mr. Wilson in case twenty-three. The truly satisfied, the gullible, and the mercenary may all appear in Burrows's testimonial ranks.

To add to the authority of his claims, Burrows takes pains to make his list of satisfied patients all-inclusive. The author's habit of referring to every man as a gentleman and every woman as a lady makes class identification difficult in some cases, but the medicine was clearly aimed at all. Five satisfied patients are identified as servants; from there the ranks rise through lighterman, coachmaker's assistant, china painter, soldier, farmer, "country gentleman," high sheriff (retired), justice of the peace, and "person of distinction." The last three do not, I should point out, suffer from venereal disease. Two of the three are identified by name in Burrows's text and both, like the unnamed person of distinction, suffer from problems related to scurvy. Burrows graphically describes the skin condition of each distinguished gentleman lest we suspect that scurvy is here a polite euphemism for venereal infection. The unnamed "country gentleman," on the other hand, along with a number of other "gentlemen" whose class remains in question, clearly suffers from syphilis. Since Burrows touts his remedy as particularly useful to those whose constitutions are too delicate to endure mercury treatments (the elderly, children, pregnant women, invalids), both the sturdy workman and the more refined aristocrat could presumably have profited from the Syrup.

Another aspect of class that emerges in the early testimonials involves a sort of noblesse oblige. Higher-class patrons or employers provide referrals for a number of the lower-class patients: a soldier is recommended by his colonel, a farmer by his minister, a servant by his master. Burrows includes scant information about who pays for treatment in such cases; indeed, the essay never discusses the financial transactions it was written to create. The cases of servants, however, are particularly suggestive. One Richard Adams conceals his difficulty for some time, "being apprehensive of losing his place, if his master should come to the knowledge of his situation." When he at last takes to his bed, the consulting surgeon "proposed to his master, a mercurial course, which was agreed to"—implying that the master made decisions about, and paid for, the treatment. The decision to switch treatments then appears to have been made collaboratively between master and man: "having heard of the vegetable Syrup, in a similar case, they were resolved to make trial of it" [53]. In the other three other cases involving servants, the sufferer clearly acted on his own, whether from a similar fear of losing his job or simply because he felt no need for assistance.

Burrows not only seeks to appeal to persons of every class but also aspires to a national market. Locations are specified in about two-thirds of the cases, sometimes by city and sometimes by district. London and Cambridge are particularly well represented, probably because Burrows's first edition was available at booksellers in those two places,[32] but testimonials also pour in from Middlesex County, Bedfordshire, and Staffordshire. As if to extend his range, Burrows carefully includes an American patient living in London and a member of the Spanish ambassador's household, nationality unspecified.

Both sexes are likewise represented in the testimonials, although not in equal numbers. Writing about female venereal patients raises peculiar difficulties in a text where the side effects of mercury treatments in one male patient "cannot with delicacy be described" [48]. Burrows's cases include only three women, and one of these is set down as a scurvy sufferer rather than a venereal patient. The scurvy victim's symptoms are recorded in gruesome detail but are, of course, nonsexual. The two venereal patients are treated as utterly unsexed, with the exception of a clinical mention of one woman's formerly suppressed menses; no reader could possibly derive titillation or offense from the description of their cures. Burrows notes that one of the two female venereal cases is a wife whose husband he has also treated, and while it seems reasonable to wonder about the occupation of the second, who has suffered for four years from "the most dreadful symptoms" and for whom no partner is mentioned, Burrows refers to her as a lady and places all his emphasis on her terrible pain and speedy cure.

Any patient, in short, could prosper by taking the "New Vegetable Remedy." Rich or poor, male or female, newly afflicted or veteran of countless mercury regimens, Burrows's magic formula offered quick and permanent relief. The reader with some scientific background might focus on the first part of Burrows's *Dissertation;* the less learned might skim over it in favor of the stories of sufferers like themselves. Those in whom the vegetable wars might have been expected to produce some alarm—whom to believe when every remedy boasts of being genuine and labels its competitors poison?—were likely too desperate to care: if one remedy failed to work, another could be tried, and if the side effects proved miserable, they could hardly be worse than those of mercury.

Patients believed. But what of Burrows? Certainly he could have had faith in his own claims. As a physician he had witnessed mercury's side effects and watched disease recur in those whom mineral medicine had supposedly healed; he had reason to wonder if plant-based medicines might do more good. From the perspective of our own time his scientific theories, while laughable, are scarcely worse than those of his mercury-advocating contemporaries. He also maintained at least the pretense of scientific experimentation, testing his Syrup first on soldiers in the Westminster Hospital and later suiting the dose to the particular case. Perhaps Burrows really thought of himself as a researcher pushing the boundaries of knowledge and healing the afflicted. My own verdict is rather different: to me he seems a small-time medical man down on his luck. Better educated than other dealers in proprietary medicine, he nonetheless employed the usual tricks of the trade, and whatever high medical ethics he may once have possessed were quickly compromised when poverty struck. His Vegetable Syrup and Anticancerous Elixir probably hurt patients no more than the remedies he had been trained to offer, but I have trouble thinking that Burrows truly believed his own assertions.

Yet whatever the truth, the case of John Burrows must not be taken as proof that eighteenth-century alternative medicine was entirely dishonest. Illnesses incurable by the medicine of our own time do indeed make us vulnerable to quackery. But Burrows rightly points out that a gap between illness and treatment can and should call forth new research. Velnos's Vegetable Syrup failed to eradicate venereal disease. Indeed, it probably did little more than make a few men—though not Burrows—rich. Still, Burrows and his fellow vegetable doctors might have been satisfied to learn of the remedy that finally became standard for syphilis: penicillin mold was plant-based.

Notes

1. John Burrows, *A Dissertation on the Nature and Effects of a New Vegetable Remedy, an acknowledged specific in all venereal scorbutic & scrophulous cases, as published by authority of his Britanick majesty's royal letter patent, granted to J. Burrows, M.D. in the year 1765. And an appendix, containing a number of cures in extraordinary cases, performed in these kingdoms; attested by persons of character, and fully proving the extraordinary merit and singular virtues of this medicine*, 3d ed. (London: printed for the author, 1780), 37. I would like to thank Dr. Betty Rizzo for first steering me toward John Burrows and for very generously sharing her research on Burrows's life and career.

2. C.J.S. Thompson, *The Quacks of Old London* (New York: Brentano's, 1928), 345. Thompson does not cite sources, and I have been unable to verify his information, but the fortunes he describes seem well within the range of plausibility. An eighteenth-

century marginal annotation in Swainson's *Observations on the Venereal Disease* estimates the price of Swainson's syrup as "2/9 per dose" (London, 1791; Woodbridge, Conn.: Research Publications, 1988, microfilm), while Roy Porter has found another vegetable syrup advertised at the extraordinary rate of eight and sixpence: *Health for Sale: Quackery in England, 1660-1850* (Manchester: Manchester Univ. Press, 1989), 117. Burrows's patients generally took two doses a day, and judging by his case studies a two-month course of treatment was not unusual.

    3. Claude Quétel, *The History of Syphilis,* trans. Judith Braddock and Brian Pike (Baltimore: Johns Hopkins Univ. Press, 1990), 90.

    4. Roy Porter has challenged the whole notion of "alternative" medicine in the eighteenth century, arguing that "quacks" closely imitated their mainstream counterparts and that mainstream doctors were as interested in profits as their less credentialed brethren; see his *Health for Sale* for more on the concept and history of the "quack." As this essay will demonstrate, however, it remains useful to distinguish between treatments accepted by the medical establishment and those that operated from outside the mainstream.

    5. Burrows, *Dissertation,* 3d ed., 32.

    6. Virginia Smith, "Physical Puritanism and Sanitary Science: Material and Immaterial Beliefs in Popular Physiology, 1650-1840," in *Medical Fringe and Medical Orthodoxy, 1750-1850,* ed. W.F. Bynum and Roy Porter (London: Croom Helm, 1987), 176-81. For more on this divide see Allen G. Debrus, *The English Paracelsians* (New York: Franklin Watts, 1965).

    7. See for instance W. Buchan, M.D., *Observations Concerning the Prevention and Cure of the Venereal Disease* (London, 1796; reprint, New York: Garland, 1985), 104-5, 215.

    8. See Owsei Temkin, "Therapeutic Trends and the Treatment of Syphilis before 1900," *Bulletin of the History of Medicine* 39 (1955): 315-16.

    9. Burrows, *Dissertation,* 3d ed., 21. Burrows cites Sydenham's opinion that the disease was introduced to the Americas from the coast of Guinea; clearly, there is interesting work to be done here on the symbolic association of the slave trade with the origin of syphilis.

    10. Buchan, *Observations,* 105-6.

    11. Swainson, *Observations on the Venereal Disease* (London: for J. Ridgway, 1791).

    12. Titles from the *Eighteenth-Century Short Title Catalogue.* The former dates from *circa* 1778, while the latter, a 1796 "description of a remedy for all scorbutic eruptions and impurities in the face," appears bound with Hoyle's whist rules and a tax table; its reference to scorbutic conditions is a common euphemism for venereal skin conditions. For more on the advertising of proprietary medicines see Helen MacGregor, "Eighteenth-Century V.D. Publicity," *British Journal of Venereal Diseases* 31 (1955): 117-18.

    13. In his *History of Syphilis,* Quétel mentions many eighteenth-century venereal remedies advertised in France as containing no mercury; among them is a "new vegetable anti-venereal remedy" offered by Velnos (90). The title page of Isaac Swainson's *Directions for the Use of Velnos' Vegetable Syrup* (London, 1786) proclaims that Swainson is the "only successor to Mr. de Velnos and Dr. Mercier." Swainson later claimed to have purchased the recipe for four thousand pounds at a time when de Velnos's "perfidious agents" were concocting their own imitations: *An Account of Cures by Velnos' Vegetable Syrup* ... (London: printed for the author, 1790), 2-3.

    14. "A Voluptuary Under the Horrours of Digestion," noted in Porter, *Health for Sale,* 150.

15. *Calendar of Home Office Papers of the Reign of George III*, 3 (1770-72): 618. The patent gave Burrows "the sole use and benefit" of his invention for fourteen years; it was granted 17 February 1772.

16. Swainson, *An Account*, 3-4.

17. Swainson admitted his lack of medical credentials in his pamphlets. Thompson believes that he was originally a woolen draper: *Quacks*, 345. Burrows should not necessarily have been embarrassed by his association with the Syrup, however: Porter believes that many legitimate physicians created patent medicines or sold proprietary medicines: *Health for Sale*, 8, 155.

18. Swainson, *An Account*, 3-4.

19. Swainson, *Observations on the Venereal Disease* (London: for J. Ridgway, 1791), 7.

20. Swainson, *An Account*, 3.

21. Wallis's *Eighteenth-Century Medics: Subscriptions, Licenses, Apprenticeships* lists a John Burrows born in 1750 and apprenticed in 1767, but this information must refer to another man of the same name, possibly even a son: Peter John Wallis et al., 2d ed. (Newcastle upon Tyne: Project for Historical Bibliography, 1988). Burrows must have been born in the 1710s or 1720s to be old enough to be a practicing physician in 1745. The date of his death also remains untraced, but he must have died between 1785, when the final edition of his work on cancers was published, and 1790, when Isaac Swainson notes that Burrows is dead: *Observations*, 44. The date and specifics of Burrows's medical training remain unknown, and it is perfectly possible that his degree, like many in the eighteenth century, was purchased rather than earned.

22. *Daily Advertiser*, Monday, 25 April 1763.

23. Betty Rizzo, "John Sherratt, Negociator," *Bulletin of Research in the Humanities* 86, no. 4 (1983-85): 426.

24. Ibid., 425, citing BL Add Mss 24,170 ff. 158-59.

25. Burrows, *Dissertation*, 4th ed., 78-79.

26. Burrows, *A New Practical Essay on Cancers*, new ed. (London: printed for the author, 1783), 74. The fourth edition of the *Dissertation* similarly plays on the lure of exotic medicines, claiming that in his recent travels in Spain, Burrows has discovered a wonderful new remedy which, "by topical application," cures ulcers in the urethra and bladder (76); Porter notes that such claims of exotic origin were common (*Health for Sale*, 108-9).

27. I have had access to the third and fourth editions of the *Dissertation*. The fourth simply resets the material of the third, with appended material (discussed above) on Burrows's new ulcer unguent and his service in Spain. Here and throughout, I will thus refer primarily to the third edition, which boasts "Improvements" on earlier editions (title page). The third edition includes cases from 1768 through 1772 (presumably those of the first edition) plus five cases from 1775; the fourth adds two more cases, one from 1784, the year of publication. The fourth edition is available on microfilm in *The Eighteenth Century* (Woodbridge, Conn.: Research Publications, 1983): reel 296, no. 17.

28. Buchan, *Observations*, 139, 157, 153, and passim.

29. W.F. Bynum, "Treating the Wages of Sin: Venereal Disease and Specialism in Eighteenth-Century Britain," in *Medical Fringe and Medical Orthodoxy*, 14-15; Peter Wagner, "The Discourse on Sex—or Sex as Discourse: Eighteenth-Century Medical and Paramedical Erotica," in *Sexual Underworlds of the Enlightenment*, ed. G.S. Rousseau and Roy Porter (Chapel Hill: Univ. of North Carolina Press, 1988), 46-68.

30. "John Ainsley, Surgeon (Attending), Cavendish Square," from case seven, is probably the John Ainslee whom Wallis cites as practicing from that location. The Dr. Morris of cases eleven and twenty-four, identified in the latter as "physician to the army and the Westminster Infirmary," could be either of two Dr. Morrises (Michael and George) who fit this profile.

31. Beddoes complains of this at the end of the century; see Porter, *Health for Sale*, 193.

32. The title page of the 1772 edition lists G. Kearsley as the London bookseller and Fletcher and Hodson as the Cambridge representatives.

Chapter 6

"And blights with plagues the Marriage hearse"

Syphilis and Wives

MARY MARGARET STEWART

I wander thro each charter'd street,
Near where the charter'd Thames does flow,
And mark in every face I meet
Marks of weakness, marks of woe.

In every cry of every Man,
In every Infant's cry of fear,
In every voice, in every ban,
The mind-forg'd manacles I hear.

How the Chimney-sweeper's cry
Every blackning Church appalls;
And the hapless Soldier's sigh
Runs in blood down Palace walls.

But most thro midnight streets I hear
How the youthful Harlot's curse
Blasts the new-born Infant's tear,
And blights with plagues the Marriage hearse.

"LONDON" FROM WILLIAM BLAKE'S *SONGS OF EXPERIENCE* (1794) POINTS TO A problem in eighteenth-century England that was seldom openly discussed—venereal disease within a marriage. This very silence created a danger for the many wives who were innocent—innocent in the sense that they had not had sex outside the marriage; innocent in the sense that they knew nothing about venereal disease and/or their possible exposure to it and did not therefore recognize the symptoms in themselves or in others. When Henry Thrale told

Hester Thrale that "he had an Ailment" and showed her "a Testicle swelled to an immense Size," she had "no Notion but of a *Cancer.*" "Poor Fool," she records. She "press'd him to have the best help that could be got—no he would have only Gregory—a drunken crazy Fellow that his Father had known: however," she continues,

> when I pressed him with an honest earnestness and kind Voice to have Hawkins, Potts or some eminent hand—he said it was nothing dangerous with a Smile; but that since I had an Aversion to Mr. Gregory he would send for one Osborne; a sort of half Quack, whose Name I have sometimes read in the papers as possessing the Receipts of a M: Daran a famous Practitioner in the *Venereal* Way: I now began to understand where I was, and to perceive that my poor Father's Prophecy was verified who said If you marry that Scoundrel he will catch the Pox, & for your Amusement set you to make his Pultices. This is now literally made out; & I am preparing Pultices as he said, and Fomenting this elegant Ailment every Night & morning for an Hour together on my Knees, & receiving for my Reward such Impatient Expressions as disagreeable Confinement happens to dictate. However tis well tis no worse—he has I am pretty sure not given it me.[1]

In part to provide information to such wives, Dr. John Profily published in 1748 *An Easy and Exact Method of Curing the Venereal Disease in all its Different Appearances: With an Account of its Nature, Causes, and Symptoms: Demonstrated By Way of Dialogue between Physician and Patient For the Use and Instruction of all Unfortunate Persons who may labour under that Disorder; by which in common Cases they may be instructed to Cure themselves, or know if they are treated according to the Art by those whom they apply to.* In the preface of this work addressed "to the President and Fellows of the College of Physicians of London," Profily clearly signals that women are an important part of his intended audience:

> The Venereal Distemper, exclusive of every Degree of Pain, has the direful Attendants of Shame, Reproach and Ridicule. It too often happens, that those injurious Attendants, totally undeserved by the blameless and innocent, attack them in a severe manner. Many of the Female Sex, incapable of Vice from virtuous Sentiments, become daily the wretched Victims of this fatal Enemy, brought upon them innocently; tho' such unfortunate Sufferers will never meet with Reproach or Ridicule but from

base and ill-disposed Minds. If Pity and Relief can any where be rightly placed, surely the properest Object to exercise them on is the melancholy Situation of a disconsolate Female, whose Body [is diseased] by the Embraces of a careless vicious Husband.

One of his cases involves a woman who has gotten venereal disease three times from her "wicked Husband" [267]. Hester Thrale Piozzi notes in her diary: "And so poor Mrs Siddons's Disorder that we have all been at such a stand about, turns upon close Examination to be neither more nor less than the P—— given her by her Husband. What a World it is!!"[2]

When the duke of Norfolk brought the charge of adultery against his wife, Lady Mary Mordant, and argued more harm is done by the wife in adultery than by the husband, Lady Mary's counsel, Sir Thomas Powys, replied: "They say the Offence is not equal, because the Man brings no children into the Family. I doubt it happens oftentimes to them that go abroad, that they bring home that to their Wives, which stick longer by them then their children."[3]

George Granville's poem "Cleora" (1712) tells the admonitory story of a young woman who weds an older peer only to put up with gross drunkenness, unwanted sex, and then venereal disease:

> What then may be the Chance that next ensues?
> Some vile Disease, fresh reeking from the Stews.
> The secret Venom, circling in her Veins,
> Works thro' her Skin, and bursts in bloating Stains,
> Her Cheeks their Freshness lose, and wonted Grace,
> And an unusual Paleness spreads her Face,
> Her Eyes grow dim, and her corrupted Breath
> Tainting her Gums, infects her Ivory Teeth,
> Of sharp nocturnal Anguish she complains,
> And guiltless of the Cause, relates her Pains.
> The conscious Husband, whom like Symptoms seize,
> Charges on her the Guilt of their Disease,
> Affecting Fury, acts a Madman's Part,
> He'll rip the fatal Secret from her Heart!
> Bids her confess, calls her ten thousand Names,
> In vain she kneels, she weeps, protests, explains,
> Scarce with her Life she scapes, expos'd to Shame,
> In Body tortur'd, murdered in her Fame,
> Rots with a vile Adulteress's Name,
> Abandon'd by her Friends, without Defence,
> And happy only in her Innocence.

Granville asserts:

Thousands of poor *Cleora's* may be found,
Such husbands and such wretched Wives abound.[4]

Writing from London in 1779, a Lydia Vernon tells the tale of an innocent Mrs. Dewars, whose husband has infected her with the "cursed disorder" of which she was ignorant. Although she asked him what her disorder might be, he not only protested he did not know but also abandoned her. After being told by a physician of Mrs. Dewars's condition, Lydia Vernon confronted Mr. Dewars, telling him she "thought he was less pardonable for Murdering the woman in this Manner (as he was now killing her by inches,) than if he Shot her through the head, that he was now the Basest of Murderers."[5]

Besides innocence, a wife faced a second difficulty: keeping her disease a secret from the servants and family as well as from her acquaintances and the public.[6] Secrecy was, of course, particularly difficult for those who did not have the means to undergo the cure outside their own homes. In fact, Profily explains in his preface that he considers cases of venereal disease in the female "and at the same time her Desire of Secrecy [is] so well satisfied, that by consulting the Monitor I here recommend to her, who cannot divulge what she would conceal, she will hereby find Refuge and Redress."

On 6 June 1742, Frances Williams's husband, Charles Hanbury Williams, settled in Bath to undergo the cure for venereal disease. His friend Henry Fox was informed of the infection and frequently reported to concerning its progress and the ineffectual treatment. But Frances Williams was not. What she had been told about his retirement to Bath we do not know, but whatever it was, it was not the truth. The longer Charles Hanbury Williams stayed at Bath, the more certain he became that his venereal infection was a serious one. His complaints of buboes ("swellings or tumours that arise in the groin")[7] and chancre (a venereal sore or ulcer; primary lesion of syphilis) plus the resistance of his infection to treatment clearly indicate to us he had syphilis. As he continued to undergo his cure during June, July, and August, Frances remained in London taking care of their two young daughters, faithfully writing to her husband the news of London and his family.

Sometime during the summer months, Frances began to develop health problems—probably beginning with violent headaches and then pains in her arms and shoulder blades, shins, and joints, as well as general languor.[8] She must have become aware of warts or ulcers on her genitals.[9] Eventually, she got a chancre on the roof of her mouth.[10] In her letters she enumerated her complaints to her husband, who gave no hint concerning what might be the cause of her deteriorating health. Still innocent, she shared her complaints with close friends and her aunt, Lady Kildare. By the end of August, she discovered the cause of her problems, and with her aunt's knowledge and approval, she placed herself under the care of Doctor J. Oldfield, a London physician.

Lady Kildare expressed her indignation. "I cant conclude this," she wrote Charles Hanbury Williams, "without telling you that though I saw her in the miserable Condition she is in, It never entered into my head that any Gentleman, or a man of the least honnor, Could doe so base, so cruel an action, to a woman whose virtue I will defie any body to touch."[11]

Frances Williams was furious, particularly after Williams cast suspicion upon her by suggesting that there was no possible way he could have gotten the disease. "What an opinion must you have of your having subdued my reason and Common Sense," she wrote her husband, "as well as master'd my affections, in writing me such a Letter, as I have now before me? To add the charge of the most *shameless* & *infamous Crime*, I could commit, to the *Cruelest injury*, I could Suffer! This you have done, without aspersion, & in the most glaring light, of your own *Guilt*. You leave me, in the hurry & confusion, that your own frightful Consciousness brought upon you, Endeavour to delude me with a thousand inconsistent Shifts & turnings; (wch. now I have laid together, make me amazed with my own, so long continued Blindness.) But, wch. is more than all, you suffer such a distemper, & the Remedy of it, without the *least intimation* of it, to the *only* Person, from whom you *receiv'd* the Injury, and from *her alone*, you are so infinitely industrious to conceal it, that you had rather she should *perish* herself, than be made acquainted with it." In that same letter she demanded that he make her "the *most Express* & *direct Acknowledgment*, & *Satisfaction*, for so *outrageous* & *horrid* an *Imputation;* & 'till that is *amply* done" she refused to have any more correspondence with him.[12]

By 15 September, Doctor Oldfield reported to Williams that his wife's "distemper advances very fast and will require the most effectual Remedy very soon, that is I believe in less than a week, to prevent its running beyond the ready and certain reach of means, and to secure against any lasting ill consequences from it."[13] On Thursday, 23 September 1742, Frances Williams, accompanied by her friend Mary Trevor, took lodgings on Fenchurch Street in the City to be in Dr. Oldfield's neighborhood. That night she began her remedy. Two days later, Dr. Oldfield omitted the treatment in the evening because of Frances Williams's "extream Languor and weakness."[14] Six weeks later, on 8 November 1742, her "weak State" required her to remain at her Fenchurch Street lodging. On 12 November, seven weeks after moving into Dr. Oldfield's neighborhood, she prepared to leave, and by Wednesday, 17 November, she was in her aunt's home on Albemarle Street.

Whatever remedy Dr. Oldfield prescribed, it would have centered on mercury, which Frances Williams could have taken orally by pills, or injection as a physic, or as an ointment rubbed into her ulcers and body by friction.[15] Most likely, she underwent a course of salivation, an operation to which Charles

Hanbury Williams resorted after all other treatments failed.[16] It was a treatment he had vowed he would never consent to undergo.[17] And for good reason. The remedy required confinement six to seven weeks and was a painful and debilitating experience.

Standing before a fire, the patient began the cure by rubbing mercurial ointment into her feet and ankles until the ointment was absorbed, the skin dry, and the ankles red. She then covered up the parts to which she had applied the ointment and got into a warm bed where she had to lie for two hours until the ointment had penetrated the body more deeply. From the beginning to the end of this remedy the patient was instructed to keep the chamber warm. On the third day, she rubbed the ointment into her skin from the ankle to the top of her calf. On the fifth day, she rubbed the ointment from the calf to the buttocks and then wrapped herself in a flannel sheet. During this time, she was not to drink wine or malt liquor and she was not to eat any solid meals but only broth and very light food. She was directed to drink an extraction of barley made with liquorice. On the seventh day of her confinement she was to rub the ointment from the buttocks up the loins and back to the neck.

During the period of friction, the patient remained wrapped in flannel and spent most of her time in bed. As early as the fifth day, patients complained of feeling faint, of headaches, and of pains in the gums and teeth. At that time, the doctor checked the mouth and tongue for redness and for signs of ptyalism (excessive secretion of saliva). By the end of the seventh day the tongue and mouth were generally red and the patient began to spit a "thick, tenacious, viscid, putrid Substance" as much as three pints within twenty-four hours. As the spitting continued, the patient lived entirely upon broth unless she had no temperature. In that case she was permitted to eat a poached egg. Dr. Profily instructed his patients to drink as much as two or three quarts of Ptisan (a drink made by boiling down barley water and other ingredients) every day. But, before drinking, the patient was instructed to rinse her mouth with Ptisan "for fear that the acrimonious viscid Phlegm which sticks in [the] Mouth should be carried with the Liquor into [the] Stomach."[18] After ten or twelve days the patient was permitted to get up and sit by the fire in the warm chamber. If too weak to sit up, she lay face down in bed as she was instructed to lie whenever she prepared for sleep.

During his treatment, Charles Hanbury Williams complained to Henry Fox that he had "nothing easy about [him] but [his] hands."[19] A patient's greatest complaint was a sore mouth, ulcers in the mouth, difficulty swallowing, and a swollen tongue that made speech difficult and slurred. Ulcers near the uvula and root of the tongue were treated with spirit of salt and a little honey two times a day until the "white *Muscus* comes off, & till they appear red, and ready to be covered with a *Cicatrix*."[20] The patient was admonished to endure the pain so that the liquid could penetrate the crust of the ulcer. Ulcers on the sides of the tongue were washed in warm milk to encourage them since they supposedly produced the saliva.[21]

After eighteen to twenty days the patient's spitting was not to exceed five or six pints each day. If it exceeded that amount, the patient was instructed to change the sheets and the flannel wrap, which retained remnants of the mercurial ointment, and to treat the ulcers on the tongue. If the patient's spit did not amount to five or six pints a day, she was told to repeat the friction with mercurial ointment two or three times.

After the patient had been spitting regularly for twenty days and after the ulcers on the body had healed, it was time to curb the spitting, to cure all the ulcers in the mouth, and to strengthen the patient so that she might leave her confinement. She was instructed to take off the "foul" flannels, to put on clean flannels, and to put fresh linen on the bed. All parts of the body where the ointment had been rubbed were then washed with oil of sweet almond and then with brandy. She must take a glyster and then, the next day, a purging physic.[22] If the spitting did not stop, the physic had to be repeated every other day until the spitting disappeared. The ulcers on the side of the tongue were treated with spirit of salt and honey; the mouth was washed with barley water and Honey of Roses and then with red wine. The patient was then allowed to eat solid food, air the chamber, and go out.[23]

Charles Hanbury Williams was particularly concerned about public knowledge of his and his wife's illnesses. When Henry Fox wrote to Williams he always refers to Dr. Oldfield as "O" and Frances Williams as "the person." In his correspondence with Williams, Dr. Oldfield refers to Frances Williams as Williams's "friend" and always uses the masculine pronoun when referring to her. Mary Trevor, who kept Charles Hanbury Williams informed of his wife's condition when Dr. Oldfield could not write, was always referred to as M——— T———. Both Fox and Frances Williams let him know, however, it was a vain wish that the affairs could remain secret. On 28 October 1742, Henry Fox told Williams, "Mr West this morning told me that He heard from Bath that You had been under the Cure You have gone through. . . . Mr Pelham indeed long ago told me that He had heard Your Illness had been of the Kind it was. I soon put Him off that Discourse whether off of the Belief of it I don't know."[24] In November, Frances Williams wrote her husband: "I should imagine, you could want no *information* from *hence* of *this* Affair's being *publicly* known, &, indeed, how could you conceive it possible, it should be otherwise, when you have continued so *long ill*, in *such* Circumstances, in, the most *Public place*, Excepting *this*, in England, & during wch. time, I have *disappeared* here, for above 6 weeks? Besides, in my 2d Letter to you, I told you, that *your* having *kept me*, in *Ignorance*, had been the *means* of *informing* others; & when it came to be *known*, what my *distemper*, was; it was not a time, for *me* to *deny*, from *whom* I had *receiv'd* it; or Scarce to be *Silent* about it, without *favouring* the *horrid Suggestion*, I tremble to relate."[25] Indeed, the condition of both Charles and Frances was widely known. On 15 November 1742, Horace Walpole wrote Horace Mann: "Hanbury Williams is very ill at Bath, and his wife in the same way in private lodging in the city: all the old women are full of it,—I don't mean, of what he and his wife are."[26] On 12 November 1742, Mary Delany wrote to her sister in a tone quite different from the comic one of Walpole: "Lady Frances Williams is dying with ye foul disease, & that monster her husband never told her what ail'd her. they are parted. such husbands and such wretched wives abound."[27] Despite Mrs. Delany's grave forecast, Lady Frances recovered from this bout of illness. In fact, she lived until 1781, surviving her husband by twenty-two years.

From the time she discovered the cause of her illness, Frances Williams's resentment was so strong that she declared she would never return to Charles Hanbury Williams. Despite his confession that there was a way he could have contracted the disease outside of marriage,[28] despite his declarations of love and deep affection (letters coached by Henry Fox), despite his threat to insist that the two girls live with him, despite the duplicity of Dr. Oldfield, who without Frances Williams's knowledge had been engaged by Henry Fox to work to bring about a reconciliation, Frances Williams remained adamant.[29] She demanded an Agreement of Separation; furthermore, she refused to see Charles Hanbury Williams again and insisted that all negotiation concerning the settlement of separation be carried out by correspondence and through their lawyers. After exchanging separation proposals by post or intermediaries, they reached a settlement or separate maintenance contract. During the negotiation, Charles Hanbury Williams told Fox he would return what Lady Frances brought to the marriage, "which," he thought, "is doing a great deal for one that parts with her husband against his consent."[30] They agreed to live separately with Williams paying his wife an allowance. Lady Frances, as she requested, was "entrusted with the Education of the Children, as they are Girls," although Williams would not be deprived "of their Company," whenever he should "think fit to Command it."[31]

We wonder how many other "wretched wives" suffered as Lady Frances did. Most would not have had the means and the support to demand or even consider a separation. They lived out their lives in shame, fear, and resentment.

Writing to Mrs. Pennington in January 1793, Hester Thrale Piozzi observed: "Poor Siddons pities my very soul to see her: an indignant melancholy sits on her fine face, and care corrodes her very vitals, I do think. God only can comfort her, and His grace alone support her, for she is all resentment; and that beauty, fame, and fortune she has now so long possess'd, add to her misery, not take from it. I am sincerely afflicted for her suffering virtue, never did I see a purer mind, but it is now sullied by the thoughts that she has washed her hands in innocence in vain! How shall I do to endure the sight of her odious husband?"[32]

Notes

I thank Paula R. Backscheider, Betty Brophy, and Betty Rizzo for suggested sources.

    1. "The Family Book," September 1776, in Mary Hyde, *The Thrales of Streatham Park* (Cambridge: Harvard Univ. Press, 1977), 165-66. Thrale's ailment lasted about one month, "most of September" according to Hyde, 167.

    2. *Thraliana: The Diary of Mrs. Hester Lynch Thrale (Later Mrs. Piozzi), 1776-1809*, 2 vols., ed. Katherine C. Balderston (Oxford: Clarendon Press, 1942), 2:850.

    3. *The Proceedings Upon the Bill of Divorce Between His Grace the Duke of Norfolk and the Lady Mary Mordant* (London, 1700), 60.

    4. George Granville, "Cleora," in *Poems upon Several Occasions* (London: J. Tonson, 1712), 114-15, lines 27-47 and 52-53.

    5. "A Collection of letters with some later papers of the Congreve family of CONGREVE and STRETTON," William Salt's Original Collection, William Salt Library, Stafford, 47/47/3.

    6. Secrecy was also important to men. Henry Thrale wanted such secrecy that Hester did not even tell her mother ("The Family Book," 7 September 1776, in Hyde, 167). Dr. Profily's male patients also wanted secrecy (*An Easy and Exact Method of Curing the Venereal Disease in all its Different Appearances*, 144), and as we shall see, Charles Hanbury Williams wished only his close friends to know of his ailment.

    7. J.H. Smyth, M.D. and Man-Midwife, *A New Treatise on Venereal Disease, Gleets, Seminal Weaknesses; The Dreadful Effects of Self-Pollution, and the Causes of Impotency; Directing Methods of Cure established by repeated Experience*, 6th ed. (London, 1771), 16. Thomas Gataker points out that a bubo "is much oftener owing to the more malignant species of the venereal disease than to a gonorrhoea": *Observations on Venereal Complaints, and on the Methods Recommended for their Cure* (London, 1754), 16.

    8. Smyth, *New Treatise*, 22.

    9. Profily, *Easy and Exact Method*, 134.

    10. BL, Add. MSS 51390, fol. 69v.

    11. Charles Hanbury Williams (CHW) Papers 26013, fol. 4., Lewis Walpole Library, Yale University. Lady Kildare's letter was dated 10 September 1742.

    12. Ibid., fols. 6r-6v. Frances Williams's letter was dated 13 September 1742. Hester Thrale records that Osborne told her Henry Thrale had consulted him "two Months ago about this tumefied Testicle, that he advised him Vomits which he never took, & that he has been neglecting himself all this while lest I sh:d think he might be *tainted* forsooth" ("The Family Book," 7 September 1776, in Hyde, 167).

    13. CHW Papers 26013, fol. 3.

    14. CHW Papers 71-11383, p. 175.

    15. Smyth explains that mercury is very good because "it opens the pores, small vessels, and ducts of the glands; resolves obstructed humours, attenuates those which are two thick and visced, especially the lymphs, dissipates concretions even in the remotest parts of the body" (33).

    16. After attending a dinner at Lord and Lady Richmond's home, Henry Fox wrote: "Mr. Digby had talk'd a great deal of an Inflammation & swelling of Your Glands which made you spitt excessively and which (& all this *bonnement*) He hoped would

do You a great deal of good; till, I was forced to turn the Discourse, lest the Dss of Richmond, or Ly Pembroke, or Lady Emily should find out from Him what He did not know Himself" (BL, Add. MSS 51390, fol. 78).

17. On 13 October 1742, Henry Fox wrote Williams: "I am only concern'd for your universal Uneasiness, but as You have never told me what Operation it is, & as I have heard Pierce & You both declare against the common one I can't tell what You mean" (BL, Add. MSS 51390, fols. 69r-69v.).

18. Profily, *Easy and Exact Method,* 205.

19. BL, Add. MSS 51390, fol. 66.

20. Profily, *Easy and Exact Method,* 208. The OED defines *Cicatrix* as "the scar or seam remaining after a wound, sore, or ulcer is healed."

21. One of Dr. Profily's patients refused to take a Course of Salivation. He complains: "Pain of Salivation, such as to be four or five Weeks without Relaxation or Sleep, without being able to swallow any thing, and by this Torture I should purchase the Cure at a very dear Rate; besides, to lose my Teeth, or have them all loosened and grown black, and the Gums worn away ... with the great Scent that Salivation leaves, so as to make all the World know, that such a Person has past through the grand Remedy, is to me of very great Consequence" (ibid., 145).

22. Physicians believed that the disease was carried away from the body through the mouth (saliva or vomit), the bowels, and sweat.

23. I have summarized Dr. Profily's method of salivation (*Easy and Exact Method,* 204-11). Not all doctors believed in salivation, although they believed in friction. George Key, a surgeon who opposed salivation, claimed, "All physicians and surgeons, deserving the title agree, that Mercury should be applied by way of friction, but differ greatly in the dispensing of it": *A Dissertation on the Effects of Mercury on Human Bodies, in the Cure of the Venereal Disease* (London, 1747), 16. William Fordyce, a surgeon who recommended friction, criticized Profily's regimen. "One is tempted to smile at the common manner of applying the mercurial ointment, first on the feet, then on the legs, then on the thighs, then on the arms, shoulders, and trunk of the body; as if there were some magic in the process, and the doctor were a conjurer. Surely the ointment rubbed upon the thighs, which can be defended from cold in winter by flannel drawers, and in summer by cotton or linen ones, worn during the whole time of the inunction, and where it can be applied without any inconveniency, is as well or better calculated to convey the mercury into the blood, though not to keep up the parade of art": *A Review of the Venereal Disease, and Its Remedies* (London, 1767), 86-87.

24. BL, Add. MSS 51390, fol. 82.

25. CHW Papers 26013, fol. 22.

26. *Horace Walpole's Correspondence,* ed. W.S. Lewis (New Haven: Yale Univ. Press, 1954), 18:104.

27. Newport (Gwent) Central Library, MS, fol. 2. I thank Janice Thaddeus for this reference to Lady Frances in the Delany correspondence. The passage was omitted from Lady Augusta Llanover's version of the letter in *The Autobiography and Correspondence of Mary Granville, Mrs. Delany,* 6 vols. (London: Richard Bentley, 3 vols. 1861, 3 vols. 1862), 2:198.

28. Fox advised Williams: "And I would advise You to take hold of the first word that either *the Person* writes; (or .O. sends You that You may own) upon which You can introduce an Assurance that Yr Letter was mistaken; & in the strongest absolutest, Manner possible take it to Yourself. The only Difficulty is how You will do it consistently with what You have already wrote. Whether You will say that having thought it impossible that way, You had not mention'd the Affairs of the two .Cs.

which You have since heard do not make it so impossible as You had allways imagin'd, & then ask pardon etc etc" (BL, Add. MSS 51390, fols. 37r-37v).

29. On 30 August 1742, Henry Fox wrote Williams: "I have seen O. He is the only Person able to do you any Service, & I never saw any body more inclin'd to it, nor could any body talk more sensibly or more affectionately & reasonably upon the Subject. But in order not to destroy His Power of serving You, It is absolutely necessary that it should not be known that I have seen Him; *the person* being in very ill Humour with me" (BL, Add. MSS 51390, fol. 36).

30. BL, Add. MSS 51390, fol. 86.

31. CHW Papers 71-11383, p. 177.

32. *The Intimate Letters of Hester Piozzi and Penelope Pennington, 1788-1821,* ed. Oswald G. Knapp (London: John Lane, 1914), 74.

Chapter 7

The Problem of Syphilitic Children in Eighteenth-Century France and England

Barbara J. Dunlap

Claude Quétel is referring to more than medical issues when, in his *History of Syphilis*, he states that by the eighteenth century syphilis in children had become "a problem on a national scale."[1] The eighteenth century, and particularly the latter part of the century, was extremely anxious about the prevalence—perhaps exaggerated—of syphilitic children. If children were victims, they might also survive to generate a "tainted posterity" of the stunted, deformed, and dull—a citizenry that would cause the Enlightenment's vision of human progress to recoil upon itself.

In *Moll Flanders* (1722) Daniel Defoe lets Moll make a prescient reflection about why she abandoned a drunken client: "how would he, if he had any Principles of honour, as I verily believed he had, how would he abhor the Thought of giving any ill Distemper, if he had it, as for aught he knew he might, to his Modest and Virtuous wife, and thereby sowing the Contagion in the Life-blood of his Posterity?"[2]

In 1724, the physician turned political philosopher Bernard Mandeville published anonymously *A Modest Defense of Public Stews, or An Essay Upon Whoring as is Now Practis'd in the Three Kingdoms* in which, with poker-faced comedic vitality, he proposed a system of public brothels. Such institutions would be the best way for the state to control the consequences of sexual activity outside of marriage. After picturing the web of infections that unregulated private whoring creates, he draws a conclusion that anticipates a theme of twentieth-century public health campaigns: "But what makes this Mischief the more intolerable, is, that the Innocent must suffer by it as well as the Guilty: Men give it to their Wives, Women to their Husbands, or perhaps their Children; they to their Nurses, and the Nurses again to other Children; so that no Age, Sex, or Condition can be entirely safe from the Infection."[3] Between them Defoe and Mandeville encapsulate some of the century's concerns about syphilis and children. Mandeville reflects the traditional perception of children as innocent sufferers, while Defoe combines a prescient understanding about the route of transmission with a very contemporary fear that syphilis could be transmitted to the third generation and beyond.

Infantile syphilis attracted attention almost from the beginning of the virulent outbreak of the 1490s. By the eighteenth century a number of doctors had written on the subject, but their concern centered mainly on the route of transmission.

In 1497, Gaspara Torella, physician to the Borgias, described the manifestations indicative of syphilis in sucklings and suggested they were acquired through contact with infected wet nurses: "In nursing children the infection first appears in the mouth or on the face; and this occurs on account of infected breasts or from the face or mouth of the nurse, either one or the other. Also nurses are accustomed to kiss infants and I have often seen infants infected with this disease by diseased nurses."[4]

Cecilia Mettler sums up the state of knowledge about syphilis by the seventeenth century: "Infection of infants was generally admitted, but it was still not clear whether they were infected *in utero*, became infected during passage through the birth canal, or, after birth, from the milk of the mother or nurse. The complicating feature in any attempt to resolve this problem was that many apparently healthy women were delivered of syphilitic infants, and that some obviously syphilitic mothers gave birth to apparently healthy children."[5]

A popular text in England and France during the seventeenth century was Jacques Guillemeau's manual for physicians and midwives, *The Manual of Nursing and Bringing Up of Children*, originally published in 1612. He includes advice about caring for infants with smallpox, "French Pocks," or syphilis, noting that the infants contract it "from the mother's womb," or from a postpartum infection—"by the Nurse's fault, who may be defiled and infected with it." He described the classic signs as "pustules, ulcers, and excoriations" on the buttocks and thighs and prescribed treatment. An infant infected by a wet nurse must be given to another who would be fed a special diet and take a "decoction" and an opiate that would "make her milk medicinal and to hinder the child from imparting the disease to her so soon, as otherwise he might do, if she took no precaution." But recognizing the difficulty of finding a nurse willing to undergo both the treatment and the risk, he added: "If you cannot find a Nurse, that will venture to give the children suck, instead thereof you shall cause him to sucke a Goate; which I have caused some to doe." He advised direct treatment of the infant through application of quicksilver (mercury) ointment and treacle water; an older child could be purged, bled, and given the same medications as a nurse.[6]

The language used in eighteenth-century descriptions of children born with congenital syphilis is often dramatic. Jean Astruc, professor of medicine at Paris, wrote in 1736 that infants born alive would be objects of horror: "Squalid, erysipelatous, half-rotten, ulcerated Foetus's, from the same cause, since the virulent disposition of the maternal Blood, ruins, wastes, and destroys the tender Body of the Embryo.... [They will be] strumous, rickety, gibbous, hectical, lean, die miserably before their time; or if they live, are short, broken-backed, large-headed, crooked, bandy-legg'd, variously distorted, and thick-jointed."[7] While the observations on stunted growth and enlarged head are accurate for some congenital syphilitics, rickets is now recognized as a condition resulting from a diet deficient in vitamin D, not from syphilis.

If Astruc presented syphilitic infants and children as objects of horror, three decades later the anonymous article in the *Encyclopédie* presented them as objects of pity whose future was hardly more optimistic:

> It is easy to forecast the illnesses of those children born to parents attacked and tormented by venereal disease. If these victims of lubricity have strong constitutions during the first years of their infancy, the disease will show itself all over the surface of the body, and particularly on the head, by means of excretions and crusts which ooze bitter and corrosive matter, so dangerous to suppress or cure.
>
> At puberty all the other signs appear: stunted growth, spitting of blood, which terminate in phthisis and death.... Generally these children are born in order to punish the fathers for their lewdness, *per libidines vages,* and they are witty, amiable and endearing. But they are born in order to die in youth at the latest, since they rarely live beyond the age of twenty-eight.[8]

As the century progressed, fear that syphilitic children would die was joined by the increasingly articulated fear that they would live to produce more syphilitic children. Variations of the phrase *hereditary taint* as a coded reference began to gain currency. Syphilis as a menace to the family line had been one theme of Claude Quillet's eugenically minded poem, *Callipaedia*.[9] The original Latin version appeared pseudonymously in Leyden in 1655, and it was several times translated into French, the last version appearing as late as 1832. In England *Callipaedia* made its first appearance in 1708, with Quillet's subtitle translated as "the art of getting beautiful children." Canto III was translated by a prolific if not inspired poet named Samuel Cobb. After warning young men away from whores, the text asserts that only healthy men should marry; the sickly—those venereally infected—will have sterile unions or wives who experience frequent stillbirths:

> How oft with vain Complaints they load the Skies,
> And guiltless Gods accuse with fruitless cries;
> When the true Cause of their repeated Blame
> From a distemper'd feeble Marriage came. [III, 429-32]

The popular pediatrician Hugh Downman painted several scenes of tender family life revolving around breast-feeding in his *Infancy, or The Management of Children* (1774-75 and many editions thereafter). But he also issued a stern warning against "hired nurses" and cautioned especially against deceiving appearances:

> Besides, who can assure the lacteal springs
> Clear and untainted? Oft disorder lurks
> Beneath the vivid bloom, and cheerful eye,
> Promising health, and poisonous juice secrete
> Slow undermining life, stains what should be,
> The purest nutriment. Hence worse than death,
> Long years of misery to thy blasted child,
> A burden to himself, by others shunn'd,
> He wishes for the grave, and wastes his days
> In solitary woe, or haply weds,
> And propagates the hereditary plague,
> Entailing on his name the bitter curse
> Of generations yet unborn, a race
> Pithless and weak, of faded texture wan,
> Like some declining plant, with mildew'd leaves,
> Whose root a treacherous insect gnaws unseen. [1:142-57][10]

Downman articulates the same concern with "contagion in the life blood of his posterity" that Defoe had articulated through Moll Flanders fifty years before. But here the infection is feared not as the result of misbehavior on the part of the father but as the outcome of allowing one of the deepest intimacies of family life—breast-feeding—to be taken over by a lower-class outsider.

Thomas Denman, a popular physician and accoucheur, reported important observations about snuffles in young infants to the *London Medical Journal* in 1790. Reporting on eight infants born to "people of rank and fortune" between April and October, he noted a condition that appeared after about two weeks which first seemed to be merely a cold but was characterized by heavy discharges from the nose, often bloody. The infants had trouble swallowing and suckling (as they had to breathe through their mouths), and could no longer take the breasts of their wet nurses. They "wasted away" and died in convulsions, despite treatment with emetics and Peruvian bark (generally considered a treatment for malaria). He did not mention using mercury ointment, then the treatment of choice for syphilitic infants, and he indicates nowhere in his letter that he even considered the condition to be a possibility.[11] Emphasizing the concerned hygienic care he and the nurses provided, he was perhaps unwilling to associate syphilis with the infants of "people of rank and fortune."

In the middle of the eighteenth century there was still disagreement on how syphilis was transmitted and how it would behave in the third generation. The influential Dutch physician Gerhard Van Swieten believed that the infant could be infected during delivery if the mother had venereal ulcers on her genital organs, and he shared the contemporary view that the disease could be transmitted directly at conception by the father or the mother.[12] Yet his descriptions of the clinical course of syphilis anticipated nineteenth-century work.[13] Swediaur was one of the first to use the term *hereditary syphilis,* meaning that the disease had been contracted in utero or from the father's semen (a route now known to be impossible). He distinguished it from what he believed to be the more common congenital form, contracted at birth, and from acquired syphilis, contracted through the nipples of a wet nurse or a kiss from someone who was infected.[14] The term *hereditary syphilis* is now considered inaccurate. Only "primary diseases" (where the agent is in the germ plasm) are truly hereditary, and the term *congenital syphilis* is commonly used to identify infants born with this chronic condition.[15]

Toward the end of the ancien régime there was a sense of national danger, not only in terms of a static or declining population but in terms of a decline in the French "temperament." By the nineteenth century the French were commonly using the term *heredo-syphilis* to connote the disease passed from parent to child. Syphilitic infants put the nation at risk for the future through the transmission of a tainted heredity if they survived to become parents. Quétel quotes Joseph Raulin, who wrote in 1768 that a syphilitic who marries knowing he is infected "cheats one's fatherland, endangers [it] by bringing into the world children who cannot serve it" (doubtless in the military), and threatens future generations with misery and premature death.[16] Here is a dramatic presentation of the fear of "hereditary taint"—the passing of the syphilitic infection though the generations with the concomitant incidence of sickly, stunted, or mentally deficient offspring—which would so grip the French imagination in the next century.

In France especially, concern with syphilis in infants was deeply interwoven with the prevalence of wet-nursing. It was not simply an alternative to maternal care. It was a business, a vital part of the economy. Upper-class infants were usually but not always wet-nursed at home where the employers

The Problem of Syphilitic Children

tried to control the nurse's sexuality by forbidding or closely supervising any meetings with husbands or lovers. But thousands of middle-class and working-class urban infants were given to wet nurses who might live up to two hundred miles from the parents' home. Economic factors in the two decades before the Revolution and social unrest and war after it are linked to the increase in abandoned infants [*enfants trouvés*] who needed to suckle a hired nurse. It is now time to look at the problem of syphilis in children in the context of the use and abuse of wet-nursing.

From the introduction of syphilis in Europe, wet nurses were considered a possible source of infection, and it was subsequently understood that the nurses could become infected by their nurslings. As the signs of the diseases do not present themselves immediately, infected infants could transmit syphilis before they actually showed symptoms themselves. These hapless beings had often been fathered by soldiers, sailors, camp followers, and customers of prostitutes, but the ability of the infection to be passed from infant to nurse and from nurse to infant created a web of infectious people.[17]

By the eighteenth century, and particularly the latter part, the use of wet nurses among the upper and middle classes was moderating. Randolph Trumbach attributes this change to the forging of strong bonds of attachment between child and mother, which strongly improved both physical and psychological health. During this period, wet-nursing was endemic in France, although later in the century influential women of the bourgeoisie and upper classes—possibly inspired by the writings of Rousseau—began to suckle their own infants. But wet-nursing was too deeply woven into the French economy to be vanquished by theory.[18]

From 1685, a complex system of requirements and record keeping had evolved intended to protect the infants from being placed with women who did not really nurse them or were infected and also to protect the nurses from infection and ensure that they were paid. Of course, the mere existence of legislation did not prevent abuse. The lack of a serologic test to detect syphilis in the newborn, the lack of any systematic method of rural oversight such as regular visitation of the nurses' homes (not surprising considering that the roads into some small villages were merely cart tracks), and human greed and dishonesty created a business steeped in moral ambiguities.

Since 1715, the lieutenant-general of police in Paris had jurisdiction over the four Parisian Bureaux des Recommandaresses where new parents (often fathers) and *meneurs* [agents for the nurses] sought each other. From 1762, the youngest living infant of a wet nurse accepting an assignment was required to be at least seven months old, a requirement often flouted as it was recognized that the milk of a recently delivered woman was the most suitable for a newborn. The fear of syphilis created an atmosphere of mutual suspicion between parent, *meneur*, and nurse, which the legislation of 1762 codified. At the time a nurse was engaged, the parents, the police inspector, or the *meneur* could request that she undergo a free medical examination, and nurses who refused were not supposed to be given infants. Equally, the nurses or *meneurs* could demand an examination of the baby to determine whether he or she was syphilitic, and the parents could request a free examination when the baby or toddler was returned.[19] But these examinations could not detect latent disease.

In the last years of the ancien régime, Jean-Charles-Pierre LeNoir, the lieutenant-general, estimated that only one-thirtieth of the 20,000 or 21,000 babies born annually in Paris were suckled by their own mothers and another 1,000 or so were suckled at home by a live-in wet nurse. For the rest, "the least wealthy and consequently the most numerous class was necessarily forced to take wet nurses at considerable distances and in some ways at random."[20] Sometimes the distances were as great as two hundred miles, as prices dropped the farther away the nurse lived from Paris. The *meneur* or *meneuse* who recruited nurses from the provinces brought them to the capital to be inspected by parents, then loaded a cart with a basket of babies and several nurses for the trip back home. Steeped in their own excrement, often too cold or too hot, subject to dehydration and infections, the children who survived passage to an unknown home faced an uncertain future. The care they might receive at their place of destination ranged from tenderness to indifference.[21]

In the 1783 edition of her *Avis aux meres qui veulent nourrir leurs enfants*, a practical guidebook for breast-feeding mothers, Marie Lerebours attacked the entrenched wet-nursing system in France on several grounds, particularly on the ground that it created both a high mortality rate and indifferent health among the many who survived: "I estimate that only half of the babies who are sent out to nurse from the provincial towns ever return; of this surviving half, those who are in the best condition are those one encounters most often. The ill and deformed are shut away and those who are dead in the country totally escape our view." While acknowledging that some infants were fortunate to fall into the hands of wet nurses who expressed affection and nursed them frequently, she also commented on the "great number of infants in a pitiable condition that one sees in country villages." Nowhere in her book does Madame Lerebours mention syphilis, but some of the conditions she attributes to poor nursing suggest syphilis—whether congenital or acquired from the nurse: "this one is knock kneed; that one has a weak back. Another stoops. . . . It is rare to see an infant at nurse who does not have some deformity or infirmity, whether apparent or concealed. Several others are tubercular. . . . Many are undersized who would not have been so if they had been nursed by their mothers. Many become consumptive. . . . Skin eruptions are also very widespread. Who knows if they may not be a consequence of bad milk taken in infancy. Finally, many infants have weak eye sight, and cannot endure broad daylight because they have been shut up indoors too much."[22] These conditions could be attributed to more than one cause, but it is more than likely that some of the children she saw had venereal disease with its attendant ills.

The moral dilemma presented by wet-nursing was even more complicated when the disease was suspected. Human milk, as the cleanest and most easily digested food, was the baby's lifeline. But if a syphilitic infant had a weak suck due to the chronically obstructed nasal passages Denman had observed, then the nurse needed to draw out her milk by hand expression or a tube and feed it by cup or spoon. Although feasible, the process is extremely time-consuming. Syphilitic infants who could suckle well might infect their nurses, who could then spread the diseases to husbands, lovers, or future children they might bear or nurse. As this became recognized, dry-nursing or even direct suckling of animals was employed, but modern knowledge about the composition of milks suggests that other problems would then have arisen. In addition to the dangers of bacteriological contamination, the proteins in bovine milk and to a lesser extent in ass's or goat's milk act as allergens and can affect the infant gastrointestinal tract, leading to vomiting, diarrhea, colic, occult bleeding, asthma, and skin disorders.[23] Already invaded by the spirochete of syphilis, these infants' compromised gastrointestinal tracts were even more adversely suited to cope with foreign proteins than those of healthy infants. Thus, the interests of the syphilitic infant and the wet nurse were on a collision course. And the true lifesaver for such infants, maternal suckling, was then erroneously thought to be unsafe for their mothers. For a foundling, of course, the idea of being suckled at the maternal breast contradicted the facts of his pitiable situation.[24]

British physicians certainly used the fear of hereditary infection to warn men against prostitutes. Moreover, the latter half of the eighteenth century saw increased emphasis on the importance of mothers suckling their own infants, and to the extent that upper-middle-class and noble women did so, more of their children survived. Randolph Trumbach's influential book, *The Rise of the Egalitarian Family* (1978), cites figures indicating a 30 percent drop in infant mortality after 1750 among this group.[25] Not only were the infants and nursing toddlers receiving the most suitable food and having their immune systems strengthened but they were also receiving more affectionate and personal care. Trumbach discusses in detail the changing family structure that encouraged such attention and the gradual recognition that wet-nursing was unnatural. Beyond philosophical or psychological principles, one reason physicians promoted maternal suckling was fear that a wet nurse was a latent carrier of syphilis.

John Armstrong's popular *Oeconomy of Love* (1736 and reprinted several times),[26] a poetic guide to sex and marriage for young men, warns against prostitutes and emphasizes the physical disfigurement that syphilis can entail, particularly the decomposition of the bridge of the nose. To men who marry and beget children, he warns against sending the child away

> from his parents' arms,
> With Nurse unpitying, unbenign, exil'd
> To squalid lodge, to find in Famine's cave
> A lingering death, or by a deadlier hag,
> Then her that rides the lab'ring night, oppress'd
> Untimely sink beneath a heavier fate. [456-61]

He alludes to spurious wet nurses who are not really lactating or do not suckle the infant sufficiently. But slow starvation is not as hard a fate as infection—the "deadlier hag."

At midcentury the relatively new Foundling Hospital in London had to respond to an Act of Parliament that instituted a policy of general reception; today we would call it open admissions. The hospital had a concerned board of governors who assumed responsibility for the infants from their arrival through to their apprenticeships to trades or domestic service. The Foundling Hospital was reasonably well run. Wet nurses were lodged near the premises in Coram's Inn Fields to succor the infants until country nurses arrived to take them. These nurses were chosen and monitored with some care; they were usually rural women married to agricultural laborers or farm servants with children of their own.[27] The general reception period, which lasted until 1760, created a massive need for nurses and inspectors. The policy was eventually revoked, but the floods of infants it attracted suggested reservoirs of social desperation and opportunism.

"No one," wrote one of the governors, the social reformer Jonas Hanway, "can form an idea of what wretched objects some of these poor infants are without seeing them."[28] Just under fourteen hundred infants were admitted in the hospital's first nine years of existence, but from 2 June 1756, when the open policy was announced, through 31 December 1756, nearly eighteen hundred infants arrived. By the end of the experiment nearly fifteen thousand infants had arrived, and many of them were sent by provincial parishes who did not want them as a burden on the rates. The mortality rates rose, but many of the infants had been near death on arrival. The welfare of abandoned infants attracted not only the interest but the active involvement of such outstanding men as Jonas Hanway, Hans Sloane, Dr. William Cadogan, and, of course, the founder himself, Thomas Coram. They knew the social reality of venereal disease and provided for the medical inspection of nurses and free treatment if a nursling caused them to become infected. Yet the transmission of infection between foundling and nurse does not seem to have been as great a concern for the London Foundling Hospital as it was in the foundling hospitals of France.

The number of children abandoned to the Foundling Hospital of Paris greatly increased in the decades before the Revolution to some eight thousand.[29] While direct exposure of children in the streets greatly decreased, the number of infants abandoned after their birth in the charity hospital—the Hôtel-Dieu—elsewhere in the city or in the provinces greatly increased. Provinces got rid of their sickest, weakest abandoned infants and toddlers, especially those in whom the symptoms of venereal disease had shown themselves, by sending them to the hospital in Paris. Illegitimate children were more likely to be abandoned. Claude Delaselle's archival and statistical study of abandonment in eighteenth-century France concludes that it was not "depravity," as moralists had claimed, but "the combined pressure of their associates, their social milieu, and the material and moral distress into which they were sinking" which led many unmarried servant girls to abandon their infants and young children. He admits to leaving the "libertinage" in the shadows.[30] The lifestyle of the libertine, however, surely increased the possibility of his contracting and spreading venereal disease. Poor married couples also abandoned their infants, particularly in times of famine or high bread prices, but abandonment of children born outside of marriage was a constant. In some locales authorities suspected that the women who turned up at charitable hospitals to work as wet nurses were often the mothers of the abandoned children, but no systematic follow-up work was done.[31]

"Illegitimate" infants were the more likely to be premature, small for gestational age, weak, or to exhibit symptoms that suggested congenital syphilis. This indicated that they would be difficult to feed and—even if they should survive—would fail to become productive workers in the parish. The concern over diseased children infecting wet nurses was great enough to result in a written statute for the Hôtel-Dieu in Montpellier, which guaranteed that it would tend women so infected.[32] The survival of these infants could depend on their receiving human milk directly from the breast to ensure it would be free of bacteriological contamination. "Illegitimate" infants were also the infants least likely to receive nourishment in adequate quantities or to receive it at all.

The last days of the ancien régime saw some attempt to mitigate this dismal picture when, in 1780, the lieutenant-general of police in Paris charged the first inspector general of hospitals with the job of providing a hospice at Vaugirard for the specific purpose of treating syphilitic children. Conceived as a facility for therapeutic treatment and not just as a refuge for paupers, the hospice encouraged syphilitic mothers to come and breast-feed their infants, as it was recognized that this could be done with no further ill effects to the infants. The authorities envisioned a "model establishment" with separate beds and cots for each baby and mother, high standards of cleanliness, and modified mercury treatments for the mothers. Passed through the milk, the mercury would also provide gentle treatment for the infants. If two-thirds of the infants still perished, this was actually a lower rate of mortality than the Foundling Hospital in Paris enjoyed. Wet nurses were provided for abandoned infants with preventative treatment for the nurses, but cow's milk was later substituted.[33] While this lessened the risk for the women who cared for the infants, it provided them with less than optimum food—again an example of the cruel dilemma of wet-nursing. In 1810, one of the physicians to the hospital published an account of its work that included detailed descriptions of symptoms, including skin lesions and affections of the mucous membranes. But he still included ophthalmia among the disorders caused by syphilis,[34] and thus no new treatments were investigated.

The intendants, who were the king's personal representatives, were able to make some headway in offering good care in their provinces because they had the authority and facilities for supervision.[35] But this humane approach could not resolve the social conditions that led to infantile syphilis or increased abandonment.

Legislation during the Revolution was intended to improve on the ancien régime's piecemeal provisions for abandoned children by placing their care under uniform jurisdiction. A decree of the National Assembly passed on 28 June 1793 provided various levels of financial support to poor working families, including support payment for the first twelve years of the child's life. Infants with "infirmities" were to receive the maximum payment. Mothers who wished to claim these pensions were to suckle their own infants. To minimize infant abandonment, each country district was to have a place of refuge where a woman could give birth and suckle. She could then receive payment to help her keep her child. "The most inviolable secrecy shall be preserved in all matters," said a provision doubtless designed to encourage mothers to claim relief.[36] There were, of course, political motivations for this largesse.

A healthy population would ensure national strength, and healthy children were symbols of hope. But the very conditions of the Revolution and the wartime society that France became militated against these noble aims. In addition to the young people who had gathered in provincial cities to work in small factories and in private homes, the Revolutionary armies created an even more mobile male population, constantly on the road between engagements, coming and going from military hospitals or hauling supplies. As casual sexual contacts increased, so did abandonment of babies. The war also increased the number of widows with children, and the pensions, described above, were inadequate. If the mother could not supplement it with other wages, she might be driven to abandon her youngest infant. As Alan Forrest has shown, the program decreed in 1793 was never really operative, and the problem of numbers grew. There were not enough wet nurses, and there was no really operative program of apprenticeships for those children who somehow survived life in hospitals he calls "*mourirs*" for babies. The fetid hospital dormitories and inadequate wet-nursing staff—some of whom were syphilitic—became a laboratory for cross-infections. Those foundlings who were farmed out traveled the longest distances to women who were themselves often undernourished, overworked, and sometimes diseased nurses.[37]

By the later 1790s, the Directory was abandoning the idea of centralized responsibility and was so badly behind in its payments to provincial nurses that the women began to return babies to the hospitals in sizable numbers. At the same time, the institutions that cared for them were often pressured to care for soldiers, too, and the manufacture of bed linens and clothing for infants was far less of a priority than supplying such articles for the army. The social disruptions of the Revolution and Napoleonic eras affected many French infants and children adversely—particularly those of the Third Estate. Abandoned infants and children suffered even more, and syphilitic infants and children with their special needs who were abandoned to the public care suffered the most, despite humanitarian and political theories which favored—and even attempted—the amelioration of their lot.[38]

Notes

1. Claude Quétel, *The History of Syphilis*, trans. Judith Braddock and Brian Pike (Baltimore: Johns Hopkins Univ. Press, 1990), 5.

2. *Fortunes and Misfortunes of the famous Moll Flanders*, ed. G.A. Starr (London: Oxford Univ. Press, 1971), 227. Jerome Schneck commends Defoe for his prescience in "Daniel Defoe's *Moll Flanders* and Congenital Syphilis," *New York State Journal of Medicine* 78 (1978): 2104-5.

3. Bernard Mandeville, *A Modest Defense of Public Stews*, intro. Richard Cook, Augustan Reprint Society Pamphlet #62 (Los Angeles: William Andrews Clark Memorial Library, 1973), 2-4.

4. Cecilia Mettler quotes Gaspara Torella in her *History of Medicine: A Correlative Text Arranged According to Subjects*, ed. Fred A. Mettler (Philadelphia: Blakiston, 1947), 629. In the first decades of Europe's virulent syphilis epidemic, "the early lesions were frequently confused with other venereal as well as non-venereal diseases," and there were probably cases of "mixed and superimposed infections." See U.S. National Communicable Disease Center, Atlanta, Venereal Disease Program, *Syphilis: A Synopsis*, U.S. Public Health Service Publication #1660 (Washington: U.S. Public Health Service, 1968), 6.

5. Mettler, *History of Medicine*, 630.

6. James [Jacques] Guillemeau, *The Manual of Nursing and Bringing Up of Children* (1612; reprint, New York: Da Capo Press, 1972), 114-15, 119.

7. Jean Astruc, *A Treatise of the Venereal Diseases in Six Books Containing an Account of the Origins, Propagation and Contagion of this Distemper*, trans. William Barrowby, M.D. (1737; reprint, New York: Da Capo Press, 1972), 52, 56. For more on rickets see Jan Riordan and Kathleen Auerbach, *Breast-Feeding and Human Lactation* (Boston: Jones and Bartlett, 1993), 114.

8. "Vérole grosse," *Encyclopédie, ou Dictionnaire raisonné des sciences, des arts et des métiers par une société de gens de lettres*, 2d ed. (Paris, 1771), 17:71-72.

9. Claude Quillet, *Callipaedia, or The Art of Getting Beautiful Children* (1733) in *English Poetry Full Text Data Base: Part II, 1660-1800* (Cambridge, Eng., and Alexandria, Va.: Chadwyck-Healy, 1994). Quillet (1602-1661) was trained as a physician at Paris and later took orders in Rome. *Callipaedia* first appeared under the pseudonym Calfidius Letus, an anagram of the author's name; the original title is *Callipaedia sive de pulchrae prolis habendae ratione*.

10. Hugh Downman, *Infancy, or The Management of Children: A Didactic Poem in Three Books*, 2d ed. (Exeter: Trewman, 1802).

11. Thomas Denman, "Some Account of a Disease Lately Observed in Infants," *London Medical Journal* 11 (1790): 374-80.

12. Quétel, *History of Syphilis*, 104.

13. David Nunes Nabarro, *Congenital Syphilis* (London: E. Arnold, 1934), 10.

14. Quétel, *History of Syphilis*, 104, referring to the French translation of Swediaur's work, *Traité complet sur les symptômes, les effets, la nature et le traitment des maladies syphilitiques* (Paris, 1786).

15. Nabarro, *Congenital Syphilis*, 1-3.

16. Quétel, *History of Syphilis*, 103. *Peurs et terreurs face á la contagion*, ed. Jean Pierre Bardet (Paris: Fayard, 1988), discusses syphilis in nineteenth-century France.

17. Valerie Fildes, *Wet-Nursing: A History from Antiquity to the Present* (Oxford: Basil Blackwell, 1988), 72. For a historical account of breast-feeding and other infant feeding customs see Fildes, *Breasts, Bottles, and Babies: A History of Infant Feeding* (Edinburgh: Edinburgh Univ. Press, 1986).

18. Randolph Trumbach, *Rise of the Egalitarian Family: Aristocratic Kinship and Domestic Relations in Eighteenth-Century England* (New York: Academic Press, 1978), 187-88; Fildes, *Wet-Nursing*, 116.

19. George Sussman, *Selling Mother's Milk: The Wet-Nursing Business in France, 1715-1914* (Urbana: Univ. of Illinois Press, 1982), 37-44.

20. Ibid., 20, quoting Jean-Charles-Pierre LeNoir's *Details sur quelques établissements de Ville de Paris* (Paris, 1780), 63.

21. T.G.H. Drake, "Infant Welfare Laws in France in the Eighteenth Century," *Annals of Medical History (New York)*, n.s., 7 (1935): 53; also Sussman, *Selling Mother's Milk*, 20; Fildes, *Wet-Nursing*, 148-49.

22. Marie Angelique Anel Lerebours, *Avis aux meres qui veulent nourrir leurs enfants*, 3d ed. (Paris, 1783), 58-59, 65-67. All translations from this work are mine.

23. Riordan and Auerbach, *Breast-Feeding*, 126.

24. The observations of Abraham Coleus, an eighteenth-century Dublin physician, were elevated by great nineteenth-century syphilologist Jonathan Hutchinson to "Colles' Law": Syphilitic infants who suckle their own mothers, even those whose own syphilis is latent, will not infect her, but they will infect a healthy nurse (Nabarro, *Congenital Syphilis*, 12-13). We now know that they will not "infect" their mothers because the mothers are already infected.

25. Trumbach, *Rise of the Egalitarian Family*, 187.

26. John Armstrong, *The Oeconomy of Love* (1736) in *English Poetry Full Text Data Base: Part 2, 1660-1800* (Cambridge, Eng., and Alexandria, Va.: Chadwyck-Healy, 1994).

27. Fildes, *Wet-Nursing*, 188.

28. Jonas Hanway quoted in R.H. Nichols, *The History of the Foundling Hospital* (London: Oxford Univ. Press, 1935), 61. The Foundling Hospital is Nichols's subject. See also Margaret McClure, *Coram's Children: The London Foundling Hospital in the Eighteenth Century* (New Haven: Yale Univ. Press, 1981). In this article I am concerned only with its approach to venereal disease.

29. Olwen H. Hufton, *The Poor of Eighteenth-Century France, 1750-1789* (Oxford: Clarendon Press, 1974), 319.

30. Claude Delaselle, "Abandoned Children in Eighteenth-Century Paris," in *Deviants and the Abandoned in French Society*, ed. Robert Forster and Orest Ranum (Baltimore: John Hopkins Univ. Press, 1978), 47-48, 78.
31. Hufton, *Poor in Eighteenth-Century France*, 328.
32. Ibid., 342-43.
33. Quétel, *History of Syphilis*, 104-5.
34. Nabarro, *Congenital Syphilis*, 11-12.
35. Quétel, *History of Syphilis*, 105.
36. Drake, "Infant Welfare Laws in France," 59-61.
37. Alan I. Forrest, *The French Revolution and the Poor* (Oxford: Basil Blackwell, 1981), summarizing 118-21, 129.
38. Ibid., 129-34. It is interesting if depressing to read about Jules Parrot's work with syphilitic infants at the Hospice des Enfants Assistes in the 1870s. At this "funeste maison de la rue d'Enfer" there was a mortality rate of 33 percent and "l'ignorance totale des réglés élémentaires d'hygiene individuelle, alimentaire." In 1878, 118 of 173 syphilitic infants who were admitted died. See Stephane Thieffrey, "La decouverte de la syphilis congenitale par Jules Parrot à l'Hospice des Enfants Assistes," *Bulletin de l'Academie Nationale de Médecube* 164 (1980): 725-29.

Chapter 8

The London Lock Hospital and the Lock Asylum for Women

Linda E. Merians

> "But as the disease, for the cure of which this Hospital has been erected, is of such a nature, as to render the persons afflicted with it, rather objects of abhorrence than compassion, at least in the eyes of many who have not cooly considered the matter, it will be needful for me upon this occasion, and on behalf of the miserable inhabitants of this house, to relate their distressed state, and then the inducement of the governors of this charity to its first institution will appear most laudable."
> —Reverend Martin Madan, 1762

THE ESTABLISHMENT OF A CHARITY HOSPITAL SPECIFICALLY FOR THE TREATMENT of venereal disease proves that at least some people understood that the poor who were afflicted with the "secret malady" had to have access to medical treatment. The number of men, women, and children treated at the hospital from 31 January 1747 to 3 March 1800—26,800 in all—demonstrates that the need for such a facility was indeed great.[1] Yet, British ambivalence to the disease and to those who had it complicated the venture from the start. The tendency to see certain of the afflicted as culpable and others as innocent victims played a pronounced role in the operations and the fund-raising campaigns of the Lock Hospital and the Lock Asylum for Women. "Cool consideration," as the epigraph to this article relates, was what the governors of the Lock Hospital desired from their countrymen and women, but they rarely received it. Moreover, as the eighteenth century drew to a close, the governors of the Lock Hospital and the Lock Asylum for Women were barely capable of it themselves. Such a shift in sentiment suggests how a wall of silence was erected around the "secret malady," thereby serving to marginalize and demonize those afflicted with it even more.

The founders of the hospital tried to frame their intentions within the public hospital movement sweeping Britain throughout much of the eighteenth century, and especially in London during the 1720s, 1730s, and 1740s: "The Utility of Public Hospitals, is of late Years too well understood to need any Recital of the Benefits that attend them. It is certain the Poor are thereby assisted with Advice, Medicine, and every Necessary to restore them to Health. All Persons labouring under the Venereal Disease are more destitute of Relief than any other Objects of Public Charity, though at the same Time their Disorder admits of Cure more frequently than most others."[2]

Meetings to establish the hospital began in July 1746, and a core group of men emerged pretty quickly. The leader of the effort, surgeon William Bromfield (1712-1792), was assisted by other medical men—namely, Thomas Williams, who, like Bromfield, would serve as a house surgeon for several decades, and two well-known London physicians, Charles Cotes (1703-1748) and Peter Shaw (1694-1763). The other eight men who exhibited leadership during the six-month planning period (William Windham, Richard Lyttelton, Vaughan Lloyd, Edward Sheppard, Maynard Guerin, James Morris, George Vandeput, and George Fettiplace) came from business, military, and political circles. In November 1746, Bromfield purchased for £350 a ninety-nine-year lease on a house and property near Hyde Park Corner. With a location secured, the planners organized themselves into committees and began writing the procedures, rules, and regulations of the Lock Hospital.

An initial group of sixty-seven subscribers and benefactors paid in amounts ranging from a guinea to £50, and by the time the hospital opened on 31 January 1747, it had received approximately £339 from its supporters.[3] The third duke of Ancaster, then the lord great chamberlain of England, gave a gift of £50; in March 1747, he agreed to be president of the society, and he would hold this honorary title until his death in 1778. The first slate of officers also featured the earl of Rochford and Colonel Richard Lyttelton as vice presidents of the Lock Hospital. Lyttelton's interest in the Lock Hospital or in venereal disease generally is demonstrated by his active participation in recruiting governors for the hospital and, as Marie E. McAllister's article shows, in serving as patron for a time to John Burrows. Despite the fact that during its first year of operation the hospital would enroll at least twenty-three new subscribers, some among the most important names in London—including Robert Walpole, the duke of Bedford, the Hon. John Grey, and Miss Fanny Murray, the celebrated London courtesan—the institution was clearly controversial.[4]

British society did not embrace this charity hospital as warmly as it did some of the others. The Lock Hospital had significantly fewer annual and lifetime governors than other charity hospitals.[5] Furthermore, judging from Lock Hospital publications, it seems that the entire endeavor was attacked as one that would condone or actually promote vice. The published accounts of

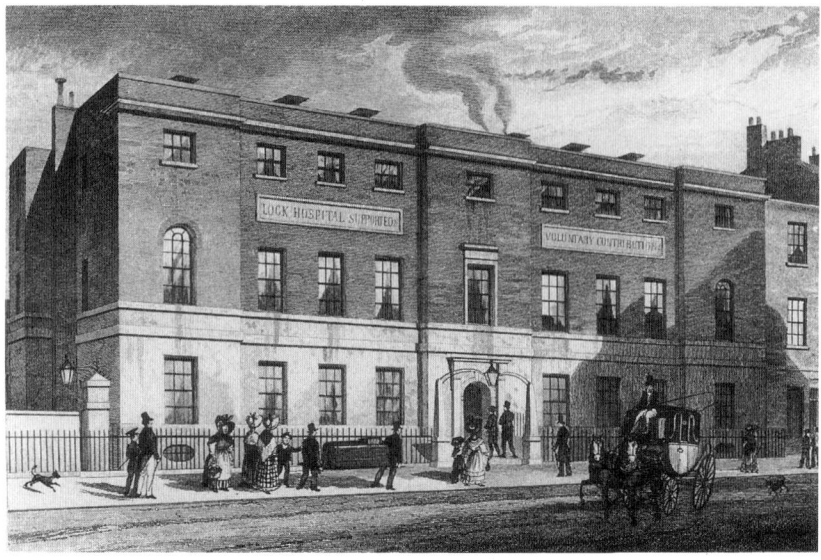

Fig. 7. Lock Hospital. Collection of Linda E. Merians.

the Lock Hospital attempt to answer the negative charges by stressing the "Christian" purpose of the place. These published reports, entitled "An Account of the Proceedings of the Governors of the Lock Hospital" and issued throughout the century, are prefaced by two citations from the Bible. The first serves as an epigraph: "And Jesus said unto them, he that is with out Sin among you, let him first cast a Stone at her." This is followed by an illustration of Jesus saying to the "adulterous" woman, "Go and Sin no More" [John 8:7 and 11].

The temptation and tendency to blame women for the spread of venereal disease was ever present and increasing during the century, and so it is important to note that the language in the Lock Hospital accounts does not aggressively mark women for condemnation. In fact, it addresses their particular vulnerability with remarkable sympathy: "Tho' the Necessity of a Charity of this Nature is obvious to many, yet some have apprehended it may prove an Encouragement to Vice; it is there-fore necessary to remove Prejudices of this Kind. *First,* We are to consider, that many poor Creatures, labouring under this Disease, are in themselves no ways culpable, as it may have been occasioned by bad Husbands, diseased Parents, suckling Children born with the Disease, or Children that have imbibed it from their Nurses."

Even more remarkably, in the subsequent paragraphs, the language used in explicit and implicit references to prostitutes is also compassionate and generous. Moreover, the rhetorical question at the end of this section strives to redefine the "good Christian" as one who supports the efforts of the Lock Hospital: "But still the Scrupulous object to those who *voluntarily* draw this Misery on themselves, as improper Objects.—In fact, these are some of the greatest, as they are, generally speaking, destitute of Friends, and consequently abandoned to Vice and Diseases. Should these then be left to rot alive, and under a kind of Necessity to communicate Contagion in order to support Life? Shall we suffer them to perish, without any Attempt made to convince them of their Guilt and Danger, and not give them another Opportunity of reforming their Lives?—Every good Christian will answer, No: It is our Part to relieve the Distressed, theirs to amend their Lives" [*An Account*, 1749, 1751, 1767 (p. 2)]. Significantly, this language stands in stark contrast to the language used in the Lock Asylum's reports later in the century, which, as we will see, tended to blame afflicted women more forcefully, especially for spreading venereal disease.

The founding members and many of the first group of governors played an extremely active role in administration during the first few years of the hospital's operation. The rules for the governors and the administration of the Lock Hospital were in keeping with the rules and regulations of other eighteenth-century charity hospitals. Annual or lifetime governorship of the hospital could be bought for five guineas paid annually or with a £50 bequest. Governorship gave one the power to sponsor patients for admittance to the hospital. It also brought with it the right to vote at the hospital's general quarterly and annual meetings, the right to have one's name listed as a governor on the hospital's published reports, the right to be an officer of the hospital, and, if the person so desired, the right to serve on one of the hospital's committees.

The Weekly Committee ran the hospital. Composed of about sixteen men, the members met every Saturday at 10 A.M. (changed to Thursdays in October 1762) to carry out their duties, which most often involved admitting and discharging patients, negotiating staff problems, and overseeing the hospital's accounts. The rules required that prospective patients come to the hospital on Saturday (on Thursday after October 1762) mornings with a letter of recommendation signed by one of the governors. Once a patient was admitted to the hospital, he or she faced a difficult four to six weeks. When the hospital first opened, salivation appears to have been the standard method of treatment. In January 1756, Lock Hospital surgeons and physicians said that "some of the cases may be cured without Salivation," and in the following year Bromfield wrote that "the torments of a salivation should, if possible, be avoided."[6]

Whichever course of therapy a patient endured, he or she certainly felt weak and miserable. The rules at the hospital were restrictive, the overcrowding was serious, and the diet would not have fortified anyone. The "low diet" allowed the patient water gruel, sage, or balm tea for breakfast; one pint of broth for dinner, and one pint of milk pottage for supper. The "milk diet" afforded the patient water gruel or balm tea for breakfast; pudding for lunch; and one pint of milk pottage for supper. The "full diet" presented patients with the same breakfast choices as the other two diets, but dinner on Monday through Saturday alternated between one pound of meat or one pound of broth, with pudding on Sunday. For supper, patients on the "full diet" could have milk pottage, butter and cheese, a fourteen-ounce loaf of bread, and a quart of beer. The amount of liquids on all these diet plans must certainly have been intended to replace the fluids the patients lost as a result of the laxatives given them as part of any course of therapy.

Not surprisingly, records reveal that throughout the century many patients elected to leave the hospital before their treatment was completed, that is, before the Lock Hospital would record them as being discharged "cured."[7] The Lock Hospital did not keep a running total of the number of patients who died while they were undergoing treatment, but examination of the yearly records shows that from January 1747 to March 1800, 294 patients died while in residence at the hospital. With sixteen recorded deaths, 1772-73 was the worst year for in-house fatalities.[8] With four exceptions, most years record ten or fewer patient deaths.

The ever-increasing number of patients treated by the Lock Hospital (see Table 1) quickly demonstrated the need for additional ward space. When the hospital first opened, there was just one ward for women and one ward for men, amounting to room for thirty patients. Creating additional wards to keep up with patient demand was a difficult and expensive undertaking. Although building improvements were often made during the early years of operation, the first major renovation did not occur until November 1755, when Carolina Williams offered the necessary funds to fit up a special ward for married women.[9] In 1766 a major reconstruction was undertaken to rearrange the assigned spaces and to raise the ceiling to create a number of additional wards. Finally, in 1795-96, four additional wards were built for fever and infectious patients.

The decisions in both 1755 and 1766 to create additional wards, especially separate wards for married women and infants, suggests that the Lock Hospital began to make distinctions among venereal disease patients. In this regard, they clearly intended to separate the women patients who might be considered "innocent" from the women patients who might be considered "culpable" in their acquisition of the disease. Moreover, the number of married women who sought treatment at the Lock Hospital was considerable enough that it was a statistic of great interest to the governors. Hospital records show a special mark next to a female patient's name if she was married. In 1754-55, for example, 53 married women were treated, "several of whom had Children Sucking at the Breast & several other Children range from six to Eleven Years

Table 1

Number of Patients Treated by the Lock Hospital,
January 1747-March 1800
(in-house and outpatients included in the total)

31 January 1747-15 March 1748: 285
March 1748-March 1750: 543
March 1750-March 1751: 362
March 1751-March 1752: 366
March 1752-March 1753: 399
March 1753-March 1754: 172
March 1754-March 1755: 511
March 1755-March 1756: 607
March 1756-March 1757: 651
March 1757-March 1758: 764
March 1758-March 1759: 567
March 1759-March 1761: 1219
March 1761-March 1762: 332
March 1762-March 1763: 343
March 1763-March 1764: 454
March 1764-March 1765: 541
March 1765-March 1766: 480
March 1766-March 1767: 491
March 1767-March 1768: 500
March 1768-March 1769: 611
March 1769-March 1770: 602
March 1770-March 1771: 629
March 1771-March 1772: 683
March 1772-March 1773: 689
March 1773-March 1774: 773
March 1774-March 1775: 752
March 1775-March 1776: 803
March 1776-March 1777: 774
March 1777-March 1778: 565
March 1778-March 1779: 690
March 1779-March 1780: 586
March 1780-March 1781: 601
March 1781-March 1782: 675
March 1782-March 1783: 809
March 1783-March 1784: 855
March 1784-March 1785: 725
March 1785-March 1786: 685
March 1786-March 1787: 708
March 1787-March 1788: 812
March 1788-March 1789: 697
March 1789-March 1790: 699
March 1790-March 1791: 675
March 1791-March 1792: 710
March 1792-March 1793: 691
March 1793-March 1794: 665
March 1794-March 1795: 633
March 1795-March 1796: 602
March 1796-March 1797: 521
March 1797-March 1798: 539
March 1798-March 1799: 531
March 1799-March 1800: 426

Note: Since some patients were admitted in one year and released in the next, there may be some double counting.

of Age."[10] In the following year, out of 607 patients (442 of whom finished a course of treatment), 83 were married women, and some of them came with their children as well.[11] There was never any attempt to record whether the male patients were married or not.

The Lock Hospital seems to have identified as its most "innocent" patients those children who contracted venereal disease as a result of sexual attack. *The Account of the Proceedings of the Governors of the Lock Hospital* (1751) reports that from the hospital's opening in January 1747, it had treated more than fifty children (ages two to twelve) who were victims of sexual attack. Such attacks on children were not uncommon throughout the eighteenth and early nineteenth centuries: they were the result of the widely held notion that having intercourse with a virgin (which is why children were "selected") could clear someone of the disease. The Lock Hospital mounted a very public campaign against this belief, which had become so common that defense attorneys and judges often used it in cases brought forward to prosecution.[12] It was commonplace for paragraphs like the following to appear in the published accounts.

> As several Children from Two to Ten years old have become Patients in this Hospital from ways little suspected by the Generality of Mankind, the Governors think it their Duty out of regard to little Innocents to publish the motives of wicked People to so vile an Act and to Assure them of the Fallacy of it.
>
> It is a received Opinion with many of the lower Class of Mankind, both Males and Females, that when infected themselves if they can procure a sound Person to communicate the Disease to, they certainly get rid of it.
>
> And from this Principle the most horrid Acts of Barbarity have been frequently committed on poor little Infants, tho' these vile Wretches have by Experience been convinced of the Absurdity of such vulgar Notions, yet this requires the utmost Publication to prevent such unheard of Cruelty and Inhumanity for the future. [1749, 1751, and 1767]

In the sermons he preached at the Lock Hospital Chapel and from other pulpits as well, Rev. Martin Madan repeatedly raised the case of these victimized children. In fact, on 28 March 1762, at the opening of the Lock Chapel, Madan acknowledged the potential indecorousness of his subject: "To what I have said concerning the objects of this charity, I must add something, that for its consequences ought to be mentioned in the most publick manner, though for its enormity I hardly know how to mention it at all. What an idea must it give us of the wickedness of the human heart, to be told, that in order to get rid of the disease, as they foolishly think on easy terms, men who have been infected with it, have, from the most weak and groundless principles, which have no foundation, but the most diabolical cruelty and wickedness, communicated this loathsome distemper to numbers of little innocents."[13]

In at least one case, the Lock Hospital did more than just speak against the practice. In November 1764, the governors decided to bear the expense of prosecuting a defendant named Edmund Thirkell for the rape of five-year-old Mary Amelia Halfpenny, who had been admitted to the hospital on 28 June 1764. In February 1765, the secretary reported that Thirkell was found guilty of the crime.[14]

In order to support the hospital's expenses as well as to pay for new improvements and construction, the governors were constantly devising fundraising campaigns. They frequently organized breakfasts and dinners at Ranelagh Gardens, which in 1755, for example, would bring in £221. Moreover, like other charity hospitals, the Lock Hospital had close ties to theater and music circles in London. There was at least one benefit performance for the Lock Hospital at London theaters in 1747, 1749, 1750, 1753, 1754, 1755, 1756, 1758, 1762, 1764, 1766, 1767, 1768, 1771, 1774, and 1776. Needless to say, these benefit performances had the potential to supplement the hospital's treasury to a considerable degree. In 1755, there were benefit performances of *The Provoked Husband* and *The Schemers* that brought in £197 and £128.[15]

David Garrick and John Lacy, two of the Lock Hospital's most faithful supporters from the ranks of the London theater circles, were given honorary lifetime governorships in return for all their help and support. Garrick and his wife (Eva Maria Veigel Garrick [1724-1822]) appear to have been particularly sympathetic to those who had venereal disease. Not only did Garrick arrange for benefit nights over the course of many years but he also paid calls on men the governors wished to become subscribers. The notes of the general meeting held on 22 November 1755, for example, reveal that Garrick accompanied six governors who were deputized to wait on Sir Jonathan Fredrick and his brother in order to make an appeal to them on the Lock Hospital's behalf.[16] Even after Garrick's death in 1779, his widow continued the family's support of the Lock Hospital, and she became a benefactor to the Lock Asylum for Women. The Lock Hospital received support from other notable London theater people, including the comedian Samuel Foote. John Rich, manager of Covent Garden, often lent the Lock Hospital a benefit night at his theater, and leading male actors Spranger Barry, Charles Macklin, and William Powell performed in benefit nights.

The Lock Hospital also looked to London's most famous composer for help. As he did for Thomas Coram's Foundling Hospital, for which he gave benefit performances of his *Messiah*, George Frideric Handel awarded the Lock Hospital a benefit performance of his *Judas Maccabeus*. The performance took place at the King's Theater on 7 May 1753, making £78 for the society.[17] Also, the popular violinist and composer Felice Giardini (1716-1796) appeared in numerous benefits for the Lock Hospital over the course of many years. The oratorio *Ruth*, which he wrote with Charles Avison, was performed in the Lock Hospital Chapel in 1768, 1771, 1774, and 1776.

The role the chapel played in the continuing survival of the Lock Hospital deserves special mention as well. In the late 1750s a campaign was mounted to build a chapel, which opened in 1762. Financially speaking, the selling of eight hundred pew spaces and the publication of the sermons preached and the hymns sung at the hospital became money-making opportunities for the Lock Hospital. Indeed, the chapel provided a venue for benefit concerts and sermons, which meant that the society was no longer so dependent on London theater companies for benefit nights. By the 1770s, the chapel was responsible for bringing in more receipts than the annual dues paid by the governors or by any other fund-raising effort. In 1773-74, for example, tickets and seats in the chapel brought in £967, the performance of the oratorio (in the chapel) gave the charity £345, the performing of sacraments brought in £81, and the sale of hymn and music books amounted to £61. Annual subscriptions, on the other hand, were responsible for just £669. The first edition of Martin Madan's *A Collection of Psalms and Hymns* appeared in 1760, and the number of subsequent editions, thirteen by 1794, suggests its popularity and money-making capability for the charity. The book could only be purchased at the Lock Hospital, and as the published reports demonstrate, the proceeds were given to the charity.

The Lock Hospital was an attractive charity to the growing number of Methodists and Evangelical Christians living in London during the second half of the eighteenth century. Part of this was surely due to Martin Madan's popularity. By the late 1760s and 1770s, many of the first group of governors had died or were no longer so active in the charity's affairs, and the second generation seem to have been more "religiously" than "medically" oriented. William Bromfield's retirement as surgeon in 1770 and his final and bitter break with the charity society in 1781 (caused by a disagreement over the salary and responsibilities of the chaplain and his assistants) can mark to a certain extent the end of the Lock Hospital's first era.

It behooves us to remember that "The Royal Proclamation Against Vice and Immorality," signed by George III on 1 June 1787, was largely the result of effort expended by William Wilberforce, who simultaneously founded his own "Proclamation Society." Wilberforce (1759-1833) is today more remembered for the active role he played in the late-eighteenth-century abolitionist movement, but his leadership in the Evangelical movement, which started with his own conversion in 1785-86, helped to create a circle of philanthropists who would help to found the Lock Asylum for Women. Present along with Wilberforce at the first meeting (18 April 1787) of the founders of the Lock Asylum were his friends, Henry and Robert Thornton from the celebrated family of Evangelical bankers, Sir Charles Middleton, and William Morton Pitt. The two Lock Hospital chaplains, Rev. Thomas Scott and Rev. Charles E. De'Coetlogon, were also in attendance. Other Wilberforce friends, like Hannah More, soon became active, albeit silent, benefactors.

The founders of the Lock Asylum well understood that many of the women patients "have no method of subsistence but by prostitution, and can procure no lodging but in a house of infamy. These have scarcely any alternative, but starving or a prison on the one hand, or returning to their former practices on the other."[18] In other words, what these women needed was a place of refuge that would accept them after they were discharged from the Lock Hospital. This is exactly what Wilberforce and his cohorts resolved to provide them. In short, their plan was to transform patients into penitents. At their second meeting (21 April 1787), they resolved the following:

> That the Object of this Institution be to receive such female Patients as having been cured in the Lock Hospital of Disorders contracted by a vicious and irregular course of Life, and during their residence there having had the opportunity of Religious Instructions, have given sufficient proof of sincere Repentance.
>
> That the design of their being received be to maintain and protect them till they can be restored, either to their Friends or to the Community at large, in a way of Industry according to their Ability.
>
> That if after their Restoration to Society, they be found to have behaved well in their respective Situations, they shall be consider'd as entitl'd to such farther countenance, protection and encouragement as the circumstances of the Institution will enable the Governors in their discretion to give.

On 26 May 1787, it was ordered that two houses, numbers 5 and 6 on nearby Osnaburg Row, be taken and fitted up to become the Lock Asylum for Women.[19]

The founders' compassion was perhaps equaled by their readiness to judge negatively the women they intended to help. The first three paragraphs of *Account of the Institution of the Lock Asylum* (1788) depict the prostitutes as pitiful and blameworthy agents of personal and national destruction. Significantly, those who are identified as their prey become, rhetorically speaking, the victims of these evil women rather than their coconspirators.

> It is generally allowed that none of the human Species are more miserable in themselves, or more mischievous in Society, than those unhappy Women, who disgrace our Streets, and subsist upon the infamous Wages of Iniquity. Their Occupations, Connections, and the Scenes which they perpetually witness, speedily obliterate every Sentiment of Virtue that they may have received from Education, and familiarize them to Wickedness; until shame and Remorse being completely banished, they are in the daily Practice of Effrontery, Deceit, and Licentiousness, prepared for any kind of Degree of Vice to which they can be tempted.
>
> Young Women, having been seduced and deserted, are banished from their Friends; excluded from their former Prospects and Satisfactions; and frequently, after an Indulgent Education, are left without other Resource, than that of entering the vile Recesses of Debauchery. When once initiated in these Seminaries, the general consequences are increasing Wickedness, a ruined Constitution, a premature Death, and, as far as we can see, everlasting Destruction.

The paragraph devoted to decrying the "malignant influence" the prostitutes have on British society is especially dramatic in its use of hyperbolic language.

> In the mean Time their malignant Influence on Society is equally deplorable. They throng our Streets and lay in wait for the inexperienced and incautious: So that a Youth can scarce walk a Mile in many Parts of this City without running the Gauntlet through at least fifty of those Temptations, which are most likely to prevail against him. Thus are the rising Generations successively corrupted; Evil Habits are early contracted, ruinous Connections formed, Conscience and the Sense of Shame subdued, and our Youth trained up for a Life of Profligacy.[20]

The emotional nature of this patriotic appeal to those who care about the "rising Generations being successively corrupted" hints at the larger political reason why British men and women should support the effort to begin such an institution.

The founders and the early supporters of the Lock Asylum for Women were extremely generous to the society, which was kept financially separate from the Lock Hospital. The earl of Dartmouth served as president of the Lock Asylum from 1789 until his death in 1801. Sir Charles Middleton, first baron of Barham (1726-1813), was also extremely active in the establishment of the Lock Asylum, serving as a vice president of the society for many years. He and his wife were responsible for bringing in substantial contributions. The first royal patron of the asylum was Frederick, duke of York. These supporters were key to the institution's secure financial start. It is noteworthy that the Lock Asylum received more money from subscriptions and gifts before its opening than did the Lock Hospital before its initial admission of patients, approximately £396 to £339.[21] By 24 April 1788, the date of its first annual General Court meeting, the Lock Asylum had eight lifetime governors and seventy-four annual governors. Moreover, sixty-five other benefactors, forty-three of whom were women, gave the society gifts of money.

The important role women played in the establishment of this charitable society is evident in the Lock Asylum's early history. Significantly, many more women donated start-up money to the Lock Asylum than did women forty years earlier when the Lock Hospital was established. The Lock Asylum was, it seems, a more "acceptable" society for women benefactors. From 6 May until 5 July 1787, the day the Lock Asylum admitted its first female penitents, twenty-six of the first hundred benefactors were women. Among them were the countess of Dartmouth, Mrs. Garrick, Hannah More, Lady Mary Fitzgerald, Mrs. Carteret, Lady Smythe, Lady Middleton, Mrs. Elizabeth Carter, and Mrs. Bouverie. A number of these women would be faithful friends to the Lock Asylum even after their deaths. In 1792, for example, the estate of Mrs. Anne Isabella Cavendish paid in a legacy of £100, and in 1799, Mrs. Bouverie, who had been giving to the charity since May 1787, also remembered the society, granting it a legacy of £100.[22] After her death in 1833, Hannah More's last will and testament announced her final gift—£200—to the society.[23]

Although women benefactors clearly played a crucial role in financing the Lock Asylum, they did not actively participate in its administration. No women were present at the initial discussions (18, 21 April; 3, 17, 26 May; 7, 14, 21, 28 June 1787), and not one of the many female subscribers, governors, or benefactors is recorded as participating in any vote. Thus, no women were appointed to the first Weekly Committee, and none were present at the first annual General Court meeting, held on 24 April 1788.[24] The administration of the Lock Asylum was similar to that of the Lock Hospital. Governorship was less expensive, however. It could be bought on an annual (2 guineas) or a lifetime basis (20 guineas).

Existence at the Lock Asylum was extremely restrictive. The rules for admission were inflexible: admittance must be immediately upon discharge from the Lock Hospital; the woman must have received a positive written recommendation from the chaplain of the Lock Hospital; and she must have been judged by the hospital's Weekly Committee as having been a "good patient" while at the hospital and as having the potential to be a sincere penitent during her stay at the Lock Asylum. Admittance and care were free of charge, but the "female penitents," as they were called in all Lock Asylum publications, had to honor a strict code of conduct.[25] They were "not allowed to converse with any Person, but in the presence of the Matron." They would "not be allowed to go out of the House and Premises on any account whatsoever, but in the Company of the Matron, or some other Person appointed to assist her." Further, "No Letters shall be written or received by them but under the Inspection of the Matron or Chaplain: And their Boxes, and every thing that comes to them, shall be liable to the Inspection of the Matron." They were expected to attend "family worship" every morning and evening, and on Sundays and holidays they were required to attend "public worship" at the Lock Chapel. They were not permitted to drink "strong Liquors" of any sort, nor could they play games or read any books not approved by the chaplain. The women rose at 7 A.M., went to morning prayers at 8, dined at 1 P.M., attended evening prayers at 8 P.M., and went to bed at 9. They were employed within the two houses kept by the Lock Asylum, generally sewing and doing other handiwork, and every woman was permitted to keep a fourth of her "clear Earnings." There was no fixed period of residence. The plan was that when employment was found or when return to one's family/friends was arranged, the female penitents would leave. More frequently, however, they ran away.

An Account of the Institution of the Lock Asylum (1796) recorded that more than half of the penitents accepted by the asylum had not been reformed:

22 Restored to, and remain with their Friends; some of them are Married, and Mothers of Families.
72 Placed out in different Services.
11 Expelled for ill Behaviour.
112 Have disappointed the Expectations of their Benefactors, by eloping from the House, or Services, in which they have been placed.
10 Have died in the House.
17 Remain in the ASYLUM, March 25th, 1796.

This rate of "success" and "failure" would not change much over the years. Indeed, by March 1802, of the 364 women who had been admitted to the Lock Asylum since July 1787, only 129 could be counted as successfully reformed: 40 had been received by their friends or family, and 89 were in service positions. Of the others, 16 died, 15 remained under the asylum's protection, and 204 are not mentioned.[26] Thus, the Lock Asylum was not able to boast of "cure" rates, whether real or imagined, as the Lock Hospital did.

Instead, the official voices of the Lock Asylum chose to focus on individual successes, and thus every early published account issued by the society (1788, 1792, 1796, 1802) includes testimonials about various patients. It is more than a little ironic that the Lock Asylum would have to use the same rhetorical strategy as did so many of London's eighteenth-century quacks. *An Account of the Institution of the Lock Asylum* (1788) included four such penitent histories, which incidentally present four different types of Lock Asylum inmates. The first two represent young women from middle-class families who were enabled to a great extent to return to their former stations in life:

> One young woman of decent family and previous good character, having been seduced, and finding herself both pregnant and diseased, was strongly tempted to destroy herself and when about leaving the Lock Hospital, upon some new aggravations of her distress, had actually formed her determination to do so. This appeared in the fixed melancholy upon her countenance, which excited attention and compassion: but being spoken to in a friendly manner, and the proposal being made to her of retirement, refuge, and needful provision, she was brought to confess and give up her desperate purpose; and has ever since behaved with such decorum, fidelity, and industry, as entitle her to the most entire confidence in a situation, in which she is enabled to support both herself, and the child of which she has since become the mother.
>
> Another young person, of reputable parents in the country, came to London, and went to service, was speedily debauched, and in a few weeks came into the Lock Hospital: when she was discharged cured she was admitted into the Asylum: and her father being applied to willingly received her, and some months after expressed his entire satisfaction in her conduct, and his gratitude to the charity in the strongest terms; his daughter having (as he said) taken care of his household affairs, ever since her return, in the most prudent and commendable manner; and had at that time a prospect of being married and settled to advantage, and the completion of his wishes on her behalf.

The next two penitent histories describe the situations—past, present, and presumably future—of reformed criminals who are now in "proper service":

> Another young Woman having for some years lived in those criminal connections which supply the means of ease and soft indulgence, appeared in the Hospital in that Style of Dress,

> which marks those thoughtless unhappy females, who having hitherto been exempted from the languishing Distress and Penury which commonly succeed: But upon being discharged cured from the Hospital, was found reluctant to return to her former course of Life: and being entirely destitute of any other means of subsistence, she was received into this ASYLUM; she was after a time taken as a Servant of all Work, and has been now above half a Year in that Situation, in which she behaves very well, and always appears very happy.
>
> We might mention another, who having for some time before her Admission been guilty of repeated Prostitution, was in the LOCK ASYLUM so affected by witnessing the Death of one of the young Women, that ever since, she hath behaved with the utmost Seriousness, and apparent Piety: She hath been in Service above half a Year.

Subsequent published accounts often included new testimonials and added in italics up-to-date information about the former penitents.

By 1796, however, the Lock Asylum had to acknowledge and contextualize why more than half of its women penitents failed to be rehabilitated. The defense was grounded on the institution's larger religious purpose.

> An impartial and scrupulous regard to truth, however, renders it incumbent on us to allow, that many disappointments continue to try our patience: but the institution appears with increasing evidence to answer important purposes, and the prospect of usefulness grows more encouraging—The success is at least adequate to the sentiment suggested in the original pamphlet—"If amidst *reiterated disappointments,* we be successful only in a *few instances,* and *a very small number* be brought to true repentance and a christian conversation: this will be an abundant compensation."—And as "there is joy in the presence of the angels of God over one sinner that repenteth;" we have certainly cause for thankfulness, and encouragement to persevere in an undertaking, which in all respects so exactly coincides with the genius and precepts of christianity.[27]

The necessity to put its mediocre results forward in a positive light was, of course, crucial to the asylum's continued survival.

The asylum's constant need to win new benefactors, as well as to reassure its proven friends, perhaps accounts for why its published reports stress—and sometimes stretch—the society's successes. The Lock Asylum was extremely dependent on the continued benevolence of its initial supporters, and thus the £273 decline in gifts and subscriptions from the first (£577) to the second year (£304) of operations was significant.[28] In subsequent years, subscriptions and gifts brought in even less. For example, the asylum received only £218 from subscriptions and gifts from March 1795 to March 1796.[29] When the fiscal year closed on 15 March 1796, the asylum had £113 cash in hand but owed £122.

Income received from subscriptions, gifts, charity sermons, and the work performed by women under the asylum's care would not, however, prevent the Lock Asylum from going into debt by the turn of the century. By 1802, the financial circumstances of the society demanded that the governors add frankness to their rhetorical arsenal, which had hitherto relied on exaggeration. *A Brief Account of the Institution of the Lock Asylum* (1802), published by the Philanthropic Society, made a direct and urgent appeal for help: "It has, however, become proper and necessary to inform the public, that the funds of this charity are insufficient for its support, and that a considerable debt had been incurred, which even endangered the existence of the institution: and though a great part of this has been lately discharged, by the extraordinary liberality of a few individuals; yet the further aid of the humane and pious is earnestly requested in order to ward off similar dangers in future" (4).

That both the Lock Hospital and the Lock Asylum chose to stress their Christian more than their medical purposes during the 1790s is evident by the fact that the words *venereal disease* appeared less and less frequently in their published accounts. In fact, the disease was named only once in the 1796 *Account of the Nature and Intention of the Lock Hospital*. In the nineteenth century, the secret malady had to be completely resituated as a serious national and spiritual problem rather than as a named medical concern. Indeed, in 1846, the year the Lock Hospital's Centenary Report was published, the name of the disease itself was never given:

> The malady, to the cure of which the LOCK HOSPITAL is appropriated, peculiarly requires medical assistance, and if neglected or improperly treated, it may terminate fatally by the most dreadful progress of lingering sufferings; while, at the same time, it is more generally curable than most other diseases. We may, indeed, consider the dire distemper itself, as a declaration how greatly an holy God abhors licentiousness; yet hath he mercifully provided medicines which seldom fail, when judiciously used, to eradicate it completely. We ought, therefore, doubtless, to imitate his compassion to the persons of the guilty, as well as his hatred of their crime.[30]

By the nineteenth century, the Lock Hospital did not dare ask its audience for "cool consideration" as it did in 1749. "Reason" was no longer seen as a help in curing the disease. Now the surest way to a real cure was through one's heart and soul.

Notes

1. This was the figure given at the annual meeting of the governors of the Lock Hospital on 15 May 1800 (see Asylum General, old reference 100, new reference 4, fol. 124). The total includes those patients who were "discharged as cured" on an out-patient status, patients who ran away, patients who left the hospital without the consent of the governors, patients who were discharged for irregular conduct, patients who died, and patients who remained in the hospital on the last day of the fiscal year. The Lock Hospital's "fiscal" year went from March to March. The records of the London Lock Hospital are held in the library of the Royal College of Surgeons, London. I would like to thank the staff at the library of the Royal College of Surgeons, especially Matthew Derrick and Ian Lyle, for their help.

2. *An Account of the Proceedings of the Governors of the Lock Hospital* (London, 1749). The same language appears in the accounts printed in 1751 and 1767. Subsequent references will be made in the text by year and page number.

3. I come up with this figure by adding together the sums listed in the Asylum General, old ref. 97, new ref. 1, fols. 1-20.

4. See Asylum General, old ref. 97, new ref. 1, fol. 29.

5. Judging by the number of subscribers and benefactors who wished to remain anonymous, there also seems to have been a "shame" factor in giving to the Lock Hospital.

6. Board Minutes #1, 24 January 1756. See also William Bromfield, *An Account of the English Nightshades* (London, 1757), 91.

7. *Cured* is the word the Lock Hospital used in relation to any patient who received and completed a course of treatment at the facility. The use of the word does not mean that when the patients were released from the hospital's care they were actually free of disease. In this regard, the hospital's statistics in regard to "cured" patients must be regarded as highly inflated and unlikely. For additional discussion of the use of the word *cure*, see Philip Wilson's article in this collection.

8. See Asylum General, old ref. 99, new ref. 3, fol. 3-4.

9. Mention of Carolina Williams's gift can be found in Board Minutes #1, 15 November 1755. By July 1772, her own circumstances were considerably reduced from what they once were. Asylum General, old ref. 97, new ref. 2, fol. 169, includes the following about her: "It appearing to this Court that Carolina Williams who has been a considerable Benefactress to this charity in fitting up a Ward for the reception of Married Women at her own Expence.—is now thro' various Misfortunes reduced to the utmost Poverty and Distress.... And whereas the said Carolina Williams, has in consideration of her former Services to this Charity, had the Privilege of recommending Patients to this Hospital, and thro' her state of indigence been tempted to sell such Letter to Persons afflicted with the Venereal Disease ... Ordered, That on the said Carolina Williams, consenting to give up her priviledge of recommendation, and in consideration of her former Generosity to this Charity, and her present very indigent Circumstances, she be allowed two Shillings & Sixpence per Week, during her Life, to commence from Thursday next."

10. Court Minutes #1, see 11 March 1755.
11. Court Minutes #1, see 30 March 1756.
12. See Anthony E. Simpson, "Vulnerability and the Age of Female Consent: Legal Innovation and Its Effect on Prosecutions for Rape in Eighteenth-Century London," in *Sexual Underworlds of the Enlightenment*, ed. G.S. Rousseau and Roy Porter (Chapel Hill: University of North Carolina Press, 1988), 193-94.
13. Rev. Martin Madan, "Every Man Our Neighbour," sermon delivered on 28 March 1762, 25.
14. See Board Minutes #3, 21 February 1765, fols. 230, 273.
15. Board Minutes #1, 30 March 1756. *The Schemers*, written by William Bromfield, was an adaptation of Jasper Maine's *The City Match*.
16. Board Minutes #1, 22 November 1755.
17. General Asylum, old ref. 97, new ref. 1, fol. 117.
18. An Account of the Lock Asylum (London, 1796), 5.
19. Lock Asylum Committee Minute Book, fols. 3-4, 18.
20. *An Account of the Institution of the Lock Asylum* (London, 1788), A2.
21. Lock Asylum Cash Book, n.p.
22. See the particular year as it appears in the Lock Asylum Cash Book. See also the Lock Asylum Committee Minute Book, fol. 50.
23. See *A Short History of the London Lock Hospital and Rescue Home, 1746-1906*, 17. The copy at the College of Surgeons has no author and no date of publication, although a photocopy at the Wellcome Institute for Medicine has a letter in the front cover dated 12 December 1906, signed by A.W. Cruikshank and addressed to F.W. Cock.
24. Lock Asylum Committee Minute Book, fol. 50.
25. Ibid., fols. 15-16.
26. *A Brief Account of the Institution of the Lock Asylum* (London, 1802), 2.
27. *An Account of the Institution of the Lock Asylum* (London, 1796), 15.
28. Lock Asylum Committee Minute Book, fols. 50 and 68.
29. *An Account of the Institution of the Lock Asylum* (London, 1796), 9.
30. *Centenary Report of the Lock Hospital* (London, 1846), 1.

Two

Representations
of Venereal Disease

Chapter 9

Decorums

BETTY RIZZO

THERE ARE AS MANY DIFFERENT EIGHTEENTH-CENTURY DECORUMS FOR DEALing with references to venereal disease, particularly in relation to marriage, as there are different types of discourse. Many of these decorums simply enjoin denial: one doesn't ordinarily expect to encounter references to the disease(s) in sentimental novels or dramas, in polite periodical essays, or in the biographies or histories of the period.[1] Other decorums enjoin particular approaches, almost all of which, however, tend to downplay the seriousness of the problem. In newspaper advertisements, as in many treatises on the disease, the crucial message is that if one takes the recommended prescription in quantity and time enough, a complete cure will speedily follow. The inveteracy and ultimately fatal malignancy of syphilis is seldom noted. In informal discourse among the men it's bad form to take the malady, often viewed as a badge of manliness, too seriously. As the discourses grow more polite, euphemisms combine with an arch coyness to fit the subject for mention in the drawing room, and heads are shaken over young men who have so recklessly (if gallantly) undermined their constitutions.

Despite the many differing and straitening decorums for discussing venereal disease, however, three general conclusions can be drawn. First, most people knew something about the disease, but secondly, few recognized the full epidemic severity of it. Finally, attitudes were heavily inflected by ideologically determined assumptions, or social decorums, about class and gender: women with the disease attracted more opprobrium and distaste than men; the ravages among children were generally ignored; the infection and consequent misery of prostitutes were regarded as morally deserved; infected wives were tendered little compassion or encouragement to express resentment, but rather were advised to practice a becoming submission to male prerogatives. A man might even *boast* of a clap or two, but silence and a deceptive secrecy often surrounded more serious consequences (paresis or infected wives or children), and deaths would almost inevitably be attributed to other causes, even in the bills of mortality, where death by venereal disease was probably greatly undercomputed.[2]

Each decorum of discourse prescribes its own method of naming the disease, which in turn prescribes a different attitude toward it. The official bills of mortality call syphilis the French pox, thus rejecting the disease as a national product. Members of the medical profession call it the venereal disease. The romantic annals of gallantry regard it as a wound or memento of the wars of love, and the lawyers label it the foul disease. The public usually employ the simplest of distinguishing epithets: the clap and the pox. In this usage they are supported by Dr. Johnson in his dictionary, which fails to include the words *syphilis* or *venereal* in the sense of disease, but does include pox as "the venereal disease. This is the sense when it has no epithet" and *clap* as "a venereal infection," with an illustration from Pope, "Time, that at last matures a *clap* to Pox."[3]

As Pope suggests, the clap and the pox (gonorrhea and syphilis) were generally believed to be different manifestations of the same infection. The belief was that the clap, if not speedily cured, would eventually transmute into the more serious pox. Thus, in *A Dissertation on the Nature and Effects of a New Vegetable Remedy* (1780), John Burrows speaks of a clap becoming a confirmed pox [45]. Signs of the confusion abound as to the origin of the diseases, such as the advertisement for *The Anti-Gonorrhoea, calculated for gradually extirpating the Syphilitic Contagion* [*Daily Advertiser*, 20 February 1764]. But there is also every indication that people knew the difference between the symptoms. For instance, in 1778 Hester Thrale forthrightly noted the story of an Anglican bishop encountering an enthusiast whom he had thought to have been a Methodist but who announced he was actually a Moravian: "you remind me of a Young Fellow I knew once at College—" the Bishop said, "his Tutour seeing him look pale one Day—Sir said he you seem quite Ill of late, I fear you are *Clap'd;* No Sir but I am *Pox'd* replied the Lad."[4]

Apart from medical writings, the most straightforward discussion of the disease was probably in the satire of the time.[5] The pox was naturalized to the satiric worlds of Butler, Pope, and Smollett and of such improper ephemera as *Satan's Harvest Home, or The Present State of Whorecraft; Adultery, Fornication, Procuring, Pimping, Sodomy, And the Game at Flatts* (actually a plainspoken moral work), in which the author, totting up the disadvantages of prostitution, notes:

> The greatest Evil that attends this Vice, or could befal Mankind, is the Propagation of that infectious Disease called the *French Pox*, which in two Centuries has made such incredible Havock all over *Europe*. In these Kingdoms, it so seldom fails to

attend Whoring, now-a-days mistaken for Gallantry and Politeness, that a hale robust Constitution is esteem'd a Mark of Ungentility and Ill-breeding, and a healthy young Fellow is looked upon with the same View, as if he had spent his Life in a Cottage. Our Gentlemen of the Army, whose unsettled Way of Life makes it inconvenient for them to marry, are hereby very much weaken'd and enervated, and rendered unfit to undergo such Hardships, as are necessary for defending and supporting the Honour of their Country. . . . And our Gentry in general, seem to distinguish themselves by an ill state of Health; in all Probability, the Effect of this pernicious Distemper. Nothing being more common, than to hear People of Quality complain of *rude vulgar Health*, and curse their *Porterly Constitutions*. Men give it to their Wives, Women to their Husbands, or perhaps their Children; they to their Nurses, and the Nurses again to other Children; so that no Age, Sex or Condition, can be entirely free from the Infection.[6]

Here in a notorious prurient pamphlet is the plainest statement of the true case to be found. Few other references are as honest.

Advertisements for quack remedies in the newspapers elucidate public awareness and confusion both and illustrate the decorum of medical reference. In 1772 the proprietor of the Vegetable Specific Pill recommended early attention to the venereal disease, warning of "the condition the unhappy victim is reduced to, when the infectious matter has lain undisturbed for a series of years, a state in itself so deplorable, that human nature shudders at the possibility of." Even "the simple gonorrhea," which might if attacked early be cured in a week, by the neglect of a few days may take months to cure. All is well, however, if the patient begins immediate treatment. Dr. Rock's Royal Patent Electuary, which cured all degrees and symptoms of a "certain disorder," rooted out all disease, yet prevented discovery because it might be taken "and business followed as usual." "Those who suspect they have received some taint from converse with an infected person, by taking a dose or two of this Electuary may have their minds set at ease."[7] Besides the calming misconception, perpetuated here, that the pox might so easily be dismissed, another implication is that marital partners might and should, for their peace of mind (and that of their spouses), be deceived as to the infection.

Most patent remedies helped to decoy patients into a false reliance and security. The *Daily Advertiser* from October 1768 to January 1769 promised cures from William Saunders, M.D., who published *A New and Easy Way of Giving Mercury to those affected with the Venereal Disease*, translated from the Latin of Joseph James Plenck of Vienna; from John Leake, M.D., who published a new edition of *A Dissertation on the Properties and Efficacy of the Lisbon Diet Drink, in the Cure of the Venereal Disease;* from Dr. Copp, F.R.S., of Leyden, who had cured deplorable cases "where no Salivation could reach, nor no Doctors in England could relieve," without alteration of diet or hindrance of business: "All Disorders cured"; from Dr. John Petit, proprietor of a "particular and infallible Remedy against . . . any kind of Venereal Disorder, if ever so inveterate, without the least Confinement or Alteration of Diet"; from Dr. Rock's Jesuit Drops, "for the Cure of all Stages of the Secret Disease, and its consequent Disorders from ignorant practice"; from Dr. Franks, who "cures effectually every Degree of the Venereal Disease, with Speed, Ease, Secresy, and Safety, on easy Terms and honourable Treatment. Note, Complete Lodgings always ready"; from the "Royal Patent Peru Drops . . . the only to be depended on, for the safe, speedy, and effectual Cure of every Degree of the Venereal Disease." Secrecy, dependent upon no confinement and no alteration of diet, was the key requirement, and the illusion of cure, in a disease which rapidly went underground, was almost a sure thing. Dr. Copp was the only practitioner during this period even to mention in an advertisement the problem of syphilitic children, of whom there were many but whose disease was perhaps not always recognized; he had entirely cured a woman who had suckled a "foul child" and was all over ulcers as broad as a man's hand and had lost the nipple of her right breast. Copp's reference seems to suggest that such an infant or child was conceived almost as a throwaway.

Both information and disinformation must have been circulated through such advertisements, which also helped on the epidemic by encouraging victims of the disease to rely on false remedies and simultaneously to spread the disease. Moreover, according to Dr. William Rowley in 1800, some husbands and wives infected one another on the supposition that the venereal discharge from the urethra was harmless.[8]

Little moral indignation was raised by the fact that men were transmitting the disease to their wives and children. It was variously reported without much affect that such women as Elizabeth Chudleigh, Susannah Cibber, Lady Sandwich, Sarah Siddons, Lady Folkestone—actresses to fine ladies—had been infected by their husbands.[9] A woman's misery was offhandedly downplayed, as in the case of Joseph Farington's remark about the profligate duke of Leeds and his duchess who, "on account of his irregular mode of proceeding, were supposed not to be very comfortable together."[10] The problem of the infection of wives was also treated matter-of-factly by the faculty. Burrows, who used a vegetable remedy, doctored a gentleman with advanced symptoms whose wife, who had refused mercury, was also in piteous condition, but Burrows claims to have effected cures in both in six weeks [59-60].

In general, the faculty seems to have believed in hiding the truth from those most closely affected—spouses—in order to maintain "the peace of families," a phrase frequently invoked. In his *Medical Dictionary* (1743), Dr. Robert James commended a presumably quack remedy that could be put into one's morning chocolate: "A husband can take his chocolate in the presence of his wife without her suspecting a thing: indeed, she herself can take it without realizing that she is swallowing an anti-venereal remedy; by this innocent means, then, peace and concord can be maintained in the household."[11] In other words, an unsuspecting infected wife could conveniently be (ineffectually) dosed without her knowledge.

A different decorum subsisted in frank conversation or correspondence between friends in which secrets about the disease might be confided. In 1741 Lady Mary Wortley Montagu noted that Lord Morpeth had died of consumption but that gossip attributed his death to "the venereal distemper which he caught in Italy and kept secret so long that it proved at last to be incurable." And in 1767 Horace Walpole noted at the death of Mons. de Guerchy, "It is said he had concealed and tampered indiscreetly with an old complaint, acquired before his marriage."[12] But these confidences were benign in the sense that, in general, suffering the disease did a man's reputation no harm—perhaps quite the reverse: in 1767 Lord Barrymore left his bride at the altar when he was taken ill. At first he was suspected of intending a permanent defection, and it was a matter of somewhat sniggering relief, therefore, that he was only temporarily *hors de combat* and that the marriage was duly performed as soon as he had at all recovered. Sarah Byng Osborn reported to her grandson, "Poor Lady Amelia Stanhope must see many matches concluded before her own, for Lord Barrymore is obliged to submit to a salivation, which he is now in, before he can be a bridegroom." Apparently his debilitation from the disease or its remedy was inconsequential to the bride's friends, though it was reported "his legs shook all the while the ceremony was performing: the state of his body is so very bad, it is not thought he can live long."[13] Venereal mishaps aside, once honorably married, Barrymore was again secure in reputation. If even women were comfortable writing such reports to their intimates, it can be no surprise that the letters of wits like George Selwyn and Horace Walpole habitually note news of the venereal inconveniences of their acquaintance.

The decorum of public gossip, as reflected in the Tête-à-Têtes and the other columns of the magazine *Town and Country,* is more complex. The Tête-à-Têtes glamorize gallantry, and as a consequence perforce treat venereal disease lightly, somewhat comically, as one of the scars of the wars of love (a persistent and revealing metaphor) and, like a duelling scar, as not at all dishonorable; female dropsies were similarly tut-tutted. "Perfection is not the lot of humanity" is a common conclusion of these columns, and elegance and lightness of language and style are all that is here required for dealing with amorous misfortunes. As the two ordinary venereal diseases are very rarely distinguished, it is common for every infection to be regarded as lightly as a gonorrhea. The countess of Modena had wounded several admirers, "among whom were some musqueteers, who thought her necessities entitled them to liberties, which she judged incompatible with good manners, and she herself has still some visible scars remaining of the wounds she received in these rencounters" [March 1770, 122]. Lord Deloraine (like a host of other privileged young men) had injured his constitution through dissipation but was recovered by a skillful physician; Lord Percy, too, had a constitution impaired by "the shock of . . . repeated attacks" [December 1770, 625; October 1772, 513]. Of Percy an earlier indictment read, "It is not surprising that the women of the present period should be so notorious in their infidelities to the marriage-bed, when there are such a number of lord P—r—ys, who had, before they came to maturity, debilitated themselves for conjugal alliances" [June 1771, 90]. A German count who made a conquest of a French countess at Versailles "discovered that the consequence of this intrigue would compel him to make a trip to Montpellier for the recovery of his health, the serenity of the air of that place being pronounced by the faculty very salutary for *love sick* swains" [August 1776, 401-2]. The editors tend to be most severe upon Frenchwomen: the earl of Peterborough meets a "French countess" at Vauxhall who picks his pocket and leaves him a "token of remembrance"; the earl of Howth escapes the clutches of a French Messalina who "afterwards died in a mad-house of a disorder she had long been troubled with, and to which it seems several had fallen martyrs, as well as herself" [August 1777, 401; September 1777, 458]. Puns and double entendres, of course, abound. In Ireland, General Scott is forced to break an engagement (at cards) with the duchess of Rutland on learning that his pretty servant girl "was only a nominal maid." He has to sail for England "without being able to take a personal leave," while the duchess consoles herself playing a party at *put*[14] with her groom-porter. Scott repairs, however, to Mr. Tomkyns in Arundel Street, and when the duchess returns, he is "enabled to renew the former Tête-à-Tête party, without any danger of a revoke" [January 1778, 31]. An honest fellow writing in to the magazine deprecates the suggestion of a crotchety old churl that a lovely clear-starcher in the house where Dr. Hauksbie's "remedy for a certain complaint" is sold is a prostitute: "Far be it from me to suppose, that the beautiful clear-starcher can have any hand in promoting the sale of the doctor's pills"—though a knowing patron praises her skill: "She gives the primitive gloss to whatever goes through her hand" [September 1769, 455-56]. Only occasionally does the magazine allow a glimpse of a more catastrophic and permanent accident, as in the reference to the French Messalina or to Ned Nasal (the name itself suggests he is of no consequence, an interloper in the privileged field of gallantry) who has by "a dire mishap in his amours" lost his nose [November 1781, 584]. Ned Nasal is something like the court scullion who tries to engage in the tourney lists and is justly trounced.

Another style of reference prevails in law reports such as those transmitted in *Trials for Adultery*, reports of a series of notorious divorce actions. Venereal infections figure openly only three times here in these particular transcripts (and more covertly in the Bolingbroke action—see below). The ailment, here the "foul disease," in these trials is relevant only as part of the grievance when imparted to the plaintiff by the offending spouse; therefore, it is typically mentioned only when the wife has infected the suing husband; nothing amiss done by the suing spouse is in any way relevant. Thus Dr. John Worgan, a well-known organist, in 1768 sued his wife, who had infected him, for divorce. Well clapped, he had visited the eminent surgeon William Bromfield, insisting the disorder could have come only from his wife whom he knew to be "afflicted with a running from her private parts." To preserve the peace of the family, Bromfield lied, declaring that Mrs. Worgan probably suffered from "the whites," a common ailment in women which could, he said, have been imparted to her husband. The effect of Bromfield's deception was unlucky. Worgan's discovery of his wife's profligacy with the household money, with which she treated her lover to various parties of pleasure, and his own consequent indebtedness, was delayed and the indebtedness much compounded. Meanwhile, his wife had induced her lover to sign a note to pay her butcher bill, whereupon he was soon afterwards imprisoned in the Fleet, where he died a year later. Subsequently, when Worgan did at last learn of his wife's lechery, profligacy, and murderous self-indulgence, he returned to Bromfield, who belatedly confessed the truth.[15] As Bromfield, an eminent practitioner indeed, seemed to entertain no doubts of his own probity throughout the affair, presumably secrecy, even to family members at risk, was the usual course. Mrs. Worgan had confessed to him that she had been raped by a man who came over the garden wall, and it would seem she had entirely won his confidence.

In 1770 Richard Heatley also claimed that his wife, Arabella, had given him the foul disease. He had at first refused to believe that he suffered from it, but he soon discovered his wife's perfidy. Moreover, two women servants testified to having seen her take medicines and pills, given to her by her lover, in private, twice a day, on rising and retiring. His divorce, like Worgan's, was granted.[16]

Though women were almost certainly more often wronged in this manner than men, only one woman memorialized in the *Trials for Adultery*, Martha Robinson, sued for divorce in 1775 on the grounds that her husband, Samuel, had several times communicated the foul distemper to her. He had at first taken her to a physician and threatened to murder her if she told anyone of the infection. She had been infected two or three times more, and on one occasion he had nearly killed her by giving her a powder in wine to cure her without her knowledge. A surgeon testified he had treated her husband and then herself three times for a fresh disease. Moreover, the man beat her. She had left him in 1769 to live elsewhere as a servant, but five years later he forced her back into cohabitation. She was nevertheless refused a divorce and awarded only a separation.[17] The discrimination on account of gender seems clear. Lawrence Stone notes the case of the Belchers in 1830 in which the judge ruled that as Belcher had infected his wife on the honeymoon and as the communication of venereal disease not contracted by adultery and not deliberately intended was not cruelty, Mrs. Belcher was denied a separation despite her husband's having given her the disease three times; she had to continue to cohabit.[18] Obviously a man's infection by his wife was considered far more of an infringement than a wife's infection by her husband.

Apart from such notorious cases as that of the earl of Rochester and Charles Hanbury Williams, it is difficult to identify with certainty deaths attributable to syphilis, despite the incidence of sudden madness among the aristocracy, which was surely far higher two hundred years ago than it is now. The editors of the Tête-à-Têtes would have considered reference to death by pox as dampening to the general esprit. Doctors, until actually summoned into court, were professionally discreet. Families supplied secondary causes of death, of which, in the case of syphilis, there was usually an ample supply. One can point with some suspicion to the terminal madness of Lord Orford [Walpole, 36:331-36], Lord Carteret's son Robert [18:501], Lord Pomfret [25:96], the duke of Dorset (said by Walpole [23:83] to have worn out his estate, his constitution, and his understanding), and the poet Christopher Smart,[19] but corroboration is hard to come by. It is therefore helpful to come upon a reasonably well documented case of the progress of syphilis in Frederick, Lord Bolingbroke (1734-88), whose problems were amply and variously discussed in the letters of his friends, in the annals of gallantry, and in *Trials for Adultery*. The case of Bolingbroke and his wife also illustrates how social decorums, which so much influenced the decorums of discourse, dictated that his sins were far more readily overlooked than hers.

"Bully" (as he was known to his fashionable cronies) was titled, adequately gifted, educated, and at his outset endowed with sufficient riches. He was a rake with an enormous early success with all classes of women. A celebrated procuress "administered to his pleasures, and promoted his success with the first-rate *demi-reps* of this kingdom. We might introduce the whole alphabet of initials in giving a list of his Dulcineas: the reader cannot suggest a Cleopatra, to whom he was not an Anthony," raved *Town and Country* in a 1772 retrospective of his career.[20] Bully was arguably more interested in demonstrating his prowess to his fellows by appropriating all the coveted women from milliners to countesses than in the women themselves, and once he had the name of conqueror, the women were eager to experience him and to enroll their names as having merited his attentions. As for Boswell, dealing with venereal disease must have been a commonplace occurrence for him, and one can understand why confinement and doses of mercury were often religiously endured in the simplest of cases by these men, as the invalids imagined their symptoms could lead, if untreated, to full-blown cases of the pox. Nevertheless, Bully, and others like him, probably contracted syphilis, which remained uncured, in their teens, and the disease may have been responsible for much of their subsequent irresponsibility and fecklessness.

Bully was anything but faithful to, but took care to carry on an ardent affair of many years with, the beautiful and silly Lady Coventry. She was the vainest, most fashionable, and most idiotic of noblewomen, a woman who could not forgo the use of white lead paint even after she knew it was killing her, even on her deathbed. Apparently she loved him, but that he was not himself swept away by passion is indicated by his terror in 1757 that Lord Coventry, then ill, would die, and that honor would constrain him to marry his much advertised paramour.[21] He delighted in the éclat of the affair and was an excellent public lover, notable for sitting in the pit at the opera leaning on one arm and gazing soulfully up at his object.[22] In the middle of the affair, however, he encountered a splendid match, Lady Diana Spencer (1734-1808), daughter of Charles, third duke of Marlborough. Lady Di was too beautiful, handsome, spirited, and gifted for Bully, but he was attracted to her as everyone was, and she offered a useful dowry, splendid bloodlines, a brilliant alliance, and protection from marriage to Lady Coventry.[23] When Walpole announced the match, he named the groom Frederick Clinton Maynard Nevil Douglas Viscount Bolingbroke and to the bride's name added those of Hamilton and West, to commemorate a few of their former flames [30:137]. The marriage took place in 1757, though Bully continued the affair with Lady Coventry until her death on 30 September 1760, an event which he famously commemorated: as Walpole noted in a letter of 14 October, "Lord Bolinbroke on hearing the name of Lady Coventry at Newmarket, affected to burst into tears and left the room, not to hide his crying, but his not crying" [9:307].

Among the courtesans of the first rank whom Bully kept was Nelly O'Brien, and according to Walpole he paid his wife the compliment when Reynolds painted her in 1763 of instructing the painter, "You must give the eyes something of Nelly Obrien, or it will not do" [10:52-53].

Lady Di had even more glamour than her husband. She was a beauty of great charm and wit, spoke in a fluted volubility, was no prude, and was a talented musician and an even more talented artist. Many men fell in love with her, but some of them, like the future Sir William Hamilton and the Hon. George West, though the grandsons of a duke and an earl, were only younger sons who had perforce to marry fortunes, and she willingly enough married the dashing Viscount Bolingbroke. He was a fashionable husband; that is, in an effort to keep up his reputation, he was conscientiously unfaithful, even though he suffered after she left him, protesting that if she were again Lady Di Spencer, he would again willingly marry her.

Husbands might be openly as unfaithful as they chose; wives who strayed had to be discreet. Lady Di had endured her husband's notorious affair with Lady Coventry for years and had had a number of children, two sons of whom had survived—in other words, she had done her marital duty—and moreover, though a duke's daughter, she had been painted at her husband's command with a courtesan's look about the eyes—when in 1764 she was at last "talked of" with Lord Gower.[24] Bully's response was to infect her with venereal disease so as to avenge himself on both lovers. The *Town and Country* Tête-à-Tête professed its incapability of relating the incident "in its full latitude: suffice it to say, that our hero sacrificed his own health to be revenged of his rival" [122]. The implication is that Bully deliberately sought out a clapped (even a poxed?) woman and contracted the disease in order to impart it to those whom the magazine would have named his "cornuters." It should perhaps be noted that his brother denied this story, claiming that the separation was "brought on by an accident originally, and afterwards continued by the foolish obstinacy of a woman, and promoted by the unfeeling behaviour and indolence of her brother."[25] Clearly women were not meant to be obstinate about such matters. The testimony of the divorce trial reveals that in September 1765 while Bully (almost certainly accompanied by his mistress) was visiting the dissolute Lord Orford at Houghton in Norfolk, Lady Di removed from his house in Brook Street and refused thereafter to cohabit with him.[26] Her friends supposed that she seized the opportunity of having been infected by him to justify her departure. Her sister's husband, Lord Pembroke, was later to deny to Boswell that he had twice given a venereal disease to his own wife, but by way of explanation for the rumor he did allow that Lady Di had had it.[27] Lady Holland wrote word of the formal separation in November: Bully opposed it, but she was to have £500 a year from him, to keep her place (and stipend) as a lady of the bedchamber to the queen, and to get something additionally from her brother.[28] In January 1766 Lady Sarah Bunbury reported Lady Di's reason: Lord Bolingbroke was the same as mad when he was drunk, which he generally was, and Lady Di "cannot live with him with safety to her health." Though repentant, Bully already had a woman in the house, while Lady Di herself was in great spirits "& seems to be very glad that she has got rid of him."[29]

Bolingbroke was briefly broken by the unexpected event of his wife's public departure, not least perhaps because it reflected on his hitherto invincible charm, but he soon continued onward in his reckless career, prepared to avenge himself further on the sex. "Bully is coming again into the world," wrote his friend the earl of March, "and swears he will seduce some modest woman." In November 1766 he appeared publicly with "his [immodest] girl" at Newmarket, and in December he refined his wardrobe and swore he would "at last be minister through Lady B., to whom he professes very amorous intentions."[30]

It was of course far otherwise with his wife, who could not flaunt the perquisites of her recovered freedom. Her new affair with Topham Beauclerk had to be conducted with discretion and without public declaration. To this point even after having left her husband's roof she had maintained her reputation, still continuing as a favorite lady of the queen's bedchamber, as she had been since 1761. Her husband, on the other hand, a lord of the king's bedchamber since 1761, had resigned the appointment in 1765. However, in August 1767 Lady Di had the ill hap to bear Beauclerk a daughter. She tried to veil the event in secrecy, but bribed, the servants told all as they almost always did, and the birth spurred the gallant Bully to warn her of her peril in a solicitous note: "Lord Bolingbroke is very sorry to hear Lady Bolingbroke has been ill, and desires to know how she does"; to which Lady Di replied, "Lady Bolingbroke is much obliged to Lord Bolingbroke, and she is a little better."[31]

Marlborough was a loyal brother and support to Lady Di. He strenuously opposed the idea of divorce with all its scandalous consequences. Lady Mary Coke noted in September 1767 that on the birth of Lady Di's child, Bolingbroke had instituted divorce proceedings, but it was thought, perhaps because of Marlborough's influence, that he could not succeed in his suit."[32] In December it was reported that the divorce proceedings had been set aside, that Marlborough and Bolingbroke were each to allow Lady Di £200 a year "and no more to be said about it."[33] Bully had, however, protested from the start that "he can't bear to think of Mr Beauclerk's Son inheriting his estate & title, in case his own two Sons should die."[34] Perhaps Lord Holland noted his true motivation, his determination "to marry a rich monster and retrieve his affairs."[35] Marlborough simply couldn't or wouldn't offer him the fortune Bully might hope to obtain with a second wife. The divorce hearing duly took place, Bully prevailed, and the divorce was made final on 10 March 1768.

The social decorum and the decorum of discourse that it controlled provided Bully, the plaintiff in the adultery trial, with full advantage. In the case of a woman suing, which was comparatively rare, it had been the opinion of Sir George Lee in the 1750s that "a wife was not entitled to a divorce for cruelty, unless it appeared she was a person of good temper, and had always behaved well and dutifully to her husband."[36] It was necessary, therefore, in a wife's suit, to testify to her good character, good temper, and submission. No such attestation was necessary in a husband's suit. Bully might be as he might, but nothing justified a wife's rebellion, and a wife like Lady Di who had rebelled could never have brought her own suit for divorce.

The evidence brought, therefore, outlined in full detail the progress of Lady Di's affair with Beauclerk: their meetings at the house she leased in the country, the assignations in the dining room with its convenient sofa, the "dropsy" from which she suffered. The fact that Bully's having infected her with venereal disease was well known if not introducible in evidence may be indicated by the introduction of a great deal of evidence about mysterious bottles of medicine brought to Lady Di by Beauclerk, bottles from which he allegedly removed the labels and from which she took doses twice daily.[37] The implication would seem to be that Lady Di was suffering from the foul disease in summer 1767, a full two years after the infection caught from her husband—evidently a new case and therefore evidence of her profligacy.

After the birth of the child, which soon died, and the trial, Lady Di's reputation was irreparably hurt. So, of course, was her husband's, but there was a great difference. Bully was still free in society to go where he liked. He could plan to court and marry a fortune to recoup the money he had thrown away at the gambling tables and at Newmarket. He had sinned to ten times Lady Di's degree, and he continued to sin, escaping with a little mild contempt for his fecklessness and ill management. When he parted in March 1768 from the fashionable courtesan Polly Jones, a friend belatedly complained, "What a turbulent life does that wicked boy lead with rogues and profligates of all descriptions!"[38] The verdict was hardly more severe than the usual tut-tut.

Lady Di, presuming on the enormous advantage of unremitting support from her brother the duke and her sister Lady Pembroke, tried to brave the storm and hoped particularly to keep her place at court, which would have meant complete social rehabilitation. Lady Mary Coke had noted on 15 September 1767, after the birth of the child, that Lady Di "said She had been very ill, but that She was now so much better that She thought She should soon be well enough to go to the Queen. But is it possible her Majesty can keep her in her Family after it is so publickly known She has lain inn?" She added on 20 September that Bolingbroke now had sufficient evidence for a divorce, which "will put it past a possibility of her keeping her Place at Court; indeed, it would have been shameful if She had." The matter was crucial, and Lady Di persisted; Walpole noted her declaration in October 1767 that she intended to come back into waiting in a week. But Lady Mary reported on 21 November that Lady Di had written to the queen "to say that She should not presume to pay her Duty to her Majesty till She had cleared her Character," and in fact a replacement for her was being sought. On 5 January 1768 Selwyn reported that Lady Di had sent her resignation to the queen, "who wrote her a very gracious letter on it. Bully kisses hand tomorrow."[39] The king and queen had decided to express their views by accepting Lady Di's resignation and simultaneously *reappointing* her husband as a lord of the king's bedchamber, a position he fulfilled until 1780, some time after his madness was known to be irreversible.

Lady Di paid in reputation more dearly than did Bully. The decorums of both private and public comment singled her out for animadversion. Dr.

Johnson, perfectly willing to keep up his close friendship with her partner in adultery, Beauclerk, gave a brutal verdict on Lady Di that was not at all singular: "The woman's a whore, and there's an end on't." Lord Chesterfield had already written to his son in February 1766, "Lord Bolingbroke having parted with his wife, now keeps another whore at a great expense."[40] Lord Harcourt's subsequent reference to her as that "corruptress of her own sex" was ironic, but it reflected the general opinion that she had provided a dangerous model [Walpole 29:254]. Hester Thrale records Baretti's "saying a thousand fine things" of her. "I mention'd her bad Character—Oh yes says he I know She is a Strumpet; had she not been so, She would have sate in Heaven next Jesus Christ."[41] The first volume of *Trials for Adultery* was published in 1779, making her again generally notorious by airing every detail of her adultery with Beauclerk, and in 1780 a scandalous pamphlet portrayed her metaphorically as on a vessel, the mariners a merciless crew, the captain's wife a pattern of evildoing, the vessel leaning toward Charybdis and already shattered by Scylla: "After having escaped from the teeth of one lord and master, she was induced, or rather the great justice of the gods impelled her to try her success with another. The sequel gave rise to the English proverb of the Frying Pan."[42]

In fact, Beauclerk, reported to have inherited nearly three thousand a year on the death of his mother in 1766, had to be bribed by the payment from Marlborough of a huge second dowry for his sister—perhaps £20,000—to marry Lady Di two days after the divorce. The triumphant lover, constrained by honor but unwilling to become the proprietor of soiled goods, made a brutal and abusive husband.[43] He was remarkably lice-ridden (one wonders if this constituted the same sort of punishment as Bolingbroke's venereal disease), and he was an opium addict. Public opinion has a potent effect on a husband, and it would appear that while an adulteress made a splendid mistress, she was an embarrassment as a wife. Lady Di no longer frequented the salons of fashionable women or went to public amusements where she might meet a rebuff. Beauclerk built an enormous addition to their house in Great Russell Street for a collection of thirty thousand books—"Everybody goes to see it," wrote Walpole. "It has put the Museum's nose quite out of joint" [33:136]. The Beauclerks mingled with such male wits as Walpole, Selwyn, and Garrick and with Marlborough and the Pembrokes, and they gave dinners to their intimates. Lady Di was too delightful for many of her loyal women friends—the duchess of Bedford, for instance—to give her up, but her position was always precarious.

Lady Di had rebelled against her first husband's infidelity by having affairs of her own, and she had rebelled against the venereal infection he had given her by leaving his house. She had behaved in an unwomanly, unsubmissive, and obstinate manner. Her punishment was a blasted reputation and an enforced marriage to a tyrannical second husband. Another tragic effect was the elopement abroad in 1789 of George, her son by Bully, with Mary, her daughter by Beauclerk.[44] But her last years, after her release from Beauclerk's abuse, were far better in quality than Bully's. Hers were spent in villas in Twickenham and Richmond among devoted friends, as an accomplished and celebrated painter. There is every evidence her spirit was unquenched, and she was quoted, on hearing that Lady Louisa Stuart was about to marry old Lord Strafford, as remarking, "Soh! . . . Lady L.S. is going to marry her great-grandfather, is she? If she can hold her nose, and swallow the dose at once, it may do very well. But most people would be apt to take a little sweetmeat in their mouths afterward."[45]

Her health appears to have been good, the lingering effects of her venereal infection, if any, not recorded. After several years of marriage to Beauclerk, at Christmas 1771 at Blenheim her life was given over "from a black vomit," but she recovered. At an unknown date, a Mrs. Ball at Bath cured her, probably of "the gallstone colic"—possibly the same disease [Walpole, 32:77, 15:270]. But she lived unimpaired in wit, presence of mind, and talent to the age of seventy-four. Beauclerk's health was far worse. He suffered from increasingly serious disorders, too difficult to diagnose from the evidence at hand, and he died at the age of forty-one. It is not unlikely that he perished, like Bully, from the effects of frequent bouts with venereal disease.

Bully's last years were spent in increasing dissoluteness, which was reflected, if faintly, in the public prints. Even in 1771 *Town and Country* displayed an edge to its jest in Bolingbroke's mock will: "To the unfortunate female patients in the Lock-hospital, many of whom I fear have entered there through the door of my seraglio, a quarter of a pound of tea each, to dilute the mercury in their stomachs" [October 1771, 530]. The 1772 Tête-à-Tête tells a lurid tale of his drugging and raping a virginal milliner lured to the suburbs with samples of her trade to the secluded villa of a procuress; like many similar victims of fashionable rakes, she had no recourse thereafter but to become his mistress.[46] In this case the magazine fails to exalt the nobleman's virtues and to excuse his gallantries as a sympathetic excess; though a certain prurience informs the account of the rape of the clergyman's daughter, Miss Vincent, the boys-will-be-boys tone falters. Still, Bully was not entirely without the pale. Nor of course did the child he begot on Miss Vincent figure in his disgrace—only in hers. At least, we are told, that "cloyed at length with variety, he found a disposition in his breast, with which he had been as yet unacquainted, *constancy*" [123]. And, probably, fatigue. It is not difficult to deduce that Bully had a vendetta against women.

Lady Di, chastened by the first opprobrium she had ever experienced and by the opposition that had bested her efforts to create her own decorums for the treatment of a wronged, adulterous wife whose sins in no way equalled those of her husband, lived a quiet, even edifying life after the divorce. By contrast, by the date of his divorce, Bully had lost all he had—including Di's fortune—at the gaming tables—£700 one night, £300 another[47]—and at the race course. Despite his quest for a rich wife to share his title and her fortune, he was unable after the divorce—now at the age of thirty-four—to engage one. His reputation as both husband and husbander of resources was no encouragement to marital prospects, and he continued to fulfill all dire predictions. In 1777, it was reported, he was still in quest of a fortune to marry, and he had fallen so low that when a creditor brought an action for debt and obtained judgment, before he could obtain execution, Bully had conveyed his estate away in an attempt to frustrate the law.[48] Whispers about him must have circulated, and not surprisingly in 1779 he was unable to convince a £43,000 fortune named Curtis of his eligibility.[49] Moreover, by June of that year he had left his senses, apparently permanently, from a "palsy in the brain."[50] In July Dr. John Warner noted that those who loved him grieved more for his frightful illness than for his imminent death.[51] By early February, Walpole reported, he was in a madhouse [25:11], where he remained, a victim of paresis, for the last seven years of his life.

The decorums of three of the discourses discussed here privilege male aristocratic sexual license. The discourses of the law available only to the rich and of upper-class social gossip both published and privately communicated naturally do so, and the fourth medical discourse at least does not controvert it. Thus, the bias of these discourses may differ from the moral, antiaristocratic, and sometimes antimonied class bias of the novel of the latter eighteenth century, discussed elsewhere in this volume by April London. Two social decorums that privilege aristocratic males can be seen at work in the manner in which the component parts of the Bolingbroke story have been selected and inflected for the record, one that women must remain submissive, the other that venereal disease must be casually regarded as a minor evil attendant on male prerogative and pleasure, to be endured, not extirpated. Both decorums, of course, contribute to or depend upon an increasingly powerful ideology about the differentiation of female sexuality from male, in fact, the suppression of sexuality in genteel women, and the insistence that genteel, proper women must be submissive and accepting of the wrongs done them by men. To mark the stern supremacy of this ideology, Lady Di had to be punished for her consistent eschewal of masochism.

These decorums about venereal disease also necessarily dovetail with the greater and overriding necessity of ideology—of which, of course, they are a part. As the disease was prevalent, and as males refused to give up their sexual promiscuity, women had to be taught to put up with "accidents" with the kind of forbearance displayed by Susannah Cibber, who actually hid the knowledge of the infection given to her by her husband "in hopes to reclaim him by generosity"—a point suggesting that a husband's embarrassment at having conveyed the disease to his wife might convert to mistreatment of her. Moreover, it was necessary that the disease be considered as trivial, curable, and as much a part of normal experience as possible, so what could be more convenient than the theory that even the pox could be easily nipped in the bud by early treatment? The denial at least in polite society of the separate evil of syphilis becomes almost a necessity, as does the denial of the evidence of its presence in its various victims, particularly in children. As a result of these prevailing decorums, Lady Di's reputation was permanently blasted in her own lifetime by her independent spirit and her "misconduct," and many of her indiscretions were laid open. But the history of Bolingbroke's (not to mention Beauclerk's) misuse of prerogative and privilege, his illness and end, though its components separately survive, has not been pieced together, to my knowledge, until now, and the components have not been the simplest of projects to gather. Many such stories cannot be established because bits are missing—the definitive diagnoses of friends, for instance—often from respect for the dead or the family. In the case of the Bolingbrokes, enough evidence exists to indict the establishment he represented, and which supported him, for an enormous misuse of prerogative and, in addition, for a criminal failure to recognize and control the effects of venereal infection.

Notes

1. In part the semiburied status of references to syphilis probably occasioned such reactions as that noted by an unnamed authority and sent to me in 1984 by Patricia Allderidge, archivist of the Bethlem Royal Hospital in Kent. He wrote, "Most people assert that disease wasn't described (and possibly not around, or at least not common at time) till c19, so there's no c18 literature on GPI."

2. In December 1745 the London bills listed 76 deaths from the French Pox as opposed to 14 from measles and 1,206 from smallpox; in December 1746 the same diseases were said to have carried off 100, 250, and 3,236. The bills for Northampton did not list venereal disease as a cause of death at all: *Gentleman's Magazine*, December 1745, 710; December 1746, 699. Deaths actually the consequence of venereal disease were often disguised, as Joseph Farington noted of the duke of Leeds and of Boswell as well: "The complaint which carried him off was, a mortification in the bladder, on which part, weakened by former injuries, a disorder which attacked him in another Shape ultimately resolved itself.—So it was with Boswell, the disorders in his constitution fell upon *those parts*, which happened to be the weakest": *The Farington Diary*, 8 vols. (London: Hutchinson, 1923-28), 1:267.

3. Alexander Pope, "The Second Satire of Dr. John Donne," 1. 47.

4. *Thraliana: The Diary of Mrs. Hester Lynch Thrale (Later Mrs. Piozzi), 1776-1809*, 2 vols., ed. Katharine C. Balderston (Oxford: Clarendon Press, 1942), 1:355.

5. For a discussion of references to venereal disease in eighteenth-century novels, drama, and satire, see the articles in this collection by April London, Rose Zimbardo, and Leon Guilhamet.

6. *Satan's Harvest Home, or The Present State of Whorecraft, Adultery, Fornication, Procuring, Pimping, Sodomy, And the Game at Flatts* . . . (London: for the editor, 1749), 31-32.

7. See for instance the *Morning Chronicle*, 1 August 1772. Rock's remedy was probably generally known to be ineffectual: *Town and Country Magazine* at this time referred to the fate of the clerk playing a macaroni (man of fashion) who would probably be compelled in a few weeks to apply to Dr. Rock, "who may ruin his constitution" (July 1772, 377).

8. Dr. William Rowley, *The Most Cogent Reasons why Astringent Injections, Caustic Boogies, and Violent Salivations Should be Banished for ever from Practice . . .* (London, 1800), 11.

9. For Chudleigh's infection by her husband see Augustus Hervey, *The Life and Memoirs of Elizabeth Chudleigh, Afterwards Mrs. Hervey and Countess of Bristol, Commonly Called Duchess of Kingtson* [sic] (Dublin: H. Chamberlaine et al., 1789), 11; for Susannah Cibber's infection by her husband, Theophilus Cibber, "which not withstanding she had the temper to conceal in hopes to reclaim him by generosity," see Mary Nash, *The Provoked Wife: The Life and Times of Susannah Cibber* (Boston: Little, Brown, 1977), 95-96, 101; for Lady Sandwich's infection by her profligate lord see *The Life, Adventures, Intrigues, and Amours of the Celebrated Jemmy Twitcher* (London: Jonathan Brough, 1770), 90; for Sarah Siddons's "P— given her by her Husband," see *Thraliana*, 2:850; for Lady Folkestone's infection by her lord, whose "wife's health suffered from his neglect & ill-treatment," see Farington, *Diary*, 5:160.

10. Farington, *Diary*, 1:267.

11. Quoted in Claude Quétel, *Le Mal de Naples: Histoire de la syphilis* (Paris: Seghers, 1986), translated as *The History of Syphilis*, trans. Judith Braddock and Brian Pike (Baltimore: Johns Hopkins Univ. Press, 1990), 89.

12. *The Complete Letters of Lady Mary Wortley Montagu*, ed. Robert Halsband (Oxford: Clarendon Press, 1965-67), 2:148n. 3; Horace Walpole, *The Yale Edition of Horace Walpole's Correspondence*, 48 vols. (New Haven: Yale Univ. Press, 1937-83), 22:551. Subsequent references to this work will be by volume and page number in the text.

13. *Letters of Sarah Byng Osborn, 1721-1773* (Stanford: Stanford Univ. Press, 1930), 121, 123; *The Granville Papers*, 4 vols., ed. William James Smith (New York: AMS, 1970), 4:9.

14. A card game that could be played by four, three, or two; also a thrust or shove: "to play at two-handed put" was a common euphemism for venery: J.S. Farmer and W.E. Henley, *Slang and Its Analogues* (New York: Arno Press, 1970), 333.

15. *Trials for Adultery, or The History of Divorces. Being Select Trials at Doctors Commons. . . . From the Year 1760, to the-present Time . . .*, 7 vols. (London: S. Bladon, 1779-80; reprint, New York: Garland, 1985), 2: 6th case. The page numbers of each case in a volume run consecutively from page 1.

16. *Trials for Adultery*, 3: 4th case.

17. *Trials for Adultery*, 4: 2d case.

18. Lawrence Stone, *Road to Divorce: England, 1530-1987* (Oxford: Oxford Univ. Press, 1990), 204.

19. For a discussion of Smart's madness see Arthur Sherbo, *Christopher Smart, Scholar of the University* (East Lansing: Michigan State Univ. Press, 1967), passim; *The Annotated Letters of Christopher Smart*, ed. Betty Rizzo and Robert Mahony (Carbondale: Southern Illinois Univ. Press, 1991), 56-68, 151-55; Betty Rizzo, "John Sherratt, Negociator," *Bulletin of Research in the Humanities* 86 (1983-85): 420-21.

20. "History of the Battersea Baron and Mrs. V———t," a Tête-à-Tête in the *Town and Country Magazine*, March 1772, 123.

21. *Correspondence of Emily, Duchess of Leinster*, 3 vols., ed. Brian Fitgerald (Dublin: Stationery Office, 1949-57), 1:49. His aunt, the countess of Guilford, also

noted her terror in 1756 lest Coventry should divorce his wife and Bully have to marry her (Walpole 9:203).

22. Walpole in 1765 so describes him (32:13).

23. For a thoughtful biography of Lady Di, see Mrs. Steuart Erskine, *Lady Diana Beauclerk, Her Life and Work* (London: T. Fisher Unwin, 1903).

24. "Since I am on the subject of scandle," wrote Lady Sarah Bunbury to her cousin Susan O'Brien in December 1764, "Lady Bolingbroke and Lord G—r go on as usual": *The Life and Letters of Lady Sarah Lennox,* ed. Countess of Ilchester and Lord Stavordale, 2 vols. (London: John Murray, 1901), 1:154.

25. Letter of Henry St. John to George Selwyn, *George Selwyn and His Contemporaries,* 4 vols., ed. John Heneage Jesse (London: Bickers, 1882), 2:80.

26. *Trials for Adultery,* 1: 6th case, 4.

27. James Boswell, *Boswell: The Ominous Years, 1774-1776,* ed. Charles Ryskamp and Frederick A. Pottle (New York: McGraw-Hill, 1963), 118.

28. BL Add. Ms. 52,389.

29. *The Life and Letters of Lady Sarah Lennox,* 1:182-83. Perhaps the woman was Nelly O'Brien, whose early death in 1768 suggests she may have had a venereal disease herself.

30. *George Selwyn and His Contemporaries,* 2:76, 62, 109. "Lady B." may have been the racketing Lady Sarah Lennox, now the wife of Sir Charles Bunbury and sister-in-law to the powerful Henry Fox.

31. *Trials for Adultery,* 1: 6th case, 82.

32. *The Letters and Journals of Lady Mary Coke,* 4 vols. (Edinburgh: D. Douglas, 1889-96), 2:126-27.

33. Historical Manuscripts Commission, 15th Report, Appendix Part VI, Vol. 42, *The Manuscripts of the Earl of Carlisle* (London: Her Majesty's Stationery Office, 1904), 222.

34. *The Letters and Journals of Lady Mary Coke,* 2:126-27.

35. *Letters to Henry Fox, Lord Holland,* ed. Earl of Ilchester (London: for the Roxburghe Club, 1915), 280. The same point is made in *George Selwyn and His Contemporaries,* 3:202, 247.

36. Joseph Phillimore, LL.D., *Reports of Cases Argued and Determined in the Arches and Prerogative Courts of Canterbury*... (Philadelphia: P.H. Nicklin and T. Johnson, 1835), 2:81.

37. *Trials for Adultery,* 1: 6th case, 112-13.

38. *George Selwyn and His Contemporaries,* 2:275.

39. *The Letters and Journals of Lady Mary Coke,* 2:127, 132, 158; Walpole, 30:250; *The Manuscripts of the Earl of Carlisle,* 226. At the same time Lord Pembroke, who had eloped from his wife with the daughter of a friend, by whom he had a child, and participated in other such adventures, was restored to his own bedchamber post *(George Selwyn and His Contemporaries,* 2:279).

40. James Boswell, *Boswell's Life of Johnson,* ed. George Birkbeck Hill and L.F. Powell, 6 vols. (Oxford: Clarendon Press, 1934), 2:247; *The Letters of Philip Dormer Stanhope, 4th Earl of Chesterfield,* ed. Bonamy Dobree, 6 vols. (London: Eyre and Spottiswoode, Ltd., 1932), 6:2713. In his essay "The Myth of Johnson's Misogyny: Some Addenda" (*South Central Review* 9.4 [Winter 1992]: 7-8), Donald Greene suggests the remark about Lady Di was possibly fabricated by Boswell, but it is conformable to the style of Johnson's situational declarations; as Greene points out, Johnson was thereafter fond and respectful of Lady Di. But he was also forthright in his description of (and subscription to) Christian standards, and he could distinguish nicely

between Christian and social decorums. In a conversation with Boswell in 1778 he exonerated Beauclerk *socially* but not morally: "As to this world vice does not hurt a man's character. . . . Who thinks the worse of —————— for it? . . . A man is chosen Knight of the shire, not the less for having debauched ladies" (*Boswell's Life of Johnson*, 3:349). Socially he had no quarrel with Lady Di either.

41. *Thraliana*, 1:46-47.

42. *The Picture Gallery. Containing Near Two Hundred Paintings by the Most Distinguished Ladies of Great Britain* (London: G. Kearsley, 1780), 13.

43. Farington, *Diary*, 1:66, where he remarks Beauclerk was the worst tempered man he ever knew. Conceivably Beauclerk too suffered from syphilis. In 1779 Walpole noted he thought both Lady Di's husbands had affections on the brain and, speaking of Bolingbroke's supposed impending death, he wrote, "It is a pity that one is not in as much danger as the other" (30:269). Beauclerk (1739-80) died at age 41.

44. Unpublished diary of Lady Mary Coke, entry for 28 June 1789 (photostats in W.S. Lewis Library, Farmington, Conn.).

45. *Lady Louisa Stuart: Selections from Her Manuscripts*, ed. Hon. James Home (New York: Harper and Brothers, 1899), 49.

46. The date of this escapade isn't established, but Bully's preservation from the law was dependent upon the ruined Miss Vincent's making the best of what had happened to her by settling down as his mistress. In 1768 Lord Baltimore was tried on a charge of a similar abduction and rape of a milliner named Sarah Woodcock who, after putting up a fight for several days, was finally overcome and when rescued turned ambivalent about returning home "ruined" to her father and fiancé. Nevertheless, Baltimore was nearly convicted and had to leave the country *(Gentleman's Magazine*, April 1768, 180-87).

47. In 1767 and 1768 Bully lost £700 at quinze at White's one night and £300 at Almack's another *(George Selwyn and His Contemporaries*, 2:165-66, 310). These losses were probably typical.

48. *The English Reports, Vol. 21 Chancery* (Edinburgh: William Green and Sons; London: Stevens and Sons, 1902), 1:377.

49. *George Selwyn and His Contemporaries*, 3:247.

50. Unpublished diary of Lady Mary Coke, entry for 10 July 1779; on 9 July 1779 Lord Pembroke described the illness in the same way (*Henry, Elizabeth, and George (1734-1780), Letters and Diaries of Henry, Tenth Earl of Pembroke and His Circle*, ed. Lord Herbert [London: Jonathan Cape, 1939], 202).

51. *George Selwyn and His Contemporaries*, 4:206.

Chapter 10

The Meaning of Venereal Disease in Hogarth's Graphic Art

N.F. Lowe

THE PAINTINGS AND ENGRAVINGS THAT WILLIAM HOGARTH CALLED HIS "modern moral subjects" were not intended to be pictorial sermons preaching simple messages about right and wrong. Ronald Paulson has argued convincingly that Hogarth's intention was to illustrate a conventional moral theme, beneath which he would then hide a deeper, more subversive reading. In this reading certain themes usually emerge, such as "the forces of society and fashion... against the natural impulses of the individual," a struggle in which Hogarth usually took the side of the natural.[1] For the same reason, Norman Bryson has called Hogarth "the great master of shifting textual levels." Bryson asserts that Hogarth achieved depth of meaning by moving between the moral message in the "official text" and the inversion of that message in the "unofficial text."[2] In this scheme of things, heroes can become villains, and villains victims, depending on which interpretation the onlooker has chosen to read.

In this essay, I will argue that Hogarth's depiction of venereal disease involves just such a complexity of moral meaning. In the official text, venereal disease is seen as one of the wages of sin. The individual chooses an immoral way of life, and the ravages of the disease follow from that choice. In the unofficial text, venereal disease is used as a symbol of a greater social corruption, and those inflicted with it are to be seen as pitiful victims of a cruel and exploitative element in society.

Hogarth's first pictorial series, *A Harlot's Progress*, uses the theme of venereal disease in both of these ways. George Vertue claimed the series, begun in 1731, developed from a single picture, the satirical study of a Drury Lane prostitute, awakening at about noon after a night's work.[3] This picture became the third in the series of six illustrations that make up the *Progress*. If the picture is studied as a single satirical portrait, it well serves to illustrate the complexities of Hogarth's thinking (Pl. 5). The conventional moral message is clearly illustrated. The seductive harlot may look contented, but she is about to reap the dreadful consequences of her immoral lifestyle. This moral message was an important one for Hogarth, rooted as it was in the Puritan ethic of the English middle class from which he proudly came. English artists in general and Hogarth in particular could not paint erotic scenes without inserting moral warnings about the consequences of uncontrolled sexual behavior. In this picture, retribution for the harlot's sins appears most obviously in the figure of Sir John Gonson, the magistrate, who is leading in his constables to arrest her for prostitution. It also lurks, less obviously, in the allusions to venereal disease hidden within the picture. Above the picture of Dr. Henry Sacheverell are two vials, suggesting she is trying to cure herself of venereal disease. In addition, the maid who is pouring her tea is in an advanced stage of syphilis. Her nose is eaten away, and the outsize beauty spot suggests a complexion blemished by the disease. These are clues to the ultimate fate of the harlot, who is facing degradation and early death because of her uncontrolled sexual conduct.

Hogarth used this simple moral message to satirize the fashionable French craze for paintings filled with hidden sexual allusions. These erotic paintings often depicted a woman in her bedroom, captured while at some highly personal activity. At a superficial level, the paintings were voyeuristic intrusions into the female boudoir, titillating but innocent. At another level, however, the paintings were filled with erotic intent. The bedrooms would have a *beau désordre*, where the apparently untidy contents would contribute to the artistic meaning of the painting, and in this disorder, the astute observer could read erotic themes that denied the apparent innocence of the scene. In this way, the artist could lead the spectator to imagine scenarios that could not be depicted with decorum.

A good example of what Hogarth was satirizing is Watteau's *La Toilette du Matin*, painted in about 1717 (Pl. 1). During the thirties and forties, the craze for Watteau and his style of French painting was increasing in England. Hogarth had admired this style fifteen years before the fashion reached its height in 1745. Watteau here captures a woman at the moment of rising. She is virtually naked and, with the help of her maid, is beginning her morning ablution in a totally unselfconscious way. Watteau, however, has provided clues to stimulate the erotic imagination of the observer. The disorder of the bed and the cupid's bow motif on the headboard leave no doubt that her washing follows a night of lovemaking. Watteau, however, makes no moral comment: the painting is simply a moment of intrusion into the personal life of the young woman that the onlooker, as voyeur, is allowed to enjoy. Hogarth ostensibly does the same thing in the bedroom scene of *A Harlot's Progress,* but the *beau désordre* conceals a message not of erotic intent but of moral and physical decay.

Another painting of the sort that Hogarth was satirizing is François Boucher's *La Toilette,* painted in 1742 (Pl. 2). In this boudoir scene, Boucher depicts a woman tying a garter onto her leg as she prepares for her evening out on the town. Her fresh face and pure expression dominate the initial impression made by the painting: the artist has apparently captured an innocent young woman at a moment of personal intimacy. In the *beau désordre* around her, however, there are numerous allusions to her real intent. The cat between her legs was a traditional symbol of sexual receptivity.[4] The word *chat* in French has the same double meaning as the word *pussy* in English. In the hearth we see a pair of tongs with an oddly phallic protuberance where the two "legs" of the tongs meet. Birds fill the picture: several on a screen behind her, one on the mantelpiece, and one on the fire brush in front of her. Birds signified male genitals, so this ornithological theme in her room instantly lends itself to a prurient interpretation of what is going on. Behind the screen hangs a portrait of a woman with a flower in her hair. She seems to be peeping over the screen, an innocent pastoral shepherdess observing the preparations of an urban temptress. When these clues are read, her posture, with her legs apart and a thigh exposed, takes on a different meaning. She is not an innocent caught in a moment of innocent *déshabillé:* she is a worldly woman planning a night of lovemaking. Like Watteau, Boucher makes no moral statement about the woman. The main purpose of these French paintings was simply to delight the onlooker by exciting his erotic imagination through a superficially innocent picture. The moment of unintentional *déshabillé* combines with the portents of sexual gratification to provide a picture charged with eroticism, a scene to be viewed, interpreted, and enjoyed by those clever and worldly enough to read the clues.

In the third picture of *A Harlot's Progress,* Hogarth adopts these conventions in order to undermine the hidden eroticism by combining it with allusions to the dangers of uncontrolled sexuality. Hogarth, in the French manner, captures the harlot, Moll Hackabout, at a moment of *déshabillé,* with her breast exposed, but the effect is not unintentional and innocent. She is portrayed looking cheekily at the onlooker, careless of her state of undress. The stolen watch she is gloating over reveals her amoral attitude toward life. Like the woman in Boucher's *La Toilette,* she also has a cat at her feet. However, her cat adopts a blatantly sexually receptive pose, suggesting nothing innocent about the sexuality of its owner. The more the disorder of the bedroom is examined, the more the theme of moral condemnation and punishment emerges. There is a birch cane above her bed. Next to the picture of Macheath is a portrait of Henry Sacheverell, who was put on trial for attacking the Revolution Settlement. The title of the sermon that led to his impeachment was "In perils among false brethren," a text highly pertinent to Moll's life in London and which is easily adapted to the deeper underlying reading of this series. In this context, the two vials to cure her venereal disease are ominous tokens of the horrible fate ahead of her.

In the fourth engraving, the Bridewell scene (Pl. 6), Hogarth cleverly reverses all the conventions of these French erotic paintings. Instead of the convention of showing a pretty courtesan dressing while her maid works or attends her, Hogarth depicts Moll Hackabout at work beating hemp while her maid is dressing. As in Boucher's picture, the woman is putting on a garter. However, the maid's ragged clothes, the hole in her stocking, and her ravaged syphilitic appearance make her anything but seductive. The glimpse of thigh is not erotic but grossly physical, especially as she is portrayed next to a woman crushing a flea between her thumb and forefinger.

This official text condemns the harlot's sexual immorality. The unofficial text, however, allows the onlooker to see her with some sympathy. This reading, which depicts the harlot as a victim, is explicit in the first picture of the series (Pl. 3). Moll Hackabout is portrayed as an innocent and naive young woman. Hogarth cleverly makes her resemble the dead goose she has brought down to London for her "Lofing Cosin." She is about to become an offering to the predators who are laying a trap for her. The disorder around this innocent, whose virgin state is symbolized by the hat firmly fixed to her head, is filled with allusions to the moral corruption and depraved sexuality of the society she has entered. Here, Hogarth is playing most mischievously with the conventions of French erotic painting. He surrounds the innocent young woman with clues to her impending loss of virginity, but the intention is not erotic titillation. Hogarth pointedly condemns the society that preys on young women. In the official text, Moll is turning her back on religion. In the unofficial text, religion is ignoring the plight of Moll and the other women like her. The clergyman is totally preoccupied with the address of the Right Reverend Father in London who will help to advance his career. He ignores the women newly arrived from York, even though they are innocents in need of protection. Their fate is symbolized by the pile of pots falling over nearby, which the clergyman also ignores. Pots, baskets, and hats were allusions to female genitalia, and falling or broken pots symbolized lost virginity, so Hogarth is depicting the clergy as indifferent to the way people are exploited all around them by a corrupt society.

Venereal disease emerges as a theme in the face of the bawd, recognizable as the notorious Elizabeth Needham, who ran a brothel for the aristocracy. The beauty spots on her face are pockmarks rather than a cosmetic affectation. While Mother Needham is seducing Moll into her brothel, Colonel Charteris, the infamous rapist, lurks in the background. He stands with his servant, Jack Gourly, in the doorway, fondling himself in anticipation of another victim. Charteris was wealthy and had escaped punishment for his crimes by using his social power. For Hogarth, he represents the evil that corrupts the innocent, and it is this evil, symbolized by venereal disease, which eventually infects and kills Moll.

In the fifth picture, Hogarth depicts her death at the age of twenty-three. She again resembles the dead goose in the first picture. The venereal disease that killed her may be retribution for her sin, but Hogarth, on the second level, again portrays her as a pathetic victim. She is being robbed of her few last possessions by an unknown woman, but the real villains are the two doctors, Dr Richard Rock and Dr Jean Misaubin, who have taken all her money in return for their useless quack remedies.

The *Marriage à la Mode* series is an extended illustration of venereal disease as a direct consequence of the social corruption created by the idle and extravagant aristocracy. Hogarth could be illustrating the following quotation from Jonathan Swift: "That, our young *Noblemen* are bred from their Childhood in Idleness and Luxury, that, as soon as Years will permit, they consume their Vigour, and contract odious Diseases among lewd females; and when their Fortunes are almost ruined, they marry some Woman of mean Birth, disagreeable Person, and unsound Constitution, merely for the sake of Money, whom they hate and despise. That, the Productions of such Marriages are generally scrophulous, rickety, or deformed Children; by which means the family seldom continues above three Generations."[5]

In the eighteenth century, venereal disorders were popularly known as the "alamode disease." In 1732, Daniel Turner wrote in his book on syphilis, "As to what relates to the Cure of this *first Injection* [sic] or *French Disease*, (which whether theirs or not, has one of its Epithets, *Alamode*, thence borrowed)."[6] A German treatise on venereal disease by Lewis Wilhelm de Knorr, published in 1717, was called *Venus à la mode*. The term *alamode disease* was common enough to appear in advertisements for cures of venereal disease,[7] so the very title *Marriage à la Mode* would have led the eighteenth-century observer to look for venereal disease as a theme. With this secret disease as his topic, it is not surprising that Hogarth should assert, in the advertisement he placed on 2 April 1743 in the *London Daily Post and General Advertiser*, "Particular Care will be taken that there may not be the least objection to the Decency or Elegancy of the whole work." Given the indelicate subject to be illustrated, he needed to point out that it would be handled with extreme delicacy and refinement. The observer was being alerted, however, to an encoded theme that would be hidden from innocent eyes.

The first picture in the series contains numerous clues to the fact that the earl and his issue are being ravaged by the disease (Pl. 7). Lord Squanderfield is obviously crippled by gout. One cause of gout was held to be syphilis, which was known in England as French gout. Jean Astruc explains, "The three Humours which are prepared by Nature to facilitate the Motion of the Joints, give easy Admittance to the Venereal Infection."[8] He goes on to explain that the "mucilaginous Glands" become enlarged, and the circulation of the blood obstructed, so that "an arthritic Pain is produced, attended with Tension, and Pulsation, Heat, Redness and Inflammation of the Joint" [2:16]. Squanderfield's bandaged foot, therefore, signals more than excess of certain foods and drink. It indicates advanced venereal disease, and his very prominent crutches, which carry his crest to show they are part of his regular way of life, signal the extent to which his health is crippled.

To make his point even more explicit, Hogarth surrounds the earl with numerous symbols and indicators of the venereal infection. The earl is pointing to the top of his family tree, which is less vigorous near the top, and which oddly grows from the stomach of his ancestor, the duke of Normandy, suggesting the entire family line is rooted in greed and excess and is dying off, like the branch that is dead and falling from the tree.

The large painting by the window is a portrait of the earl as a young man. He is depicted as Jupiter, but he holds a ridiculously small thunderbolt in his hand. From the region of his groin, a cannon emerges, firing a peculiarly small cannonball, significantly about the same size as the round mark on his son's neck. If there is doubt that this cannon is meant to be a phallic symbol, firing inadequate ammunition, another clue reiterates the message. The earl is staring at a portrait of Medusa. Athena changed Medusa's hair into serpents, and as a result all who looked on her turned to stone. After Perseus beheaded Medusa, Athena placed her likeness in the center of her shield or breastplate. She was a virgin divinity whose heart was inaccessible to the passion of love. The fact that Medusa now stares out from the center of the earl's wall, not from the breastplate of Athena, suggests the family is also impervious to love.

Athena was the daughter of Jupiter, who symbolized power, and Metis, who symbolized wisdom, and so she was the harmonious blend of both qualities. It was Athena who gave the state strength and prosperity. The lonely earl, the Jupiter figure in the portrait, has lost his wife. He is Jupiter without Metis, power without wisdom. He is, however, a sickly figure whose power is in rapid decline because of excess and sickness. Hogarth leads the observer to conclude that the earl has lived a life without love and that his excesses have left him and his sperm (the puny cannonball) enfeebled. His gout shows the debilitation caused by sexual dissipation, and his scrawny son reveals a further decline in the strength of the line.

The prominent mark on the viscount's neck also indicates the taint of venereal disease. Robert Cowley, in his book on the *Marriage à la Mode* series, describes the beauty spot as "a large plaster on his neck." He goes on to explain:

> Scrofula attacks the lymphatic glands of the neck as a consequence of the malnutrition of the tissues which then become

vulnerable to the spread of tuberculosis carried in the infected milk. The disease also attacks the nerves of the eyes (as Dr. Johnson knew to his cost), a weakness which could conceivably lie behind the Viscount's fatal lack of perception. Scrofula was a baffling evil in the eighteenth century. Subscribers would have seen the son's sore as an inheritance of the father's excesses and many would have interpreted it as a sign of congenital venereal disease.[9]

Of the viscount's child in the sixth picture (Pl. 10) Cowley comments:

> The boy has a sore on his cheek, a depressed forehead, blubber lips, an enlarged head, a weak leg and a stunted body. The weakness would be a sign of rickets or, more probably, tubercular osteitis caused, like his father's scrofula, by infected milk. The patch is not directly over the child's lymphatic glands so that it may have been meant as a symptom of a congenital disease rather than a scrofula. A depressed forehead can also be a symptom of either rickets or a congenital defect.... The symptoms are consistent with each other and a range of common disabilities which contemporaries were likely to regard as inherited "sins" and this must be Hogarth's essential point. [150]

Cowley could have been more explicit. Two works by Jean Astruc, whose influential work on venereal disease was first translated into English in 1737, make it quite clear that Hogarth was portraying venereal disease in both Viscount Squanderfield and his child. In his discussion of the "pocky degenerative virus," Astruc notes that some authors claim that the "*lues venera,*" or French pox, "ill cured in the father may degenerate into the rickets in the son."[10]

The viscount's beauty spot is a "Venereal bubo, or tumour" of the lymphatic gland. Astruc points out that "Venereal Buboes" are caused by an "old Venereal Taint," or a "Venereal Infection just admitted." The gland affected is determined by the laws of circulation. Apart from the neck, armpits, and groin, he specifically cites "the side of the lower jaw," the location of the black spot on the child (1:338).

The location of the black spot on the child's cheek in Hogarth's picture is not random but exactly placed over the salivary gland. Astruc's reasoning would lead to a diagnosis of a venereal bubo developed from sucking. The advanced age of his nurse would suggest that the infected milk would have come from the mother. As Steele's essay [*Spectator,* no. 246] implies, the practice of the mother breast-feeding her own child was being recommended to protect the child from the Evil, scurvy, and other infections, so the irony of this child being doubly infected by the parents may well be Hogarth's intention, for it is also clear that the child was born with syphilis.

The rickets, which Cowley suggests might be tubercular osteitis, was also strongly linked to congenital syphilis in the eighteenth century and long after. Astruc asserts that syphilitic mothers bring "puny, broken-backed, large headed, crooked, bandy-legged, variously distorted, and thick jointed" children into the world [2:37].

The argument whether rickets and syphilis were linked continued throughout the nineteenth century and has even surfaced recently. For example, J. Parrot, a pioneer radiologist, argued in 1886 that syphilis affects every bone of the infant skeleton and that rickets was a later lesion of congenital syphilis.[11] As recently as 1969, Robinson revived the argument by suggesting that the absence of bossing in the cranium was due to unrecognized rickets.[12]

There is good reason for this controversy. Congenital syphilis, like rickets, leads to craniofacial malformations that include a high cranium or "tower skull," sloping skulls, beetled brows, and collapsed saddle nose deformities. Involvement of adjacent structures can also lead to a short maxilla and a high palatal arch. The result is a face with a "dished out look." The tibia suffers anterior bowing because of periostitis of the long bones, and the teeth are affected in terms of structure, size, and enamelization, which Murphy and Patamasucon conclude "undoubtedly contributed to the historical confusion of the disease with rickets."[13]

It is quite clear, then, that Hogarth was depicting in the child an accurate picture of congenital syphilis. The child is the center point of the final picture, clinging pitifully to its dead mother. It is a moving illustration of Swift's remark that "the Productions of such Marriages are generally scrophulous, rickety, or deformed Children; by which means the family seldom continues above three Generations."

There are two other children blighted by congenital disease in Hogarth. The first of these is Moll Hackabout's son, who appears in the fifth and sixth pictures of *A Harlot's Progress*. Though he is sturdy in comparison to Viscount Squanderfield's son, his domed forehead and uncomprehending manner suggest he has not escaped the consequences of his mother's way of life. The second is the young boy in the illustration for *Evening* (Pl. 14) in the *Four Times of the Day*. In his book *Hogarth and the Times-of-the-Day Tradition*, Shesgreen notes that "he carries empty symbols of male supremacy in the ironically phallic cane and the gingerbread king, changed from a cookie in the painting to underline the picture's theme of male impotence."[14] However, his weak little legs and domed head suggest that the cause of his impotence is venereal disease, the result of his mother's adultery.

The second picture of the *Marriage à la Mode* portrays Viscount Squanderfield as a handsome and bored young man, and his wife is depicted at her nubile best (Pl. 8). Hogarth, however, provides several clues to the venereal disease attacking them both within.

The Viscount's pose, as Cowley points out, "was a well known metaphor of sexual intercourse in the sixteenth and seventeenth centuries" [58]. The pose implies sexual exhaustion, but the broken sword gives a different message. It has been broken without being drawn, a symbol of the owner's impotence. Again the black mark on his neck links his state to venereal disease. A further clue is above him on the mantelpiece. In the center is a Roman bust with a broken nose. Astruc wrote in his book on venereal disease, "The Mucus of the Nose is affected in the same way . . . from hence the whole Arch of the Nose being destroyed, and the Bridge of it falling in, those who before had an aquiline Nose become flatfaced like an ape" (2:14). The statue looks like the bust of a syphilitic and hints at the syphilis eating away at the couple below. Behind this statue is a painting of a cherub playing the bagpipes, a traditional symbol of discord and again intended to comment on the atmosphere in the Squanderfield household.

In his pocket, Squanderfield has stuffed his mistress's bonnet, and the family dog is sniffing at it. This is a delightful use by Hogarth of one of the conventions of French erotic paintings. Dogs were the traditional symbol of fidelity, but dogs were also used to suggest sexual excitement. A frisky dog alongside languid lovers was frequently used to suggest the hidden sexual arousal and tension. Here, Hogarth depicts such an excitable little dog, but its excitement comes from its discovery of the illicit mistress's bonnet, itself a symbol of female genitalia. It is a tableau depicting fidelity gone wrong. It is a fine example of how Hogarth can gain additional effect by playing around with standard images.

Lady Squanderfield's pose, with her knees apart and her stays revealed, conveys her increasing sensuality and immodesty. The pocket mirror she holds above her head looks like a halo which has slipped and which she is removing. A red mark on her lip is possibly the first hint of a venereal sore.

This scene is Hogarth at his artistic and satirical best. The profligate ways of the aristocracy, their poor taste, and their sexual indulgence are all satirized. In the disorder of the room, we witness the debt, disease, and confusion that this way of life has brought about. In Lady Squanderfield, we see the portrait of a fallen woman, reveling in all the vices that come with the aristocratic way of life, and we also see the first hint of venereal disease, which she has acquired from the same source.

The third picture in the series reiterates how the aristocracy are a source of degeneracy and disease. In a room full of the images of illness and death, Viscount Squanderfield is set apart. He alone is seated, and he alone has a carefree and grinning face (Pl. 9). The pill box he is holding out to the quack, with the lid significantly near his groin, are clearly useless remedies for venereal disease. Given his long history of infection, with the disease being passed to him at conception by his father, it is not unlikely that the pills were a quack remedy to prevent reinfection and transmission. Astruc attacked all such methods of prevention, as they not only did not work but also led people to risk the dangerous effects of promiscuous sex. "Once," he wrote, "the Fear of Infection by which Men are restrained from Intemperance, is removed, then the Reins of Lust will be let loose" [1:283].

In this case the aristocrat has infected the whore. The young girl, possibly procured for him because she was a virgin, is dabbing at a syphilitic sore on her lip. The implication is that the viscount has infected her in the same way he has infected his wife.

The viscount is threatening the quack, though not very seriously. He would seem to be blaming the inefficacy of the medication for causing the infection of the young girl, rather than his own degeneracy. Cowley points out that the tall woman is holding "a folding scalpel or bistoury," but suggests there is no evidence it was intended for surgery. In fact, textbooks abound with references to surgery for venereal disease. Turner, an English doctor, in his book on syphilis, wrote, "These accidents being likewise attended at some times with great Fluxion and Inflammation, as appears by the feverish Disorder with which they are affected, it is requisite at such times . . . to empty their veins by bleeding" [256]. There is a brass shaving and bleeding dish available on the top of the glass cabinet, so such a procedure is part of Dr Misaubin's repertoire. Given that both the doctor and the tall lady are annoyed by the attitude and antics of the viscount, and the young girl is clearly ill and distressed, it is likely that they realize how severely she has been infected, and the scalpel may suggest drastic procedures are envisaged. The tall woman may be annoyed because the viscount seems to see it all as a joke.

Cowley concludes that the tall woman is angry because of the "insinuation that the common miss, presumably sold to her patron as a virgin, gave the viscount the disease which the doctor's pills fail to cure" [87]. It makes better sense, given what we know of Viscount Squanderfield, to see him as the source of contagion. He is the cause of the corruption of the young woman's health and morals, just as his aristocratic taste for luxury and indolence have corrupted his wife and left her infected with the same disease.

Luke Sullivan explained the mark on the tall woman's chest as a brand marking her as a convicted prostitute. Cowley reads them as "FC" for female convict or criminal, and he compares her to Mrs Needham in the first picture of *A Harlot's Progress*. I have suggested in an earlier article that Hogarth frequently used beauty spots as an emblem of venereal infection.[15] Beauty spots were, of course, a fashion in the eighteenth century. In *Spectator*, no. 50, Addison poked fun at the way women changed their spots: "The women look like Angels, and would be more beautiful than the Sun, were it not for little black

Spots that are apt to break out on their Faces, and sometimes rise in very odd Figures. I have observed that these little Blemishes wear off very soon; but when they disappear in one Part of the Face, they are very apt to break out in another, insomuch that I have seen a Spot upon the forehead in the Afternoon, which was upon the Chin in the Morning."

Now these "little blemishes" are nothing to do with the loosely disguised sores that Hogarth sometimes depicts. Again, contemporary medical texts give clues as to what Hogarth is doing. Turner describes the face of one young woman suffering from venereal disease as follows: "A Gentlewoman six Months gone with Child, most part of that time incommoded with *Tubercles* on several parts of her face, a *Serpigo* on the chin, with two or three others upon the Cheek and side of her Nose, giving her great Uneasiness by the Trouble, as also disfiguring her countenance, sent for me to give Directions to her Surgeon" [256]. A few pages later, he describes "a Gentleman having a small Pustule broke out above his Eyebrow, and in Company with the Surgeon belonging to his Family, desir'd a Patch, who accordingly applied a Bit of Common Plaister upon black Silk" [271]. The pustule turned out to be a venereal sore.

Several Hogarth characters acquire beauty spots that may signal the secret disease. The most obvious ones are the prostitutes in the third painting, the Tavern scene, in *A Rake's Progress*. Six women have large black spots. The one stealing Tom's watch has two large spots on her cheek and a large spot and a small spot on her forehead above her nose. The woman behind Tom has four large spots, which tend to dominate her face rather than draw attention to her better features, and the three women at the table also have prominent facial marks. In the front left of the picture, Hogarth again uses the style of French erotic painting for satirical purposes in portraying "the posture woman," who is preparing for her performance (Pl. 11). She is in the pose of the women in French boudoir paintings, like the one by Boucher discussed above. She is putting on her shoe and seems unaware of her exposed breast. Unlike the woman in Boucher's painting, however, she looks the reverse of innocently erotic. Her tired and bored expression suggests fatigue rather than sexual excitement, and the large beauty spot on her forehead is unsightly enough to have a venereal connotation. At her feet is a chicken, the remains of their late night feast. A dead bird was a conventional symbol for lost virginity, just as a living bird was a symbol of male sexuality. This bird, however, is anything but a virile and fertile emblem of male sexuality. It is a dead carcass stabbed through the abdomen with a fork. The pregnant woman in rags behind her, singing bawdy songs, is another portent of the fate that lies ahead of the prostitute who has lost her marketable value.

Similarly, the woman lying in a faint in the engraving called *Enthusiasm Delineated* has two huge black marks on her cheek. This woman has been identified as Mother Douglas, a notorious bawd from Covent Garden, so both these women of ill repute are marked out in the same way. It is possible that Hogarth is simply illustrating the tasteless makeup of lewd women, but a comparison between these outsize spots and the cosmetic beauty spots discreetly decorating the actresses in the print *Strolling Actresses in a Barn* suggests Hogarth intends a deliberate ambiguity.

At least two kinds of plaster could be taken for beauty spots. One kind was a patch of material with an adhesive substance that was placed over a sore to hold a curative unction in place. Turner described one such plaster using black silk. Hogarth sometimes draws these as rectangular to denote that they are plasters. There is one below Tom's right nipple in the final scene of *A Rake's Progress* (Pl. 12), and the man sprawling in the foreground of *A Midnight Modern Conversation* wears two geometric plasters on his head. The other plaster was formed by adding wax to the unction to give it "a due consistence," and this wax patch would hold the curing agent, normally mercury for the pox, over the sore. Mercury was mixed with turpentine in a mortar until a brown or black powder was obtained, which was then mixed with hog's lard until the ointment was of the right consistency. Wax replaced some of the lard for a plaster, and when applied to the sore it could resemble a beauty spot.

The woman walking through Covent Garden in *Morning*, the first of the *Four Times of Day* series, is an interesting example of this ambiguity. She has two spots above and two below her left eye (Pl. 13). Shesgreen suggests that her prudish exterior masks her real intent, which is a clandestine sexual assignation in the church.[16] There are other clues to suggest she is not as respectable as she seems. Just behind her is an advertisement for a cure by Dr Rock, who made his money by selling useless cures for venereal disease. He appeared in Plate V of *A Harlot's Progress*. In a literal sense, the woman has a venereal cure behind her, so Hogarth may wish the observer to draw the obvious conclusion. The beauty spots on her face might hide a darker secret. The woman begging in front of her is also enigmatic. David Dabydeen thinks she represents a crouching black beggarwoman. "Shivering in the cold," he writes, "and wrapped from head to toe in an old blanket, she is far removed from her reputed nakedness in the tropical climate of Africa." Dabydeen points out that this black woman is paired off from her white social superior for satirical purposes. One eighteenth-century convention used blacks to illustrate the two extremes of existence, "the black representing obscenity and paganism, the middle-class white representing civilized religion, moral rectitude and so forth."[17] The black woman's nose, however, is markedly collapsed, so she might be a prostitute reduced to begging and ravaged by venereal disease. The white woman, as Dabydeen asserts, is a portrait of fraudulent piety because of her indifference to the cry for charity. Everything about her is fraudulent. She represents Aurora, the personification of the birth of the day, who had come to be associated with youth and fertility. Hogarth's Aurora is an aging figure pretending to be young, whose bony flat chest suggests anything but fertility. She is going to the church, but her lack of concern for the freezing page carrying her prayerbook and her lack of charity for the beggar suggest she is not a real Christian. If she has been treated for venereal disease and is off to a sexual tryst in the church, then her apparent respectability hides a profounder obscenity than is to be seen in the pitiful black. The only real difference between these two women may well be the poverty of the black woman, who cannot mask her state behind a hypocritical exterior.

Hogarth, then, can use beauty spots as a sexual allusion. At times they signal prurience, and at other times they are an emblem of venereal disease. The tall woman in the third scene of the *Marriage à la Mode* series may be such a character. Most commentators take her to be a procuress, an ex-prostitute tainted and branded by the profession.

In the glass case, a skeleton is propped against an anatomical model so that it appears to be sexually groping the model while whispering in its ear. Cowley points out that this tableau offers "a precise and extensive comment on the central situation," but he reads it as a symbol of the viscount's experiencing "the first caress of contagious death" [93]. Death, in the form of venereal disease, has kissed three of the main characters, and the skull of a victim of the contagion on Dr Misaubin's table signifies how he lives off these deaths. The skull, incidentally, is marked with black spots. Cowley takes these to be holes in the skull, which has been eroded by syphilis [91].

As it happens, Viscount Squanderfield is killed by his wife's lover before syphilis can complete the task. The lover is executed, and his wife commits suicide, but the dance of death continues as his sickly child will be the last of the line. A skeletonlike dog apparently whispering into a dead pig's ear is a clever reworking of the skeleton in the closet in the third scene. The pig's head, with its gaping mouth, also resembles the expression on the face of the dead Lady Squanderfield, who is being embraced by the pitiful child, who is also kissed by death (Pl. 10). As Swift wrote in the passage quoted above, "the family seldom continues above three Generations."

Ronald Paulson believes that Hogarth's sympathies are always on the side of the common people. He attacked the luxury of the aristocracy and the decadence of the social institutions that maintained them. While he attacked the middle classes for aspiring to emulate and enter into the aristocracy, he admired the tradition of hard work and clean living that existed in the trading classes of Protestant England. Moll Hackabout, the innocent young girl who comes to London as a dressmaker, fell because she tried to acquire wealth without work. The same is true of Lady Squanderfield, who is made wealthy by the hard work of her alderman father but who becomes corrupted by the aristocratic way of life. They both acquire venereal disease from the higher classes, whose idle decadence is the source of their downfall.

Tom Rakewell in *The Rake's Progress* also uses his father's accumulated wealth in dissipation, but in the eighth picture, the Bedlam scene (Pl. 12), it is not venereal disease that has destroyed his mind. The connection between syphilis and mental illness was not discovered until the nineteenth century. In the eighteenth century, madness and sex were linked because of excessive stimulation of the brain. In his 1758 *Treatise on Madness*, William Battie proposed that the nervous system and its connection to the brain at the medulla caused "laxity in the overloaded vessels." He cites "many instances of madness occasioned by praemature, excessive or unnatural venery, by Gonorhoeas ill cured with loads of mercury and irritating salts, by fevers and such like convulsive tumults."[18] Overloading the nerves and medullary substances could also be caused by the endless thinking of "infirm and shattered philosophers" and by gluttony and idleness. The latter causes madness by failing to give "due propulsion of the fluids" and adequate stimulation to the nervous system. Tom, then, goes mad because of overindulgence and consequential overstimulation of the brain and its nervous system. His fine physique in the picture contrasts with his diseased and disordered mind. His head has been shaved to cool the brain and relieve the pressure caused by this overstimulation, but he remains raving mad.

In conclusion, Hogarth, in his representations of the manners and morals of English society, used allusions to venereal disease to make a satirical attack on various forms of decadence and immorality. At the simplest level, he used it as a warning against unrestrained sexual behaviour. He vividly depicted the disease as the terrible consequence of promiscuity. At a deeper level, Hogarth used venereal disease as a symbol of a wider social corruption in society, presided over by an idle and profligate aristocracy who, in satisfying their excesses, exploited and corrupted poor and innocent people in the process. Finally, Hogarth used venereal disease to satirize the French fashion for erotic paintings, which used partially clad females and suggestive nudes to advocate the delights of uncontrolled sexual indulgence. In Hogarth's system of morality, fashionable trends of questionable taste received as much censure as immoral conduct. Both offend against decency, and Hogarth attacked them relentlessly throughout his life.

Notes

1. Ronald Paulson, *Hogarth: His Life, Art and Times*, 2 vols. (New Haven: Yale Univ. Press, 1971). See esp. 1:474-75.

2. Norman Bryson, *Word and Image: French Painting of the Ancien Régime* (Cambridge: Cambridge Univ. Press, 1981), 148-49.

3. George Vertue, *Notebooks*, 6 vols. (Oxford: Walpole Society, 1934-55), 3:58.

4. For a full discussion of these sexual allusions see Mary D. Sheriff, *Fragonard: Art and Eroticism* (Chicago: Univ. of Chicago Press, 1990).

5. Jonathan Swift, *Gulliver's Travels*, 2d ed., ed. Paul Turner (Oxford: Oxford Univ. Press, 1986), 261.

6. Daniel Turner, *Syphilis: A Practical Dissertation on Venereal Disease*, 4th ed. (London, 1732), 68.

7. British Library, *Collection of 185 Advertisements*, C112. f.9, 41. See also Roy Porter, *Health for Sale: Quackery in England, 1660-1850* (Manchester: Manchester Univ. Press, 1989), 150.

8. Jean Astruc, *A Treatise of Venereal Diseases*, rev. ed., 2 vols. (London, 1754), 2:15.

9. Robert L.S. Cowley, *Marriage à la Mode: A re-view of Hogarth's narrative art* (Manchester: Manchester Univ. Press, 1983), 39-40.

10. Jean Astruc, *A general and compleat Treatise on all the Diseases Incident to Children* (London, 1746), 216.

11. J. Parrot, *La syphilis herreditaire et la rachitis* (Paris, 1886).

12. R.C.V. Robinson, "Congenital Syphilis," *Archives of Dermatology* 99 (1969): 599.

13. F.K. Murphy and P. Patamasucon, "Congenital Syphilis," in *Sexually Transmitted Diseases*, ed. King K. Holmes, Mardh Per Anders, P.F. Sparling, and M.D. Wiesner (New York: McGraw-Hill, 1984), 352-74.

14. Sean Shesgreen, *Hogarth and the Times-of-the-Day Tradition* (Ithaca: Cornell Univ. Press, 1983), 113.

15. N.F. Lowe, "Hogarth, Beauty Spots, and Venereal Diseases," *British Journal for Eighteenth-Century Studies* 15 (Spring 1992): 71-79.

16. Shesgreen, *Hogarth*, 116.

17. David Dabydeen, *Hogarth's Blacks* (Manchester: Manchester Univ. Press, 1987), 121.

18. William Battie, *A Treatise on Madness* (London, 1758), 56.

Chapter 11

Satiric Representation of Venereal Disease

The Restoration versus the Eighteenth-Century Model

Rose A. Zimbardo

The Restoration period in England (1660-1700) is what the philosopher Hans Blumenberg calls a "zero point," a moment in cultural history when an epistemology is collapsing and simultaneously a new epistemology is arising: "the zero point of the dissolution of order and the point of departure of the construction of order."[1] For the Middle Ages and the Renaissance, the center of reality is the mysterious still center of the turning world: God. Each creature, like each planet, circles around that center in a ring of *caritas,* a cosmic *harmonia.* If any creature mistakes his own Self for the center, s\he is guilty of the sin of pride. On the other hand, for late-seventeenth-century/eighteenth-century modernism, the new epistemology in the process of construction at zero point, the *locus,* and the font of truth is the human Self. Moreover, from that cohesive unity emerge increasingly expanded enlargements of the human self: the nation, the empire, the world.

In the new eighteenth-century modernist coding, among the systems over which natural reason has control and for which it has responsibility is the physiological. To maintain a sound "constitution" (i.e., "the inner stock of vitality and strength, the vigor that flowed when all one's organs worked effectively together") it was deemed "vital to order each department of life—clothing, environment, the ensemble of activities making up the day, and so on—in the light of their health implications, so that each element should be beneficial, and the whole would provide a balanced and varied economy of living. . . . Each individual had the power . . . to further healthy living—or equally to jeopardize it."[2] Moreover, since "nation" is an enlargement of the self, maintenance of one's individual "constitution" is directly related to maintenance of the British Constitution. Therefore, good health habits are a duty of citizenship and, conversely, to engage in irresponsible activity that is detrimental to one's health threatens not just one's own body but the body politic as well.

In the new eighteenth-century modernist epistemology, ordered and ordering human natural reason imposes order upon the body, the nation, the world. Consequently, to maintain one's constitution, to discriminate right living from dissolute, and therefore unhealthy, living, becomes one's political as well as one's moral responsibility.

When self becomes discursively central, satire becomes mimetic, morally emendatory, and binary. No longer an instrument for exploding the postures of pride and mocking the singular self's pretensions to sovereignty, the new modern satire becomes a careful delineator of boundaries, a nice weigher of moral judgments, and a sharp instrument for discriminating "right" from "wrong"—and also "us," the respectable, from "them": the rake, the harlot, the criminally irresponsible "others."

The new satire regulates and reforms its reader/viewers by its own cause-effect, linear designs, its clarity, its "reasonable" line of argumentation. Rationally ordered, it makes its reader/viewer rationally ordered. The new satire is prescriptive, and if its reader/viewer chooses not to follow the prescription, then she deserves to be sick. According to John Dryden, "They who endeavor not to correct themselves according to so exact a Model [as the new satire provides]; are just like Patients, who have open before them a Book of Admirable Receipts, for their Diseases, and please themselves with reading it, without Comprehending the Nature of the Remedies, or how to apply them to their Cure."[3] Discourse, and most particularly the discourse of satire, is a means by which the sovereign self, or natural reason, governs and regulates itself and its body.

Comparison between the representation of venereal disease in the dramatic satire of the Restoration period and the pictorial satire of the eighteenth century, when venereal disease could no longer be pictured on the morally reformed stage, can illuminate the radical epistemological transformation that occurred at Restoration "zero point." Generally speaking, in the transition from premodern (i.e., Restoration) to modern (i.e., eighteenth-century) coding, the discourse of venereal disease went from being public and comic to being private—indeed, secret—and serious, and the representation of venereal disease went from being semiotic—a sign of our common human frailty—to being empirical evidence of the personal immorality and social/political degeneracy of the marginalized "other." In the new discourse and coding of modernism, all health and illness involved a moral dimension. Venereal disease, of course, was particularly morally charged, an evil for which the individual subject was responsible.

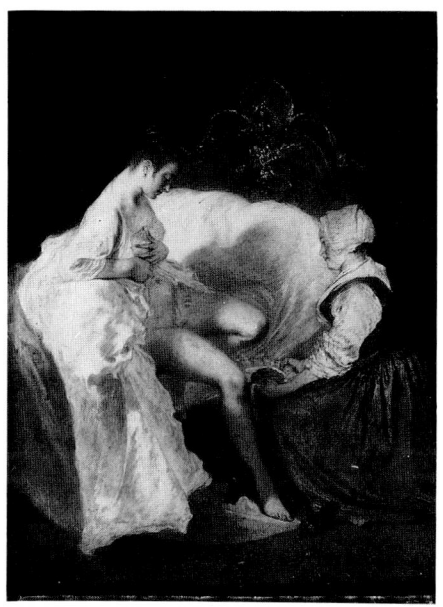

Plate 1. *Above,* Antoine Watteau, *La toilette du matin* (The Morning Toilet), c. 1715. Watteau's version of the female bedroom is elegant, sensual, and tasteful. Private collection (Bulloz, Paris). **Plate 2.** *Below,* François Boucher, *La toilette,* 1742. Oil on canvas, 52.5 x 66.5 cm. Boucher's bedroom scene seems innocent enough, but the erotic intent of the young woman is manifest from the symbolism in the *beau désordre* of the room. Copyright © Fundacion Coleccion Thyssen-Bornemisza, Madrid.

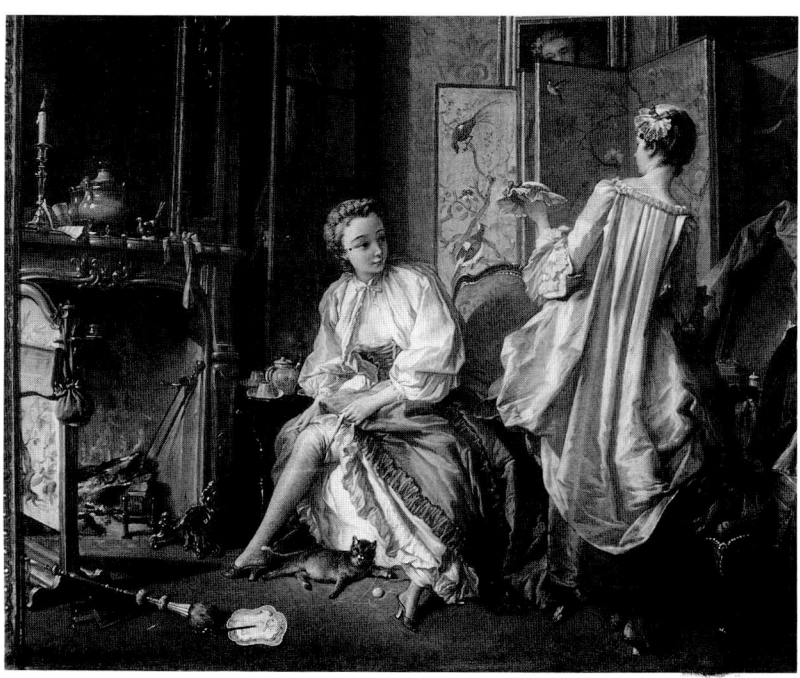

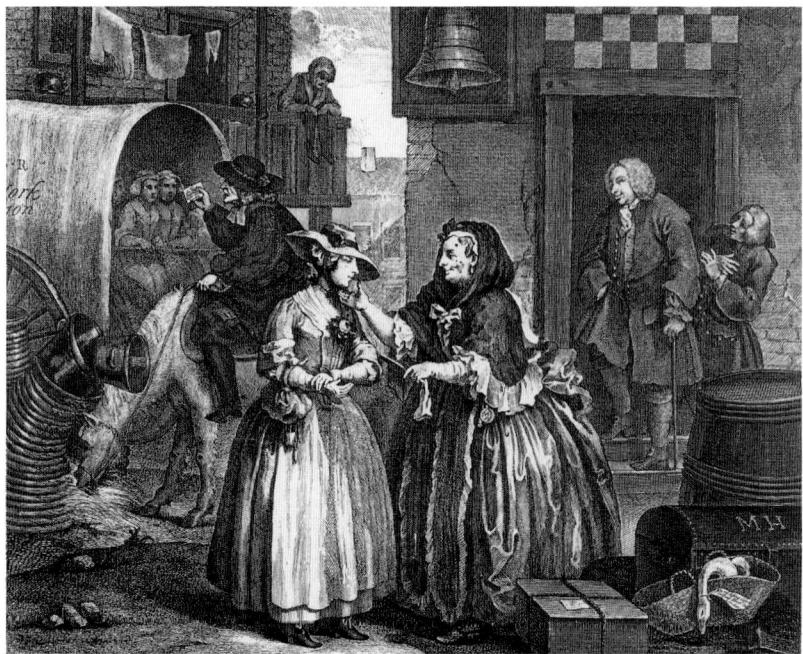

Plate 3. *Above,* William Hogarth, *A Harlot's Progress,* plate I. Beneath the obvious symbol of a bell with a clapper, the virgin Moll is being propositioned by the notorious bawd Mother Needham, whose face bears signs of advanced venereal disease. With Col. Charteris in the doorway and the mounted clergyman carrying a letter of preferment, Hogarth shows the source of corruption to be the privileged classes. **Plate 4.** *Below,* William Hogarth, *A Harlot's Progress,* plate II. Moll creates disorderly movement all around her. On her forehead and breast are the marks of venereal disease.

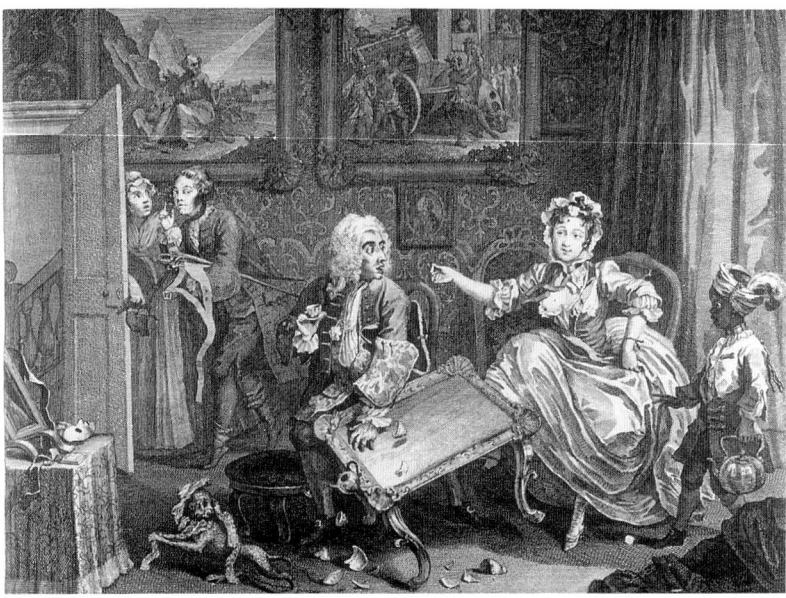

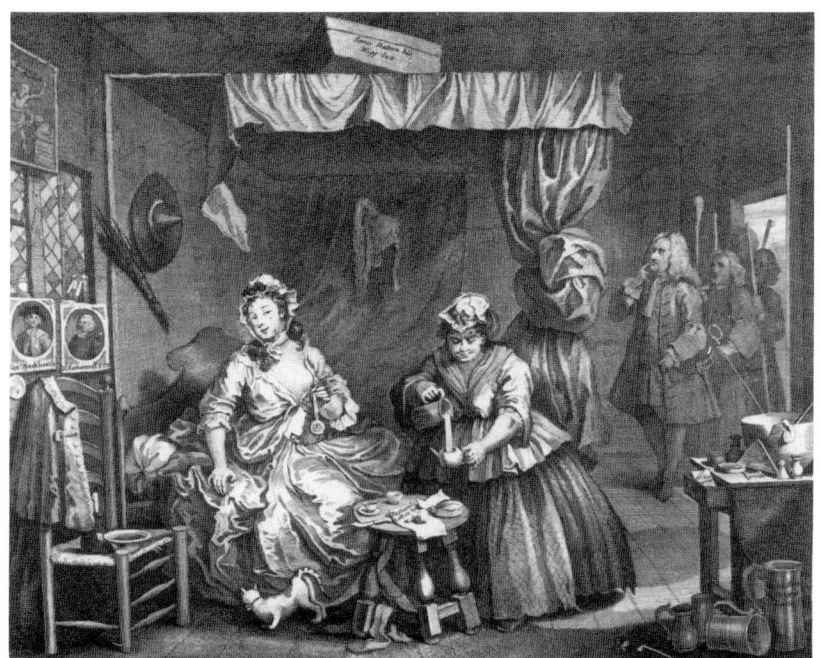

Plate 5. *Above,* William Hogarth, *A Harlot's Progress,* plate III. Moll rises after a night's work. The vials on the window sill and the syphilitic maid show venereal disease as the inevitable consequence of her way of life. She is about to be arrested by Sir John Gonson, a magistrate notorious for prosecuting prostitutes. **Plate 6.** *Below,* William Hogarth, *A Harlot's Progress,* plate IV. Moll and other women in Bridewell. Moll's syphilitic maid adjusts her garter, but her ragged clothes and exposed flesh are the reverse of erotic.

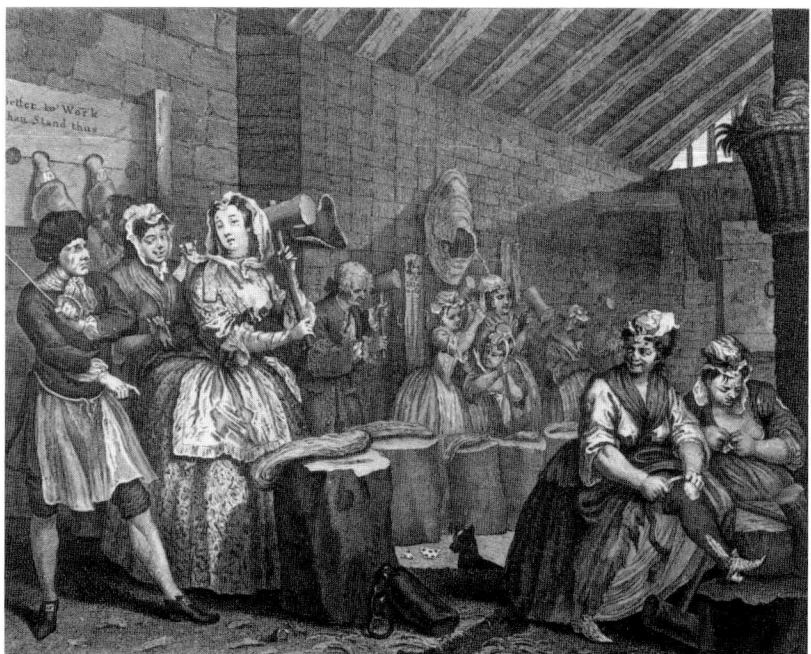

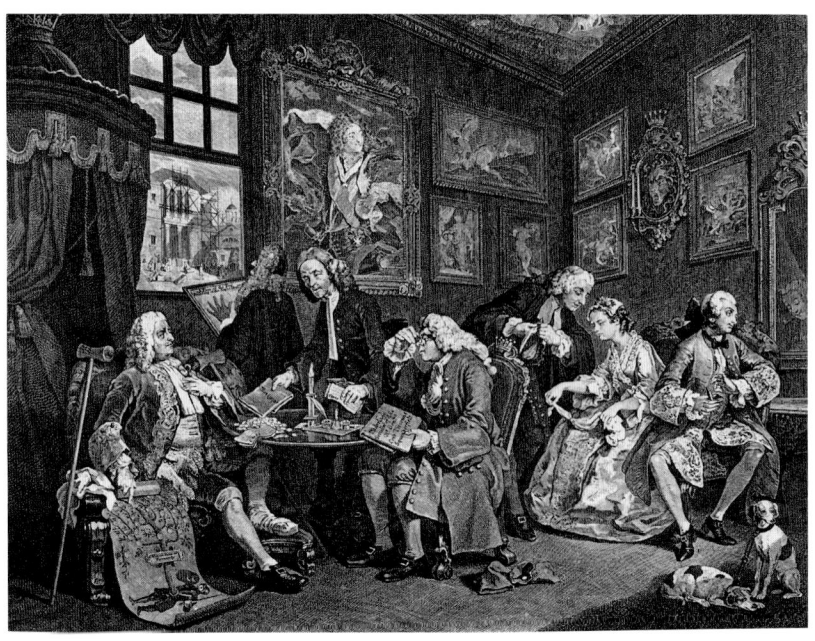

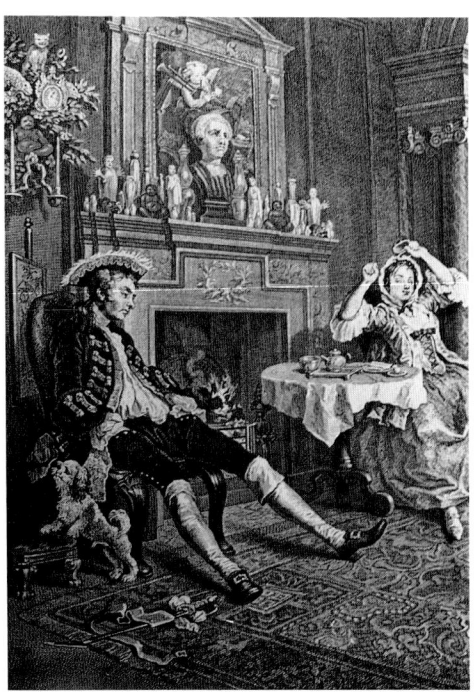

Plate 7. *Above,* William Hogarth, *Marriage à la Mode,* plate I. Hogarth's concealed theme is venereal disease as a consequence of the excesses of the aristocracy. Lord Squanderfield points to the increasingly unhealthy family tree, and his gout, and the mark on his son's neck, show that both are blighted by the disease.

Plate 8. *Left,* William Hogarth, *Marriage à la Mode,* plate II (detail). Both partners are exhausted by their sexual indulgence. She seems to be removing a halo, and his broken sword symbolizes his waning powers.

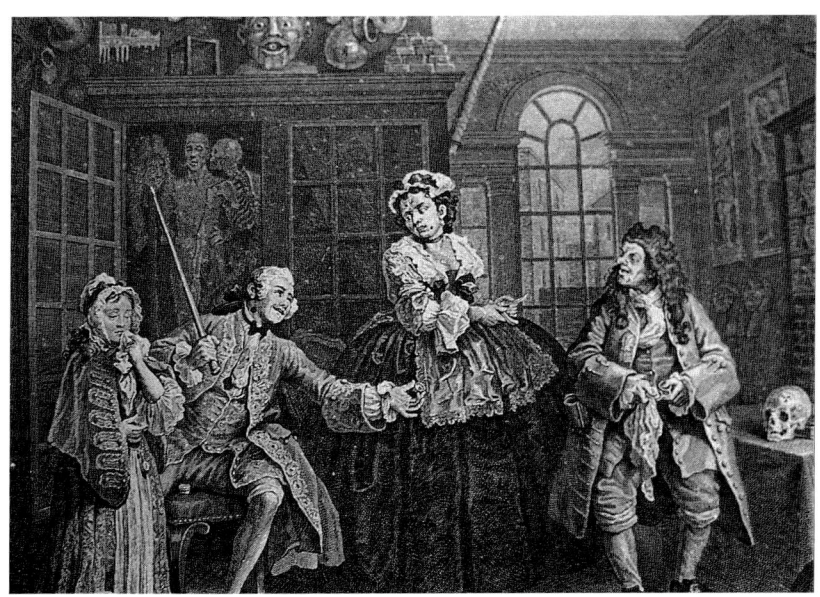

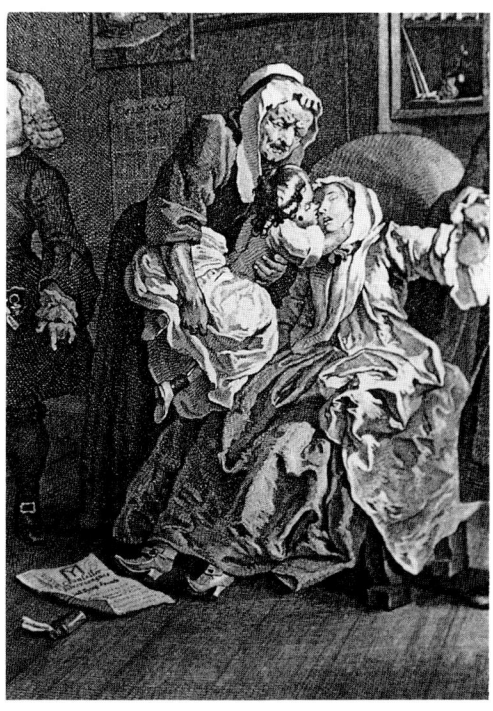

Plate 9. *Above*, William Hogarth, *Marriage à la Mode,* plate III (detail). Amid images of death, Squanderfield argues with the quack about the uselessness of his cure for venereal disease. He has infected his young mistress, to the annoyance of the older woman, a harlot also bearing the signs of infection.

Plate 10. *Left*, William Hogarth, *Marriage à la Mode,* plate VI (detail). The last of the Squanderfield line kisses the dead mother. The symptoms of congenital venereal disease are evident from the child's domed forehead, the spot on her cheek, and her pitifully crippled legs.

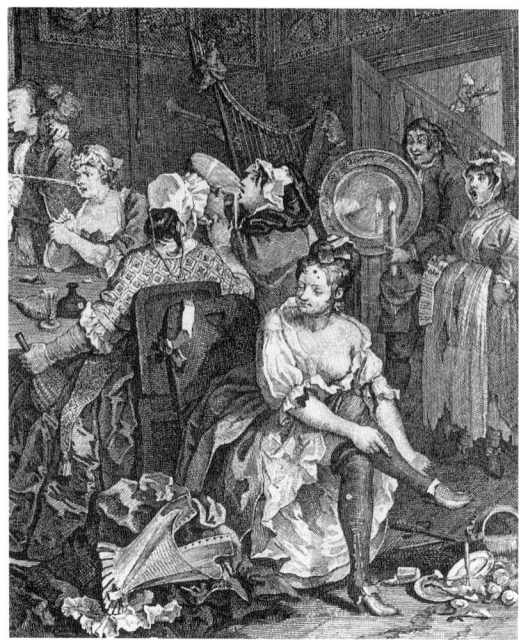

Plate 11. *Above,* William Hogarth, *A Rake's Progress,* plate III (detail). The "posture woman," depicted here getting dressed, is a parody of paintings of women at their toilet. Her decadence kills all sensuality, and tne dead bird at her feet, with a fork thrust in it, is a symbol of her sexuality done to death. **Plate 12.** *Below,* William Hogarth, *A Rake's Progress,* plate VIII (detail). The rake has been driven mad by his debauchery and sexual excess.

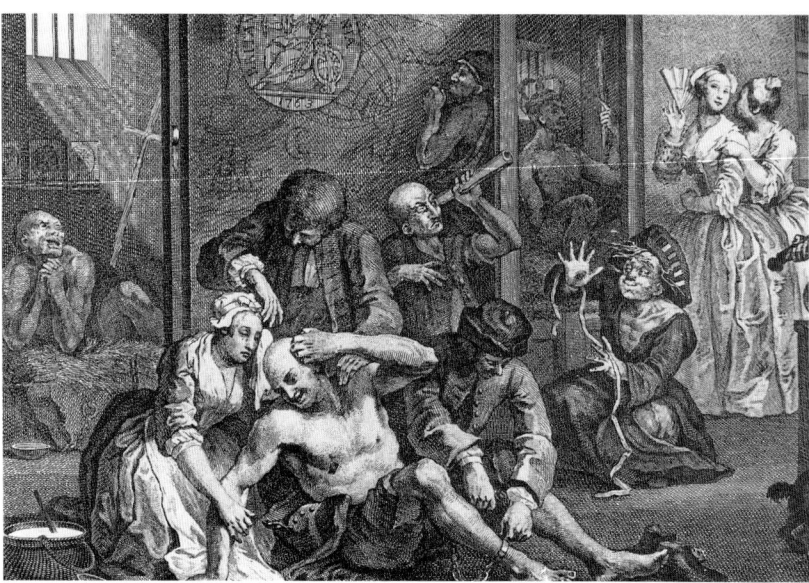

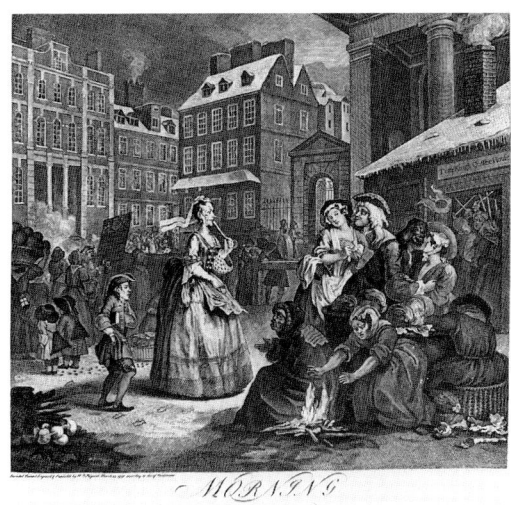

Plate 13. *Above*, William Hogarth, *The Four Times of Day: Morning*. The middle-aged lady on her way to an assignation is linked to venereal disease by the spots on her face, the placard behind her advertising Dr. Rock's cure, and the syphilitic beggar woman, an image perhaps of the fate that awaits her. **Plate 14.** *Below*, William Hogarth, *The Four Times of Day: Evening*. The horns above the head of this London dyer signal that this depiction of an evening stroll is really a study in the hypocrisy of the middle-class family. The wife and the pregnant bitch in front of her carry the results of sexual encounters. The boy's domed forehead and feeble legs suggest that he is the victim of congenital venereal disease.

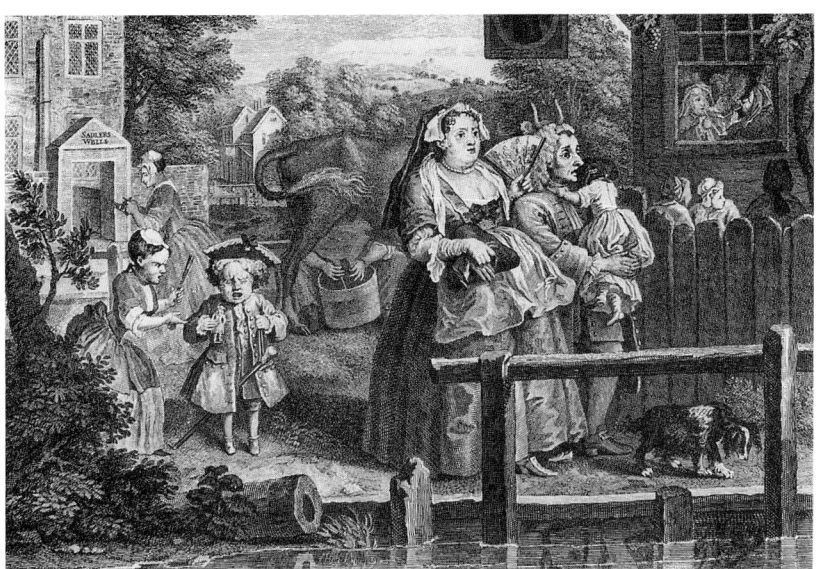

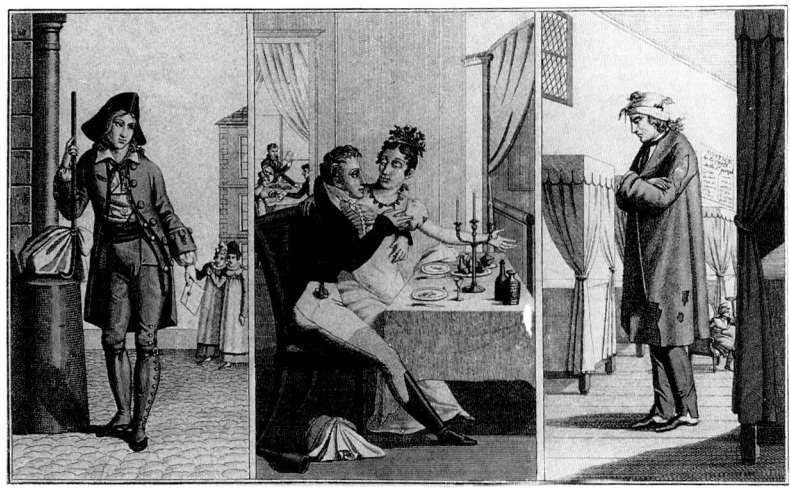

Plate 15. *Above,* La Vie d'un joli Garçon à Paris ou Le Paysan perverti. Carnavalet Museum, Paris. **Plate 16.** *Below,* La Vie d'une jolie Fille à Paris ou La Paysanne pervertie. Carnavalet Museum, Paris. These two prints do not derive from the illustrations done by Louis Binet and others for the 1784 editions of the two novels. The artist and date of composition are unknown, but the costumes suggest an early nineteenth-century date.

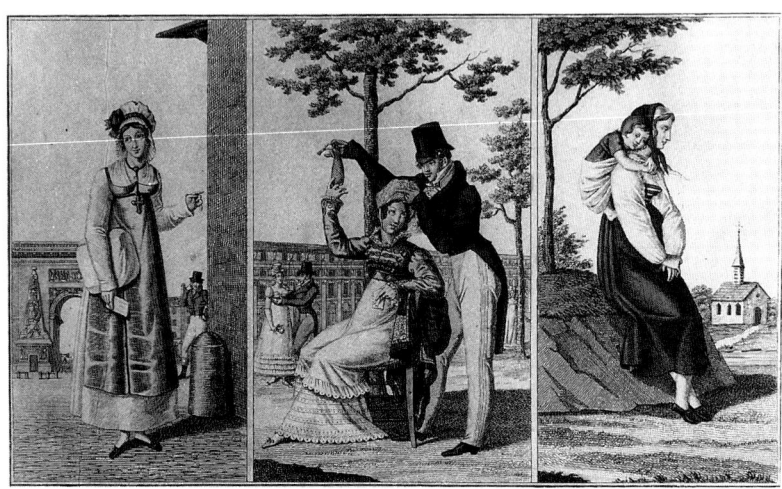

In the Restoration drama venereal disease is always treated comically, as a sign of our common human frailty, a reminder that however inflated our sense of self-importance and self-sovereignty, however elevated our heroic aspirations, we are poor, weak creatures—essentially ridiculous. At one level, reference to venereal disease is purely discursive, common in ordinary discourse, and comparable to the manifold uses of the word *fuck* in contemporary parlance. Such references—as, for example, when one character wishes a "pox" upon another, or talks about his last "clap"—thread through the fabric of a number of social discourses. For example, when Snap, the servant of Loveless in *Love's Last Shift*, is given a particularly generous tip by Worthy, the play's most admirable character, he facetiously asks what services he may perform for Worthy to repay such generosity: "Bless my Eye-sight! a Guinea!—Sir, is there e'er a Whore you wou'd have kickt? any Bawd's Windows you would have broken? Shall I beat your Taylor for disappointing you? or your Surgeon, that would be paid for a Clap of two Years standing? If you have occasion you may command your humble Servant" [I.i].[4]

In the Restoration comic world the discourse of venereal disease is common public discourse; the illness itself is common and publicly acknowledged. This passage, for instance, makes clear that one among many activities in the daily experience of a young man is having the clap and being cured, or not cured, of it. Neither the sickness nor its cure is secret or serious; rather, it is as common in a man about town as dressing well, consorting with whores, dealing with bawds—all the little businesses of ordinary life. Most frequently, references to venereal disease are used as a satiric device to undermine the pretensions of hypocrites and poseurs. For instance, Horner in *The Country Wife* mocks Pinchwife's jealousy (a trait considered to be a form of pride in the Renaissance and early Restoration) by asking whether the reason that Pinchwife is loath to have men kiss his wife is that he was not fully cured of his last clap. Loveless, in *Love's Last Shift*, argues that railing against vice is the infallible sign of hypocrisy: "I have known a jolly red-nos'd Parson, at three o' the Clock in the Morning, belch out Invectives against late Hours, and hard Drinking; and a canting hypocritical Sinner protest against Fornication, when the Rogue was himself just crawling out of a Flux" [I.i].

Florio, in *City Politiques,* pretends to be dying of syphilis as part of a scheme to seduce the wife of the man he has helped to make mayor of Naples: "Has the worthy Citizen whom I have elected to be my cuckold attained the other dignity of Podesta of Naples yet? . . . For when he is chief magistrate of Naples, I shall be ———of his wife, dispatch his domestic affairs, and receive all the fees of that sweet office" [I.i].[5] *City Politiques* is, of course, a satire on Restoration English, "true Protestant" Whigs. The Whig Citizen is coded in the play as Politician: power-hungry and money-hungry, hypocritical and pretentious—the very image of proud self-sovereignty that Restoration satiric discourse was designed to overthrow. Tory, on the other hand, is coded as Lover: for whom sexual satisfaction is more important than money and sexual appetite is more important than the drive for political status. Indeed, the Tory libertine is the Restoration's version of the clever clown of Renaissance comedy, the servant of nature and enemy of pride. Florio mourns the fact that his ruse requires him to keep company with the hypocritical "saints," true-blue Protestants who pretend to be above human frailty:

> Florio. Then I part with all the society of my witty lewd friends,
> to keep company with dull lewd saints.
> Pietro. Not saints, sir, but Whigs.
> Florio. That's as bad—and so lose my reputation of my loyalty
> and good affection to my prince. [I.i]

Imminent death from venereal disease, far from marginalizing the lover, Florio, or rendering him a despised "other," evokes the pity and affection of his many mistresses:

> Florio. And do they lament me?
> Pietro. All, all, sir. The virtuous ladies sigh and cry 'Tis pity,' the
> other run distracted; the very common whores abstain from plays,
> and bawds neglect their brandy bottles. [I.i]

Like death, venereal disease makes brothers and sisters of us all. Only when Florio is pretending to be a Whig, a "true Protestant" hypocrite, does he say that his venereal disease is punishment for a life of libertinism, anticipating as he does eighteenth-century modernist coding, which at its foundation, of course, was a product of triumphant, Glorious Revolution Whiggism.

As venereal disease is used to unmask religious and political hypocrisy in Restoration dramatic satire, so too is it used to puncture the pretensions to knowledge and command over nature of the "New Science," another bulwark of Enlightenment epistemology. In D'Urfey's play *The Fond Husband, or The Plotting Sisters* (1676), Cordelia and Sir Roger go to visit Sneak, an aspiring young Cambridge student and pretender to expertise in the mysteries of the new science. They find him in a nightgown with an apothecary in attendance, and Cordelia discovers that a "sweating chair," commonly used in the treatment of venereal disease, is part of his furniture. Sir Roger tries to pass the sweating chair off as an esoteric instrument of the new learning. "'Tis a Mathematical Engine they use at Cambridge," he says.

However, among the most interesting figurations of venereal disease in the Restoration satiric drama is Shadwell's Crazy in *The Humourists*. Crazy is not a "character" in the post-Enlightenment, novelistic sense of the term; rather, he is an exaggerated, emblematic sign. The dislocation and dissonance that are figured in Crazy make him a kind of comically conceived Everyman: the very image of high heroic aspiration and low comic grotesquerie that Restoration satire conceives to be our human nature and condition. Heroic imagination drives Crazy to extremes of daring self-sacrifice for love and valor, but the effects of that daring flight are ludicrously registered on his syphilis ravaged body:

> Craz. Beauty, Heav'ns brightest Image, the thing which all the World desires and fights for, the Spur to Honour and all glorious Actions, without which no Dominion would have been priz'd or Hero heard of.
> Errant. Oh dear Mr. Crazy! . . . thou art a sweet man. (She claps him on the shoulders.)
> Craz. Oh death! What have you done? You have murder'd me; oh you have struck me just upon a Callous Node, do you think I have a body of Iron. [I.i][6]

When the bailiffs come to arrest Crazy at the suit of Pullin, the French surgeon, whom Crazy refuses to pay because his cures have been ineffective, Raymond, the man of wit in the play, comes to Crazy's rescue. Together they fight off the bailiffs:

> Raym. Come on Crazy, thou behav'st thy self bravely.
> Craz. O Sir, I should have fought better, but for some damn'd Pustles upon my Arm, and some Arcochordones upon my right Shoulder; but really Mr. *Raymond* this is such a deliverance, that nothing can shew my Gratitude, but to bring you to see a Person of Honour hard by. [II.i]

The "Person of Honour" (i.e., aristocratic woman) to whom Crazy introduces Raymond is Theodosia, the heroine of the play whom Raymond will end by marrying.

Crazy's aspirations to heroic bravery, figured in Renaissance/early Restoration "love and honor" coding, are driven by his commitment to heroic love: "Dear Madam . . . let me but kiss this fair hand, and that will inspire me to kill twenty . . . Rascals in an afternoon—But where shall I have the Honour to wait upon you by and by?" [III.i]. His venereal disease is a satiric device that is used to undermine those pretensions to heroic singularity, a reminder that our common human frailty is our passport to the comic *harmonia*. When Crazy is about to climb over the garden wall to keep his romantic assignation, his syphilis brings him abruptly down to earth:

> Craz. The Coast is clear on this side, if my Mistress be but in the Garden, I am safe—My Dear.
> Lady Lovey. Hear I am.
> Craz. Now I come wer't as high as *Grantham-steeple!*
> Death I have broke both my Shins: I am murder'd:
> *Oh, I see these leaps are not for men that have fluxed thrice.* [ital. mine] [IV.i]

I wish to make two points by these examples: (1) Crazy is not crazy because he has venereal disease; he is crazy because he is human. An emblem of each of us, Crazy demonstrates how crazy we are when we pretend to self-sovereignty and heroic singularity and how inevitably our common frailty brings us crashing down to make us "even" with all other "earthly things" and in tune with all our fellow creatures in the great cosmic harmonia. (2) Having venereal disease neither isolates nor marginalizes Crazy. He is happily aswim—and in active courtship—in the best society.

We have always known that marriage assumes a privileged position in the English drama from the early eighteenth century onward—that sentimental, "conscious lovers" replace witty, combative ones as objects of our approval and admiration, that rakes may from time to time "relapse" but are always brought back to good, matrimonial behavior by the absolute fidelity and devotion of their virtuous wives, and that the new masculine ideal finds definition in the *husband* (in every sense of the term) rather than the sexually heroic, libertine lover. In the past we attributed this change to the inexplicable birth of a new sentimental sensibility, a new warmheartedness that arose in England toward the beginning of the eighteenth century, or we have traced the genesis of the "man of feeling" to the latitudinarian doctrine of a benevolent human nature. We have not looked for the political and economic ideological underpinnings of the change to sentimental sensibility largely because, until fairly recently, we have tended to compartmentalize discourses and to read literary and philosophical discourses in isolation from other discourses. Discourses were not so compartmentalized at the end of the seventeenth century.

Henry Abelove finds an interesting correlation between the rise in economic production and the almost exactly similar increase in population during the long eighteenth century. He demonstrates the relation between "the privileging of production" and "the privileging of intercourse" in eighteenth-century culture and explains the threat that unproductive and transgressive forms of sexual behavior came to be considered in that period: "While production increases importantly it also becomes discursively and phenomenologically central in ways that it had never been before. Behaviors, customs, usages which are judged to be non-productive come under extraordinary and ever-intensifying negative pressure."[7] There is strong evidence to support Abelove's theory in Charles Davenant's *Essay upon the Probable Methods of making a People Gainers in the Ballance of Trade* (1699): "The People being the first Matter of Power and Wealth, by whose Labour and Industry a Nation must be Gainers in the Ballance, their Increase or Decrease must be carefully observ'd by any Government that designs to thrive; that is their Increase must be promoted by good Conduct and wholesome Laws, and if they have been Decreas'd by War, or any other Accident, the breach is to be made up as soon as possible, for it is a maim to the Body Politick affecting all its parts."[8]

Sexual adventuring of any kind must be sharply curbed and penalized because any kind of libertinism, any sexual behavior unamenable to state control, threatens stable marriage, and marriage is the best mechanism for the production and maintenance of "hands" for "Mr. Bounderby"—the captains of capitalism who were first coming into ascendance in the last decade of the seventeenth and early decades of the eighteenth centuries. Defoe, prime spokesman for the trade-empire-science-nationalism nexus that was the central pillar of early modern culture, put the matter concisely: "Multitudes of People make Trade, Trade makes Wealth, Wealth builds Cities, Cities enrich the Land around them, Land enrich'd rises in Value, and Value of Land enriches the Government."[9] The discourse of capitalism and the discourse of marriage meet and intersect in the official language of nationalism. The atmosphere of moral reform that followed upon the Glorious Revolution, the atmosphere that bred "conscious lovers" and "men of feeling," then, is a product of the new capitalist culture. Charles Davenant advocates "virtue"—by which he quite openly says he means *heterosexual behavior strictly confined within the bounds of marriage*—exclusively to the end that it promotes and ensures nationalism, class stability, and growth in the gross national product: "We shall venture to affirm that if this Nation should ever be under any great Disorder, the truest course to mend it, will be to plant *in the Minds of the better sort* Morality, and Shame of doing ill to their Country, and we shall presume to assert that observing the Rules and Dictates of Virtue does not only lead to Heaven and a blessed State hereafter, but is the very best way of securing to a People in general, Prosperity, Peace, Safety, Power, and happiness in this present World" [ital. mine].[10]

When "the Minds of the better sort," infused with the new ideology, project their norms as the "universally applicable ideal for humanity,"[11] the discourse of venereal disease abruptly changes. (It also proliferates but becomes secret.) The new discourse *publicly* represents venereal disease as a condition suffered by those "others," who richly deserve their suffering, since they brought it upon themselves by their own irregular behavior; *privately*, the disease is as widespread as ever, but cure for it must be secretly sought if the respectable are to maintain their separateness from, and superiority over, those "others." Daniel Turner, in his exposé *The Modern Quack, or The Physical Imposter Detected* (1718), devotes almost half his book to those quacks who pretend to treat venereal disease. They get away with their imposture, Turner says, because their quackery is conducted under the cloak of secrecy. The victims of their imposture pay the enormous fee of "twenty five Guineas of which fifteen were paid for *Secrecy*, and ten for a pretended cure."[12]

The discourse of venereal disease goes underground, so to speak, and therefore the comic language and comic figuration of venereal disease that had prevailed on the Restoration stage is no longer possible. The subject had become a "dirty" secret, shocking to the sensibilities of the virtuous, respectable men and women whom the eighteenth-century drama presumes to be its audience. Moreover, as I have demonstrated elsewhere,[13] from the turn of the century, the conception that a drama imitates nature was replaced by the converse conception that a drama draws audiences (especially the impressionable youth) to emulate the characters it represents. The theory, best expressed in Addison's conception of associationism, postulates that young men watching libertine characters on stage will be led to imitate their behavior. Given the widespread belief that young men become what they watch, it was unthinkable that they should watch attractive young men like themselves who joke about their callous nodes and fluxes and pepper their speech with references to the clap and the pox.

Since theatrical representation of venereal disease does not exist in the eighteenth century, I have chosen for comparison with the Restoration model the eighteenth-century mode of satiric representation that comes closest to dramatic representation, the narrative print satire. Like the drama, the serial print satire is a visual mode—a "show" of action—that has plot and characterization.

Among the most illuminating examples of the new, semitheatrical satiric representations of venereal disease is William Hogarth's *A Harlot's Progress*. "Etched and engraved from paintings, April 1732," this narrative satire "tells the story of the fall and speedy destruction of a girl who comes from the country to London to earn a livelihood. The work is primarily didactic; Hogarth's intention was to reveal through the girl's life the follies and miseries of vice with a view to providing his audiences with a negative example for their own conduct."[14] The aim of the new eighteenth-century mode in satire was to discriminate right from wrong behavior—which, in turn, meant socially useful and productive from socially threatening and unproductive behavior. The new satire was expected to provide an "exact Model" and "Book of Admirable Receipts" for right living. If the reader/viewer chose the negative path that so exact a model delineated, then his fall into disease and death was inevitable.

In *A Harlot's Progress* the binary opposition between "good" and "evil" is rendered mimetically and entirely in socioeconomic terms. Hogarth's Plate I (Pl. 3) makes evident the new Enlightenment equation discussed above between individual moral action and political/social action. It presents youth with a clearly defined choice between two paths in life. The scene, a morally charged but mimetically imitated city landscape, is divided precisely in half. Centrally positioned on the dividing line are a young girl from the country, Moll Hackabout, who will become a harlot by virtue of the choice she is making, and Mother Needham, "the keeper of a notorious brothel patronized by the aristocracy" [i.e., not by the virtuous Whig merchant class].[15] To the left of the dividing line, in the upper quadrant presented to the viewer, is a poor but "respectable" dwelling, what we might call "the house of decency." A good housewife with modestly drooping head is engaged in the labor suitable to her station and gender; she is hanging out clothes on a balcony situated above Moll's plane of vision. Hers is the *right*, productive role for a woman. To the right is the "house of indecency," Mother Needham's brothel. Its walls are cracked to emblematize its moral decay, and a patron (or bawd) stands in the doorway leering at his new prey. Mother Needham, who offers the young woman the fatal choice, is richly dressed. Her satin dress and lace-edged furbelow stand in contrast to the young woman's kersey, plain cambric collar, and long, white apron, and from her waist hangs a fat gold watch. Mother Needham's face, however, the nature which no rich adornment can disguise, is pitted by the lesions of venereal disease. The picture, proclaiming its mimetic fidelity in the abundance of its careful detail (i.e., this is the way things actually are in the world; this is no metaphor), is nevertheless laden with allegorical figuration that enlarges its moral dimension. For example, the horse, traditionally a symbol of high mettle, is driven by appetite to stray from his proper path and useful function. Ravenously eating hay, he knocks down—and disorders—a stack of household basins. The cracked bell and the strangled goose are emblems from the Middle Ages of fallen chastity. Even the juxtaposition of light, which brightly illuminates the house of decency, and darkness, which envelops the house of indecency, points the nature of the moral choice the young girl faces, a choice which will mold her self—both body and soul—and inevitably shape her progress.

In Plate II (Pl. 4) Moll has crossed the dividing line and has become a denizen of the marginal world of the "other." Her keeper is a "wealthy Jewish businessman."[16] Her servant is a West Indian slave. Their natures and her own are emblematized in the monkey who scurries across the foreground wearing Moll's hat. The monkey's expression parodies the Jew's. That is to say, the inhabitants of the world Moll has chosen are not quite human; they fall below the "norm" which the new culture of English modernism imposes as "the universally applicable ideal for humanity." The most salient feature of the harlot at this stage in her progress is her disorderly movement. She is chaotic herself, and she creates around her all chaotic motion. She kicks the table over with her foot; she snaps her fingers in her keeper's face; she sends the tea china (another emblem of ruined chastity) crashing to the ground. Her dress is rich but disordered; her breast has broken the confines of her bodice. Not only is her movement purposeless but she performs no productive labor. Rather, her richly but fantastically dressed servant boy, wearing the garb of the exotic, Oriental "other," carries the tea kettle to no purpose, since the teapot is crashing to the floor. To the far left of the picture, standing as a marker to us of how we should "read" the scene, is a masquerade mask and a mirror. These pointers tell us that all the richness we see is mere disguise. Because he is a Jew and "other," Moll's keeper is not a real, solid *English* merchant but merely the masquerade appearance of one. Moll is not the vigorous young woman that her romping movement would suggest, for on her forehead and on her breast are the marks of venereal disease. Her high spirits, then, are not the outward signs of a vigorous constitution but a mere simulation of energy and health.

In Plate III (Pl. 5), "her marketability reduced by disease, Moll is forced to live in a slum in Drury Lane and serve the population at large."[17] Her occupation, "common whore," has now obliterated any other identity she might have had; the bed upon which she plies her trade dominates—indeed, incorporates—the whole scene. Moll has stepped further into the darkness in her progress, for her "sign" is now a witch's hat and broom. Moreover, the instruments that she uses to disguise her deformity are now crudely obvious: the wig box on the canopy above her bed and the jar of makeup. In place of the richly framed pictures that hung on the wall in Plate II, the content of which—Jonah admonishing Nineveh and David dancing before the Ark—suggested a possibility of reform, Moll's new icons are a medallion of the Sacred Heart, a picture of Macheath, and another of Dr. Henry Sacheverell. The religious picture is, of course, a sign of irreligion, of superstition—even demonism. In the atmosphere of post-Glorious Revolution Protestantism, "Catholic" is par excellence the radically different "other." Macheath is, of course, the highwayman libertine lover of Gay's *The Beggar's Opera,* and Dr. Sacheverell is a charlatan preacher of the day. Dangling a watch that she has obviously stolen from one of her johns, Moll has become fully an outlaw. The law, in the person of Sir John Gonson, a prominent leader in the Societies for the Reformation of Manners and Morals and a notorious prosecutor of defendants indicted on morals charges, has just broken in upon her with two bailiffs. Interestingly, venereal disease in this plate has assumed a figure. Moll's companion-servant, whose nose has been devoured by syphilis and who is pictured pouring drink for Moll, is, I think, a personification of venereal disease. Vice and its necessary punishment have merged into a single figure who will stand beside Moll through the rest of her progress.

In Plate IV (Pl. 6) Moll is in Bridewell Prison beating hemp, a beadle with a rod keeping her to her pace. Her face, spotted by the lesions of venereal disease, is tired and drawn. She stands, barely able to hold her mallet, but she is richly dressed. On the right side of the picture, almost as a parodic reflection of her, are two whores. They are similarly marked by the disease, but their faces are bestial and leering; their bodies are grotesquely deformed, and their clothes are ragged and tattered. They might be said to figure the "inner" Moll, the beast beneath the finery. The moral of plate IV—for the new binary satire must point an openly declared positive antithesis to the scene of corruption it depicts—is emblazoned on the stocks from which a prostitute hangs by her hands: "Better to Work than Stand Thus." Hogarth's satire, and, indeed, eighteenth-century satire in general, perfectly serves the function for which the macroeconomist Charles Davenant had called as early as 1699: "to plant in the Minds of the better Sort Morality and Shame of doing ill to their Country." Sexual transgression does harm not only to the body of the transgressor but to the body politic as well.

In Plate V Moll is dying of venereal disease. Her face is stark white, and she is clothed in a loose, white, shroudlike garment. To her left two quacks violently argue the merits of their respective cures; one holds a bolus and the other a vial of mercury. Both are oblivious to the presence of the victim they have failed to cure. In the extreme right and left of the picture are signs of the inheritance Moll leaves. At the left her landlady steals from Moll's trunk the props of her trade—her high-heeled shoes, her witch's hat, and her masquerade mask. These, we presume, will be handed on to the next young girl from the country who chooses to follow the harlot's progress. To the right of Moll is a child whom we assume to be her son. He scratches his head in puzzlement about how to use a common cooking pan. His mental defectiveness is, as the telltale spot on his cheek attests, the effect of congenital syphilis passed on to him by his mother. An interesting detail in the picture, about which I disagree with Shesgreen, is a matzo nailed above the doorway. Shesgreen says that it was common in the eighteenth century to smear a matzo with honey and use it as a flycatcher. I believe, rather, that it is a sign of Moll's damnation, which is figured at the beginning of her progress by her keeper's Jewishness and now, at the end, stamps her for eternity as the "alien other." Once Moll crossed the line between "us," the respectable, middle-class English Protestants, and "them," the criminal, disordered, degenerate "others," which this satire so carefully delineates, she was doomed.

Plate VI, the last of *A Harlot's Progress,* pictures Moll's wake. Her coffin, the central object in the room, is ringed by a circle of underworld types, all of whom are engaged in the activities that brought Moll to this end. They include on the far left a respectably dressed priest who is groping beneath the skirt of the swoony-eyed prostitute beside him while his other hand "spills" (a visual pun) the liquor in his glass. There is a crowd of prostitutes all drinking and a bawd who has obviously inherited Moll's ring, which, tellingly, is being placed upon her finger by Moll's maid, the personification of venereal disease. In the background one of the prostitutes stands before a mirror attempting to disguise her venereal lesions with patches. At the end of the line, to the far right, is a prominently figured prostitute, who resembles Moll as she appeared at the beginning of her progress. She reaches toward the coffin as though reaching toward her fate, while her keeper draws a silken glove onto one of her hands and she uses her other hand to steal a handkerchief from his pocket.

In front of the coffin sits Moll's son, dressed in full mourning and playing with a top, which is traditionally a symbol of idleness. On the cracked wall behind him is a coat of arms blazoned with what seem to be three tops. The conclusion of *A Harlot's Progress* nails down the satiric antithesis, or moral, of the whole narrative satire. In the new eighteenth-century culture of modernism, idleness and the desire for pleasure and luxury without the will to pay for it in productive labor are a cardinal crime for which disease and death are the only fit punishment. As Blackmore put it in his essay against wit, "the Labours of the meanest Persons, that conduce to the Welfare and Benefit of the Publick, are more valuable, because more useful, than the Employments of those, who apply themselves only, or principally, to divert and entertain the Fancy [the imagination]."[18]

NOTES

1. Hans Blumenberg, *The Legitimacy of the Modern Age*, trans. Robert M. Wallace (Cambridge: MIT Press), 220.

2. Roy Porter and Dorothy Porter, *In Sickness and in Health: The British Experience, 1650-1850* (London: Fourth Estate, 1988), 28, 30.

3. John Dryden, *A Discourse Concerning the Original and Progress of Satire: The Works of John Dryden, Poems 1693-1696*, ed. A.B. Chambers and W. Frost (Berkeley: Univ. of California Press, 1974), 75.

4. Colley Cibber, *Love's Last Shift: Three Sentimental Comedies*, ed. Maureen Sullivan (New Haven: Yale Univ. Press, 1973).

5. John Crowne, *City Politiques*, ed. John H. Wilson (Lincoln: Univ. of Nebraska Press, 1967).

6. Thomas Shadwell, *The Humorists* (1671), *The Complete Works of Thomas Shadwell*, ed. Montague Summers (London: Fortune Press, 1927).

7. Henry Abelove, "Some Speculations on the History of Sexual Intercourse during the 'Long Eighteenth Century' in England," *Genders* 6 (Nov. 1989): 128.

8. Charles Davenant, *An Essay upon the Probable Methods of Making a People Gainers in the Ballance of Trade* (London, 1699), 24-25.

9. Daniel Defoe, *Giving Alms no Charity* (London, 1704).

10. Davenant, *Essay*, 226-27.

11. See Karlis Racevskis, "Geneological Critique: Michel Foucault," in *Contemporary Literary Theory*, ed. G.Douglas Atkins and Laura Morrow (Amherst: Univ. of Massachusetts Press, 1989), 234.

12. Daniel Turner, *The Modern Quack, or The Physical Imposter Detected* (London: J. Roberts, 1718), 10.

13. Rose A. Zimbardo, *A Mirror to Nature: Transformations in Drama and Aesthetics, 1660-1732* (Lexington: Univ. Press of Kentucky, 1986).

14. Sean Shesgreen, introduction to *A Harlot's Progress: Engravings by Hogarth*,

ed. Sean Shesgreen (New York: Dover, 1973), 18. All references to Hogarth are to this edition.

15. Ibid.
16. Ibid., 19.
17. Ibid., 20.
18. Sir Richard Blackmore, "Essay on Wit," *Essays Upon Several Subjects* (London, 1712), 191.

Chapter 12

Pox and Malice

Some Representations of Venereal Disease in Restoration and Eighteenth-Century Satire

Leon Guilhamet

When Sir Carr Scroope attacked Rochester by telling him to "Sit swelling in thy hole like a vex'd toad, / And all thy pox and malice spit abroad,"[1] it is unlikely that he realized he was touching on a serious issue for satire in the next century. If we are to believe the burden of Rochester's satire against him, Scroope was too ugly to be a successful rake. And, if Rochester was correct that ugliness could save a man from infection, that fact might have encouraged Scroope to employ the accusation of the pox in his answer to Rochester's attack.

Of course, such assumptions are simply satiric posturings. For Rochester, venereal disease is indicative of what he regards as manly behavior. Rochester's satire, which deals freely with a broad range of sexuality and obscenity, is therefore relatively free of references to venereal disease. It never occurs as a moral persuasion against adultery or other sexual excesses. Not surprisingly, Rochester takes the rake's perspective in viewing such disease as something to be taken lightly:

> If you needs must have flesh, take the way that is noble:
> In a generous wench there is nothing of trouble.
> You come on, you come off—say, do what you please—
> And the worst you can fear is but a disease,
> And diseases, you know, will admit of a cure,
> But the hell-fire of marriage none can endure. [ll. 9-14][2]

George Farquhar, with a reputation as a rake and comic dramatist, takes much the same position in the following triplet:

> Take Heart howe're, 'tis my desire,
> You will revive, the P——x expire;
> Then rise like Phoenix from the Fire.³

It seems reasonable that rakes, at risk themselves to venereal disease, should not take a strong moral stand against those who are infected. And such seems to be the case. Satirists, who were also rakes, such as Donne and Churchill, as well as Rochester, do not make extensive references in their satires to the pox and clap. Pope's relative silence on the issue may have more to do with the time frame in which he wrote, when references to venereal disease were becoming rarer. Pope, for whatever reason,⁴ only mentions the pox and the clap in two of his major satires: one is in strict imitation of Donne,⁵ and another is a thrust at Lady Mary Wortley Montagu.⁶

Though gonorrhea had been known for centuries, the venereal infection that came to be known as syphilis was post-Columbian and began to ravage Europe in the late fifteenth and early sixteenth centuries. Erasmus was hardly the first to comment in print on this new and terrifying affliction, but when he does express his viewpoint in *A Marriage in Name Only, or The Unequal Match* (1529), he raises issues that would reverberate for centuries to come.

Since the relationship between the new disease and illicit sexual contact was not established, Erasmus is not censorious with regard to its victims.⁷ Rather, his moral indictment is reserved for those who, having contracted the disease, knowingly communicate it to others, especially within the bonds of marriage.

Thomas More's striking passage in the *Utopia* where marriageable men and women are examined naked for signs of the disease⁸ was clearly a concession to the ravages of what was variously called the French, Spanish, and Neapolitan disease or pox. Of course, *pox* later became the usual term, qualified by *greater* when a confusion with the smallpox was possible.

In *A Marriage in Name Only*, Erasmus directs his ire particularly toward the greedy parents of the young girl about to be married off to an infected knight. In addition to his pathos for the plight of the young girl destined to infection and early death, however, Erasmus takes a broader view of the consequences to the ruling class. Speaking through one of the interlocutors, Gabriel, Erasmus perceives trouble for the state: "But this outrage—than which you could find nothing more barbarous, more cruel, more unrighteous—is even a laughing matter with the governing class nowadays, despite the fact that those born to rule ought to have as robust health as possible. And, in fact, the condition of the body has its effect on mental power. Undeniably this disease usually depletes whatever brains a man has. So it comes about that rulers of states may be men who are healthy neither in body nor mind."

Petronius, the second speaker, elaborates further on Gabriel's contention that this terrifying threat is "a laughing matter among the governing classes": "It's amazing that princes, whose duty it is to look out for the commonwealth, at least in matters pertaining to the person—and in this regard nothing is more important than sound health—don't devise some remedy for this situation. So huge a plague has filled a large part of the globe—and yet they go on snoring as if it made no difference at all."[9]

Girolamo Fracastoro's Latin poem *Syphilis* (1530) is one of the most interesting and elaborate commentaries on the ravaging new disease and its possibilities of cure. Fracastoro writes both as a physician and a mythologist, identifying the disease with a shepherd named Syphilis who angers the gods for giving his primary allegiance to an earthly king. When the gods destroy the entire nation for its pride, Syphilis is the first to be struck down by the sickness for which he becomes the eponym.

Assuming the role of physician, Fracastoro praises guaiacum for its curative powers. It is primarily in this role that he views the disease to which he gave a name as having serious consequences for all of Europe.

Erasmus's statist concern was to be realized in England during the Restoration and eighteenth century among such humanist writers as Swift and Johnson as well as by such Whigs as Locke.[10] Through the medium of satire, the theme of venereal disease would have the impact of discrediting the monarchy and weakening its position with Parliament and the other competitors for rule.

Yet additional factors enter in to nullify the accusation of sexual impropriety as proved by the occurrence of venereal disease. First, ironically, is the knowledge that syphilis, as well as gonorrhea, is communicated by sexual contact. Once this is realized, there are attempts to exploit this insight for satiric purposes. But quickly limits are set, and the thematic use of the imagery of venereal disease in satire, the most vitriolic and restraint-free of genres, seems to limit itself from within. The reasons for this are largely unstated, but the trend toward reformation of manners, which affected the stage and, indeed, every facet of life at the century's turn and throughout the eighteenth century, imposes limits on satire. Even by 1700, following Collier's influential attack on the stage, references to the clap and pox in literature generally and satire in particular are in decline. Eventually venereal disease becomes nearly unmentioned and, one might assume, unmentionable. It gives way as a potentially devastating satiric thrust to accusations of promiscuity and homosexuality, which, of course, had always been employed but seemed to become indictments more acceptable to a society concerned with the appearance of moral rectitude.

Second, the potency of venereal disease as a satiric topos seems also to have been deflected in some measure by a decline in antifeminism. As misogyny became less popular when the ranks of readers and writers swelled with women recruits, references in satire to venereal disease associated with female prostitution began to disappear.

Third, those satirists who were rakes or would-be rakes were less likely to belabor the issue of venereal disease, since they themselves either suffered from it or admired activities in which the risk was high. Among such satirists, it must have proved difficult to indict others for a misfortune to which they were exposed by their own behavior.

A fourth reason for the imagery of venereal disease gradually receding from satire was probably related to the advance of medicine and the success of practitioners dedicated specifically to the cure of the clap and pox. Quotations from Rochester and Farquhar, cited above, suggest that there was confidence that venereal disease could be manageable if treated promptly and skillfully. Later victims, such as Boswell and Byron, for example, seem to have been deterred only minimally by the consequences of their respective infections. The early death that was so terrifying to Erasmus and his contemporaries was a rare by-product of venereal disease by the early eighteenth century.

A final reason, I believe, for the change in attitude toward venereal disease, which was reflected in satiric use of the motif, had to do with a changing and more humanitarian view of illness based on better scientific knowledge. The sufferer was no longer the sinner being punished by God, or if he was, God's vengeance did not belong to man. The rise of sensibility promoted the view that the sinner is one of us. Needless to say at such a point of insight and concomitant forgiveness, venereal disease no longer serves as a whetstone to a satiric point.

But that sentimental time is still far from the historical point from which we have set out. Though never a dominant motif in satire, the topos of venereal disease would nonetheless serve a number of purposes while it survived somewhere between frankness and scurrility. Eventually satirists would have to look elsewhere for themes with damning implications. The reality that venereal disease was a laughing matter to the ruling classes, as Erasmus clearly saw, was an attitude that would be hard to change.

In 1597 Joseph Hall published a collection of satires, *Virgidemiarum,* in six books. He called the first three books "toothless satyrs," poetical, academical, and moral. The last three books contained "byting satyres." Hall announced himself as an innovator with the lines: "I first adventure, follow me who list, / And be the second English satirist."[11] Only a year later, John Marston took up the challenge by publishing two volumes of satires that did not blush to name each sinner by his sin and to represent those sins in striking imagery and pungent language. These were *The Metamorphosis of Pigmalion's Image and Certaine*

Satyres and *The Scourge of Villanie: Three Books of Satyres*. Marston's satires, unlike Hall's, make liberal references to venereal disease and denounce sex as well as lust. In the following verses, for example, lovemaking leads directly to loathsome infection:

> What should I say? Lust hath confounded all,
> The bright glosse of our intellectuall
> Is fouly soyl'd. The wanton wallowing
> In fond delights, and amorous dallying,
> Hath dusk'd the fairest splendour of our soule:
> Nothing now left, but carkas, lothsome, foule. [ll. 165-70][12]

But Hall's commitment to cleanse poetry of all obscenity,[13] though not aimed specifically at satirists, would in the long run win the day. The reformation of language had begun.

Despite Marston's excesses and Hall's almost stoic purity, there is evidence that satire may have been poised to consider venereal disease as a significant moral issue and to present it as part of a larger reforming social vision. Even before the civil conflict that would divide England and leave the nation in a moral quandary, John Earle, the best of the English Theophrastan character writers, saw the problem of the "lascivious man" in persuasive social terms: "Nothing harder to his persuasion than a chaste man, no eunuch; and makes a scoffing miracle at it, if you tell him of a maid. And from this mistrust it is that such men fear marriage, or at least marry such as are of bodies to be trusted, to whom only they sell that lust which they buy of others, and make their wife a revenue to their mistress."[14] This language of commerce, veiled in part, is clear enough. Earle is pointing to the fact that males infected in the stews inevitably passed the disease on to their wives. If the reader questions that this is Earle's meaning, the next passage is more explicit: "They are men not easily reformed, because they are so little persuaded of their illness, and have such pleas from man and nature. Besides it is a jeering and flouting vice, and apt to put jests on the reprover. The pox only converts them, and that only when it kills them" [98]. Earle's language is direct and striking. Unfortunately, his assessment is entirely accurate: the unchaste man thinks the jest is on his side, even apparently after having been infected. Only in death does he comprehend the enormity of his crime.

Unfortunately, too, the fate of the good wife, infected by her husband, is not traced. Her illness and eventual death would provide yet another moral lesson, but one that was to be ignored in large measure by a society that would not grasp the implications of such behavior. And if there were children, and they too were infected? . . .

Earlier in this remarkable "character," Earle touches upon yet another issue that would tend to neutralize the thrust of his own moral outrage. He writes of the lascivious man: "A bawdy jest enters deep into him, and whatsoever you speak he will draw to bawdy, and his wit is never so good as here. His unchastest part is his tongue, for that commits what he must act seldomer" [98]. Moral outrage against illicit sexual activity can always be countered by the jests of the lascivious. Here in Earle we see the dilemma of the satirist. He wants to denounce vice, but he is forced to accept limits with regard to the depiction of that vice. Despite a strong moral position, there is a failure to draw out the full horror of what may follow, as if, somehow, restrictions are being observed or imposed. The final effect is to require the satirist to rely on indirection or to remove the offensive theme entirely.

Nonetheless, in *Hudibras,* Samuel Butler's mock-heroic masterpiece, venereal disease motifs seem to imply larger social issues. Hudibras sees female appetite as the source of virtually all social aberrations:

> 'Tis this that Proudest *Dames* enamours
> On Lacquies, and *Varlets des-Chambres:*
> Their haughty *Stomachs* overcomes,
> And makes 'em stoop to Durty *Grooms,*
> To slight the *World,* and to disparage
> *Claps, Issue, Infamy,* and *Marriage.* [bk. II, canto i, ll. 405-10][15]

In Hudibras's antifeminist view, it is this same love that visits venereal infections on the world:

> 'Twas he, that gave our Senate purges,
> And fluxt the *House,* of many a Burgess;
> Made those that represent the *Nation*
> Submit, and suffer *amputation:*
> And all the *Grandees* o' th' *Cabal*
> Adjorn to *Tubs,* at *spring* and *fall.* [II.i.361-66]

Butler here strikes at the members of Parliament for their supposed sexual excesses leading to venereal disease. But perhaps his most elaborate metaphor involving venereal disease comes in the first canto of the third part:

> For jealousie is but a kind
> Of *Clap,* and *Grincam* of the mind. [III.i.701-2]

In these lines Butler distinguishes between the clap and "grincam," or pox. But jealous folk (green-men) are worse than the Chinese who lie in for their ladies if they

> fall in labour of a Clap,
> Both lay the Child to one another,
> But who's the *Father*, who the *Mother*,
> 'Tis hard to say in multitudes,
> or who imported the *French Goods*. [III.i.712-16]

The ambiguity of Butler's use of the imagery of venereal disease is typical of Royalists of the period. More usual than not, their ire is, at least in part, antifeminist, in blaming women for the spread of infections among males of the ruling classes. However, they do see psychological aberration as the proximate cause of social disaster marked first by an irrational choice and followed later by an infection.

An example of this antifeminist viewpoint is found in the satire of Robert Gould. Gould's work is often reminiscent of John Marston's. Here are some of Gould's lines from his "Love Given O'er," written in 1680 and published in 1683, a vigorous attack on an actress named Bewley, satirized for her uncontrolled lust, who

> when she found that she could do no more,
> When all her Body was one putrid Sore,
> Studded with Pox, and Ulcers quite all o're;
> (Which show'd most specious when they most beguil'd)
> Sh'enrolled more Females in the List of Whore,
> Than all the Arts of Man e're did before.
> Prest with the pond'rous guilt, at length she fell,
> And through the solid Centre sunk to Hell.[16]

Gould's moral force and pungency, however, were unusual for his time. Royalist satirists, like Butler and Dryden, do not explore the ugly consequences of venereal disease, much less revel in it. It is more common for them to compose elaborate metaphors to reveal larger social or political issues. Gould's excesses are like Marston's. They sometimes suggest an unusual preoccupation with pathological aspects of sex and the morbidity to follow. Thus, it is understandable that Gould's stunning denunciations, anymore than Marston's, could not serve as a model for satire in the next century.

Dryden, though constantly ridiculed for his extramarital affair with the actress Anne Reeves, was never considered a rake. Nonetheless, it is unusual to find references to venereal disease in his satire. Yet in *The Medal* he constructs one of the most effective metaphors of this kind in a powerful attack on Shaftesbury:

> But thou, the Pander of the Peoples hearts,

> (O Crooked Soul, and Serpentine in Arts,)
> Whose blandishments a Loyal Land have whor'd,
> And broke the Bonds she plighted to her Lord;
> What Curses on thy blasted Name will fall!
> Which Age to Age their Legacy shall call;
> For all must curse the Woes that must descend to all.
> Religion thou hast none: thy *Mercury*
> Has pass'd through every Sect, or theirs through Thee.
> But what thou giv'st, that Venom still remains;
> And the pox'd Nation feels Thee in their Brains. [ll. 256-66][17]

Although venereal disease is very likely the pox cited, Dryden characteristically leaves the issue somewhat ambiguous. Dryden's heroic tones, even in his satire, would seem to be at odds with the vulgarity implied by the subject of venereal infection.

Most court satire is politically partisan, and it should come as no surprise that Charles II's ostentatious keeping of mistresses galvanized moral outrage by the Whig opposition. The influential Louise Keroualle, duchess of Portland, known as Madam Carwell to the London mob, was a particular target of scurrilous anticourt and antimonarchist attacks. The king's constant demands for more money were met with complaints that his mistresses were an unnecessary and immoral expenditure. "An Essay of Scandal" (1681) unites misogyny and xenophobia to discredit the monarchy:

> Why art thou poor, O King? Embezzling cunt,
> That wide-mouthed, greedy monster, that has done't.
> Thee and three kingdoms have thy drabs destroyed,
> Yet they are still uncured and thou uncloyed.
> Go visit Ports[mouth] fasting if thou dar'st,
> (Which well thou may'st, at the poor rate thou far'st)
> She'll with her noisome breath blast ev'n thy face,
> Till thou thyself grow uglier than her grace.
> Remove that costly dunghill from thy doors;
> If thou must have 'em, use cheap, wholesome whores. [ll. 10-19][18]

Probably the most sustained satiric attack against the monarchy took the question of succession as its focal point. The Whig opposition was particularly distressed over the prospect of James, duke of York, Charles's younger brother, succeeding to the throne. In the vicious satires inspired by this situation, hatred of the monarchy united with hatred of foreigners and Catholics. It became particularly scurrilous based on the unproved assumption that James had contracted the pox. The following passage from "Advice to a Painter to

Draw the Duke by" (1673), possibly by John Ayloffe, focuses on the fifteen-year-old Mary of Modena, who married James in 1673:

> Then draw the Princess with her golden locks,
> Hast'ning to be envenom'd with the pox,
> And in her youthful veins receive the wound
> That sent Nan Hyde before her underground;
> That wound wherewith the tainted Churchill fades,
> Preserv'd in store for a new set of Maids.
> Poor Princess, born under a sullen star
> To find this welcome when you're come so far!
> Better some jealous neighbor of your own
> Had call'd you to some sound though petty throne,
> Where 'twixt a wholesome husband and a page
> You might have linger'd out a lazy age,
> Than in false hopes of being once a queen
> Die before twenty, rot before sixteen. [ll. 41-54][19]

The anonymous satire "Hodge" (1679) assumes, erroneously, that James's daughter Mary is a Catholic and was married to William of Orange with the clandestine purpose of introducing popery into the Lowlands:

> His pocky brat, got on adult'rous Nan,
> With Orange join'd the Belgians to trepan,
> Goes to the Hague for the same holy end
> As Rome to us does spurious Este send. [ll. 68-71][20]

The standing assumptions that James had the pox, that his first wife, Anne Hyde, died of it, that their children were all infected, and that his second wife, Mary of Modena, had contracted it as well served to fuel Whig opposition sentiments during the whole of Charles's later reign. Elias Mengel sums up the incredible libel about how James came to catch the pox: "York conducted intrigues with the wives of Sir John Denham and Robert Carnegie (Carneig), Earl of Southesk. It was popularly believed that Southesk in 1668, to avenge himself, deliberately contracted 'a virulent distemper' in the brothels and passed it on to James by way of his wife."[21]

An Historical Poem (1680) repeats the libel: "But now York's genitals grew over hot / With Denham's and Carneig's infected pot" [ll. 45-46].[22] But the most scurrilous satires on the issue of succession were either authored by the poetic joiner, Stephen College, or attributed to him. College reveals no pretensions toward propriety as he attacks Louise Keroualle as the source of all evil:

> This French hag's pocky bum
>   So powerful is of late,
> Although it's both blind and dumb,
>   It rules both Church and State. [ll. 21-24][23]

The exceptional venom and scurrility of College's satires reveal why their unfortunate author was executed for his troubles.

After the vulgarity of College, Dorset, who during the debate on James's succession voted with the Whigs on most issues, merits attention for his references to venereal disease in his satire.[24] In his "A Faithful Catalogue of our Most Eminent Ninnies" (1688), Dorset focuses on the anti-Jacobite libel regarding James's putative clap:

> Poor Father Dover has got a gonorrhea,
> Was e'er, dread James, so much affection shown:
> He'd save thy soul, but cares not for his own.
> How Sedley prays, the old adult'rous fop
> May find it a Carnegan-swinding clap!
> And sure 'twill in the bones and marrow stick,
> And must be damnable to soul and pr——
> The pocky jade was a damn'd heretic! [ll. 245-52][25]

After James was deposed, Henry Mildmay summed up the whole of his reign in terms of venereal disease:

> When man was subject to mishap,
> And woman had the gift to clap;
> When *Morbus Gallicus* gave place
> To that deriv'd from Scottish race;
> And countesses were grown as common
> And pocky as night-walking women. [ll. 74-79][26]

With the accession of William and Mary, the frequency and virulence of satire using the venereal disease motif diminish. There are signs also that even in such poems as use the motif its attractiveness is waning. Attention often turns from the victim of infection to the rising profession of clap doctor, as in "Advice to a Painter" (1697), where the lord chancellor, John Somers, is accused of having the pox and consulting "his friend Tom Hobbs / Who vamps him up with his Mercuriall Jobs" [29-30].[27] This famous "clap doctor," Hobbes, is also memorialized in the sixth canto of Samuel Garth's *The Dispensary* [ll. 162-79].[28] In yet another poem, "The Court" (1700-1701), the barber James Wall is satirized: "Let *Ratcliffe* Cure the feaver, *Wall* the

Pox."²⁹ More than thirty-five years later in *London* (1738), Johnson fastens on the art of curing the clap rather than on the venereal disease itself:

> All that at home no more can beg or steal,
> Or like a Gibbet better than a Wheel;
> Hiss'd from the Stage, or hooted from the Court,
> Their Air, their Dress, their Politicks import;
> Obsequious, artful, voluble and gay,
> On *Britain's* fond Credulity they prey.
> No gainful Trade their Industry can 'scape,
> They sing, they dance, clean Shoes, or cure a Clap;
> All Sciences a fasting Monsieur knows,
> And bid him go to Hell, to Hell he goes. [ll. 107-16]³⁰

In imitating Juvenal's *Third Satire,* Johnson evokes the same gallicized English fop that Ben Jonson had satirized over a century earlier in his poem "On English Mounsieur":

> That he, untravell'd should be *french* so much
>   As *french*-men in his companie, should seeme *dutch?*

> Or had his father, when he did him get,
>   The *french* disease, with which he labours yet?
> Or hung some *Mounsieurs* picture on the wall,
>   By which his damme conceiv'd him clothes and all? [ll. 7-12]³¹

The only difference, however, is significant. Instead of having the clap, the new fop is more likely to be a medical quack with a ready cure.

Johnson's rendering of a familiar motif is interesting for yet another reason. Brief though this passage be, it reflects the kind of broad but serious social comment that was replacing the abusive scurrility of some Restoration satire. Concern about the transmission of venereal disease to future generations, particularly those to whom England was looking for leadership, was a concern of many satirists and other thinkers.

Swift's concern about this took the form of satire directed against the nobility in *Gulliver's Travels.* As an admirer of "old illustrious Families," Gulliver is able to trace the lineage of those families, including "Who first brought the Pox into a noble House, which hath lineally descended in scrophulous Tumours to their Posterity. Neither could I wonder at all this, when I saw such an Interruption of Lineages by Pages, Lacqueys, Valets, Coachmen, Gamesters, Fidlers, Players, Captains, and Pick-pockets."³² The concern for the corrupting of blood, often by means of the pox, was not, of course, limited to Swift. Butler had voiced it through *Hudibras*, and Defoe also chimed in on the issue in his long poem *Reformation of Manners* (1702):

> Casco's debauched, 'tis his Paternal Vice;
> For Wickedness descends to Families:
> The tainted Blood the Seeds of Vice convey,
> And plants new Crimes before the old decay.
> Thro' all Degrees of Vice the Father run,
> But sees himself out-sin'd by either Son;
> *Whoring* and *Incest* he has understood,
> And they subjoyn Adultery and Blood. [ll. 463-70][33]

Later in *Gulliver's Travels*, there is further reflection on the communication of diseases, not just venereal, to the present generations, and Gulliver's admiration for Houyhnhnmland is at least based partly on there being no "strolling Whores, or Poxes."[34] It seems clear to me, however, that the model for disease in Swift's comments is drawn from his knowledge of venereal infection. Also his knowledge that it is sexually transmitted accounts for his seeing it as generational and as particularly allied to moral decline.

Although Swift uses these observations in *Gulliver's Travels* to satirize the nobility, the many references to venereal disease in his poetry show that he did not see the nobility as the source of all trouble or as the only class susceptible. For Swift the real trouble seems to lie in class mixing, brought about by improvident marriages. In "The Progress of Marriage," for example, the young widow of an elderly dean comes to a sad end by choosing a second husband unwisely. After her first husband's death

> The widow goes through all the forms;
> New lovers now will come in swarms.
> Oh, may I see her soon dispensing
> Her favours to some broken ensign!
> Him let her marry for his face,
> And only coat of tarnished lace;
> To turn her naked out of doors,
> And spend her jointure on his whores:
> But for a parting present leave her
> A rooted pox to last forever. [ll. 157-66][35]

For Swift, I believe, the pox or clap provide a kind of justice to those who make immoral choices, particularly with regard to sex and marriage. There is, of course, always a tinge of misogyny in Swift, but it is important to point out that it is not always the woman who is at fault for communicating the infection. The problem is one of class and of moral choice within a rigid class setting. Women, like Phyllis in the poem "Phyllis, or The Progress of Love," who make stupid choices will live to rue the day. Having been made a prostitute to earn necessary money for herself and her husband, John, Phyllis is successful for a time,

> Till swains unwholesome spoiled the trade;
> For now the surgeon must be paid,
> To whom those perquisites are gone,
> In Christian justice due to John. [ll. 91-94][36]

Venereal disease hastens the moral decline by worsening the economic consequences. When that fall is complete, the couple now falls below John's former social level (he was a butler). Having submitted to the moral compromise with no economic advantage, the couple is then completely defined by their circumstances, moral and economic:

> When food and raiment now grew scarce,
> Fate put a period to the farce,
> And with exact poetic justice;
> For John is landlord, Phyllis hostess:
> They keep, at Staines, the old Blue Boar,
> Are cat and dog, and rogue and whore. [ll. 95-100]

From Swift's use of venereal disease in his prose work and poetry, there is the clear sense that something in society is decidedly wrong, that behavior leading to terrible physical consequences is proceeding untrammeled, without deliberation or heed. Some die; some live. But all are reduced in human stature. There is no mistaking the fact that society, for Swift, is in crisis.

For other satirists, including Pope, venereal disease has no such significance. As the century continues, the pox and clap make largely sporadic and euphemistic appearances in satire.

Some indication of why this came about may be found in one of the few passages in Charles Churchill's satire to deal directly with the issue of venereal disease. This is the portrait of the parson in *The Ghost:*

> The PARSON too (for now and then,
> PARSONS are just like other men,
> And here and there a *grave* DIVINE
> Has passions such as your's and mine)

> Burning with *holy* lust to know
> When FATE Preferment will bestow,
> 'Fraid of detection, not of sin,
> With circumspection sneaking in
> To Conj'rer as he does to *Whore,*
> Thro' some bye Alley, or Back-door,
> With the same caution *Orthodox*
> Consults the *Stars,* and gets a *Pox.* [bk. I, ll. 321-32][37]

It should be noticed that the parson is "like other men" and in many respects is excused. It is also interesting that, though this is perhaps Churchill's most explicit treatment of venereal disease in his satire, the issue of the conjurer, appropriate to this poem, is foregrounded, and venereal disease is secondary, though not entirely metaphoric. Can the satirist's apparent sympathy for the parson be related to the fact that within a year of writing this, Churchill himself was to show effects of the pox?[38]

Only in the later century does Blake have the moral acuteness and poetic fire to employ the imagery of venereal disease, the way the Hebrew prophets might have done. But decorum does not permit him to call it by its name or subject it to repeated condemnations. Nonetheless, it is a brilliant and powerful image:

> But most thro' midnight streets I hear
> How the youthful Harlots curse
> Blasts the new-born Infants tear
> And blights with plagues the Marriage hearse.[39]

Indeed, Blake sees the problem in terms of the context of social and moral decay, much as the best writers of the early eighteenth century viewed it. He, like them, follows the tradition begun by Erasmus and continued by John Earle and Jonathan Swift. It is a noble indictment, but one all too seldom made in satire of the later eighteenth century.

It is likely that references to venereal disease began to disappear from English satire in response to the continuing refinement of manners and language throughout the eighteenth century. There is, however, an additional explanation, which in a sense is part of the larger cause. As we have seen, the Restoration use of imagery related to the pox and clap is mainly in the service of Whig satirists who use it to attack Tory monarchists and, indeed, all aspects of aristocracy. Since the aristocrats were the most ostentatious in their display of mistresses, they made easy objects for such attacks.

From the beginning, however, other prime candidates for this treatment were not aristocrats at all but men whose manners and sexual mores seemed to imitate those of their betters. As such behavior patterns extended from the gentry to lower levels of the middle class, it became clear that venereal disease was not a class affliction limited to the rich and powerful.[40] In such a situation the imagery of venereal disease began to lose its power. Churchill's parson who gets the pox may be read almost as an apology for infection. The parson is like other men, and his passions, like those of other men, led him to the pox. There is nearly as much pathos here as satire, and pathos is destructive of satire. As the incidence of such pathos rose and venereal disease was seen to transcend class, satiric concern with it began to wane. It became more and more the dirty secret that fewer and fewer wished to expose. Indeed, venereal disease became so much accepted at every level of society that few could muster the boldness to single it out as the stuff of satire. In many ways this conspiracy of silence was similar to that promoted by the satirist rakes. It came about, however, for societal reasons more complex than they could have imagined.

Notes

My thanks are to Betty Rizzo and Linda Merians for providing me with some valuable references and materials before I began work on the essay. Also I have benefited greatly from reading the essays by Betty Rizzo and April London included in this volume.

 1. *Anthology of Poems on Affairs of State: Augustan Satirical Verse, 1660-1714*, ed. George de Forest Lord et al. (New Haven: Yale Univ. Press, 1963-75), 1:373. Hereafter abbreviated as *POAS*.

 2. John Wilmot, earl of Rochester. *Complete Poems*, ed. David M. Vieth (New Haven: Yale Univ. Press, 1968), 159.

 3. George Farquhar, "To a Gentleman that had his Pocket pickt of a watch and some Gold by a Mistress: A Burlesque Letter" in *The Complete Works*, ed. Charles Stonehill (New York: Gordian Press, 1967), 2:301.

 4. My own opinion is that Pope thought of himself as a rake or, more painfully, a would-be rake. See Norman Ault's account of Pope's quarrel with Cibber in *New Light on Pope* (1949; reprint, Hamden, Conn.: Archon, 1967), 298-307.

 5. Pope's "Time that at last matures a Clap to Pox, / Whose gentle progress makes a Calf an Ox" is in his imitation of Donne's second satire. See *The Twickenham Edition of the Poems of Alexander Pope*, ed. John Butt et al. (London and New Haven: Methuen and Yale Univ. Press, 1939-1969), 4:137. Donne's lines read: "Whom time, (which rots all, and makes botches poxe / And plodding on, must make a calfe an oxe)." John Donne, *The Complete Poetry and Selected Prose*, ed. Charles M. Coffin (New York: Modern Library, 1952), 94.

 6. *Poems of Alexander Pope*, 5:301.

 7. Craig Thompson points out that at this time "its sexual origin was not yet sufficiently understood." Desiderius Erasmus, *The Colloquies*, trans. Craig R. Thompson (Chicago: Univ of Chicago Press, 1965), 403. See also Gabriel's speech at the top of page 410.

 8. Sir Thomas More, *Utopia*, ed. Edward Surtz, S.J. (New Haven: Yale Univ. Press, 1964), 110.

9. Erasmus, *Colloquies*, 407, 408-9.

10. Locke's view does not focus on venereal disease, though he is clearly concerned about the moral decline of the gentry. See Neal Wood, *The Politics of Locke's Philosophy: A Social Study of "An Essay Concerning Human Understanding"* (Berkeley: Univ. of California Press, 1983). See also Wood's *John Locke and Agrarian Capitalism* (Berkeley: Univ. of California Press, 1984).

11. Prologue to *Satires by Joseph Hall* (London: Chiswick, 1825), 2.

12. *The Poems of John Marston*, ed. Arnold Davenport (Liverpool: Liverpool Univ. Press, 1961), 155.

13. See the concluding line of his First Satire of the Second Book: "For shame! write cleanly, Labeo, or write none." *Satires by Joseph Hall*, 29.

14. John Earle, *Microcosmographie, or a Piece of the World Discovered in Essays and Characters* (London: J.M. Dent, 1899), 98.

15. Samuel Butler, *Hudibras*, ed. John Wilders (Oxford: Clarendon Press, 1967).

16. Robert Gould's "Love Given O'er," cited in Felicity A. Nussbaum, *The Brink of All We Hate: English Satires on Women, 1660-1750* (Lexington: Univ. Press of Kentucky, 1984), 29.

17. *The Medal*, in *The Works of John Dryden* (Berkeley: Univ. of California Press, 1956), 2:50-51.

18. John Harold Wilson, ed. *Court Satires of the Restoration* (Columbus: Ohio State Univ. Press, 1976), 63-64.

19. "Advice to a Painter to Draw the Duke by," *POAS*, 1:216-17.

20. "Hodge," *POAS*, 2:148.

21. *POAS*, 2:157n.

22. "An Historical Poem," *POAS*, 2:157.

23. "A Satire" (1680), *POAS*, 2:291.

24. See *POAS*, 4:199-201.

25. "A Faithful Catalogue of our Most Eminent Ninnies," *POAS*, 4:203.

26. *POAS*, 4:333.

27. "Advice to a Painter," *POAS*, 6:16.

28. *The Dispensary*, in *POAS*, 6:123.

29. "The Court," *POAS*, 6:252.

30. Samuel Johnson, *The Complete English Poems*, ed. J.D. Fleeman (New Haven: Yale Univ. Press, 1982).

31. Ben Jonson, *The Complete Poetry*, ed. William B. Hunter Jr. (New York: Norton, 1968), 37.

32. *The Prose Works of Jonathan Swift*, ed. Herbert Davis (Oxford: Basil Blackwell, 1939-68), 11:198-99.

33. *Reformation of Manner*, in *POAS*, 6:417-18.

34. *Prose Works of Swift*, 11:253, 277.

35. Jonathan Swift, *The Complete Poems*, ed. Pat Rogers (Harmondsworth, Middlesex: Penguin Books, 1983), 246-47.

36. Ibid., 192.

37. *The Poetical Works of Charles Churchill*, ed. Douglas Grant (Oxford: Clarendon Press, 1956), 73.

38. See Wallace Cable Brown, *Charles Churchill: Poet, Rake, and Rebel* (Lawrence: Univ. of Kansas Press, 1953), 77.

39. William Blake, *The Poetry and Prose*, ed. David V. Erdman (Garden City, N.Y.: Doubleday, 1965), 27.

40. An example of this social complication can be seen in a rare reference to venereal disease in Crabbe's poetry:

> Nor are the nymphs that breathe the rural air
> So fair as Cynthia's, nor so chaste as fair;
> These to the town afford each fresher face,
> And the clown's trull receives the peer's embrace;
> From whom, should chance again convey her down,
> The peer's disease in turn attacks the clown. [*The Village*, Book 2, 49-52)

Further, given the long tradition of satire in which the privileged took the brunt of outrage for moral dissipation, Crabbe feels constrained to explain his viewpoint on working-class crimes:

> Yet why, you ask, these humble crimes relate,
> Why make the poor as guilty as the great?
> To show the great, those mightier sons of pride,
> How near in vice the lowest are allied;
> Such are their natures and their passions such,
> But these disguise too little, those too much:
> So shall the man of power and pleasure see
> In his own slave as vile a wretch as he;
> In his luxurious lord the servant find
> His own low pleasures and degenerate mind:
> And each in all the kindred vices trace,
> Of a poor, blind, bewilder'd, erring race;
> Who, a short time in varied fortune past,
> Die, and are equal in the dust at last. [*The Village*, Book 2, 87-100)

George Crabbe, *Tales 1812 and Other Selected Poems*, ed. Howard Mills (Cambridge: Cambridge Univ. Press, 1967), 10-12. Crabbe is a moral censor who eschews class warfare in favor of a universal Christian application and benevolence. There is little room here for damning satire in the style of Juvenal or Swift.

Chapter 13

Avoiding the Subject

The Presence and Absence of Venereal Disease in the Eighteenth-Century English Novel

APRIL LONDON

IN THE THIRD VOYAGE OF *GULLIVER'S TRAVELS*, GULLIVER'S MOURNFUL SURVEY OF the dead roused by the magical powers of the governor of Glubbdubdrib identifies "the Pox under all its Consequences and Denominations" as the source of national decline.[1] Venereal disease, modern historians speculate, had in fact reached "epidemic" proportions by the eighteenth century.[2] The contemporary signs of its public presence—from Hogarth's visual representations to the verbal sources furnished by the burgeoning market in medical manuals and in pornographic journals and directories—offer further evidence for the relationship Swift details between disease and "the Force of Luxury" [202]. To Swift as satirist, its ubiquity marks the infiltration of courtly "Vice and Corruption" into the body politic. But in the novel, the genre whose emergence coincides with that of the new commodity culture, detailed allusions to venereal disease are relatively rare. Paradoxically, such authorial circumspection argues for a tacit awareness of the ways in which the disease appears metaphorically a constitutive feature of both the novel and the culture that produced it. For the satirist who defines his moral position through notions of difference, venereal disease could be read as an image of the other. For the novelist whose success derives from the very conditions that were seen to foster venereal disease—luxury, emulativeness, individuation—allusions to it have a potentially dangerous double edge. The suggestive clusterings of women, power, money, and venereal disease that recur in eighteenth-century narratives express characteristic ambivalences about the nature of change and the relation of elite to popular culture in the period. In the variety of representations of venereal disease, from the covert references of sentimental texts to the more explicit ones of whore biographies, we find a common thread of anxiety, one often resolved (at least superficially) by the novels' concluding reversion to the nuclear family as paradigm of sexual stability. Examining canonical and noncanonical works, this essay will argue for the significance of both the absence and presence of venereal disease in registering such anxieties within contemporary fiction.

At the end of Henry Mackenzie's immensely successful 1771 novel, *The Man of Feeling*, the hero dies after hearing that his love for the virtuous Miss Walton is reciprocated: "He seized her hand—a languid colour reddened his cheek—a smile brightened faintly in his eye. As he gazed on her, it grew dim, it fixed, it closed—He sighed, and fell back on his seat."[3] In its wordlessness and pathos, this highly wrought sentimental scene characteristically focuses on the emotional at the expense of the physical. Its apotheosizing of male distress echoes an earlier moment in the novel in which the repentant prostitute, Emily Atkins, similarly induces extreme suffering in another man of feeling. In the account of her father's grief and shame "at the death of her honour," her story is turned into the occasion for an elaborate enactment of male sorrow and commiseration in the face of female iniquity [73].

These two scenes refer to a number of narrative and cultural conventions that reached their apogee in sentimental novels of the late eighteenth century: the recontextualizing of both death and prostitution in emotional terms designed to elicit sympathy, rather than in religious terms directed to consciousness of sin; the privileging of the fragmented and inarticulate; the spectatorial fascination with the sufferings of the man of feeling; and, finally, the latent but pervasive misogyny that identifies women as the source of this affecting male distress.[4] In sentimental novels, the enlightening possibilities of feeling stirred by the male desire for communion with a woman are almost invariably made subordinate to her associations with pain and mortality.

In the domestic realist tradition following Samuel Richardson, codes of decorum dictate that this desire, as in *The Man of Feeling*, be identified with the family: Harley wishes to marry Miss Walton, and Atkins wants to reclaim his daughter Emily. From the historian's perspective, such novels confirm the emergent sexual paradigm that Lawrence Stone denominates "affective individualism."[5] So powerful is this familial model of relationship that even those who repudiate its ethos reproduce its structures. Thus, Mother Sinclair and her harlots in Richardson's *Clarissa* appear as a sinister parody of Clarissa's own family, the Harlowes. And this perhaps explains not only the curious choice of a broken leg over the more likely venereal disease as the cause of Mother Sinclair's death but also why *Clarissa*'s reticence about the disease is characteristic of polite literature.

The grotesquely detailed account, sent to Lovelace by Belford, of

Sinclair's mortified, fractured leg identifies the raving, unrepentant bawd with the "contaminated carcasses" of the women who surround her in order to draw the rake's attention to the more fundamental distinction between "a neat and clean woman [who] must be an angel of a creature" and the "sluttish one [who] is the impurest animal in nature."[6] In associating Mother Sinclair's death with, but not making it a consequence of, the disease that afflicted most eighteenth-century prostitutes, Richardson identifies instead a generalized "animal" nature with the bestial end appropriate to such "profligate women" who, in Belford's view, are nothing more than "Yahoos."[7]

Such techniques of avoidance or circumspection are the norm in the domestic realist tradition of the novel and in its eighteenth-century sentimental variants. When Emily Atkins, for instance, invites the "daughters of virtue" to spare some pity for those prostitutes whose bodies are "tortured by disease," Mackenzie does not number her among the latter, preferring to focus first on the denial of appetite implicit in her emaciated state and then on her father's mental anguish.

Occasionally, sentimental novelists will subject minor villains to summary deaths whose terms evoke without specifying venereal disease, as in Agnes Maria Bennett's *Anna* (1785), where Lord Sutton, "whose whole life had been one continued scene of wickedness," finds himself at last a "martyr to disease, unconnected with any of those blessed tyes that, in soft sympathy and respectful love, can sooth the stern approach of death, drawing near to that omnipotent being, whose commands had all been broke, but from whose awful sentence of retribution his soul shrunk with terror."[8]

In Mary Ann Hanway's *Ellinor* (1798), the "*ci-devant* Lady Fanny Oswald," similarly represented as a "martyr" to her profligacy, endures the ignominy of a lonely and unlamented death: "repudiated by her relations, forsaken by her lover, shunned by her former acquaintance . . . she gave an unbounded scope to the licentious dictates of a depraved heart, and vicious imagination. Her amours were as numerous as the crimes that were the consequences of them; these ultimately led to poverty and sickness, and she died in obscurity, a martyr to those propensities, to whose gratification she had sacrificed health, beauty, fortune, rank, and fame."[9]

While the villains are incorrigible to the end, reformed sinners fear that the diseases of the past may continue to infect the future. Both possibilities clearly serve a monitory function in relation to susceptible readers. Sir George Hendon in *The Fruitless Repentance, or The History of Miss Kitty LeFever* (1769), a novel which borrows heavily from *Clarissa*, writes on his wedding day, "I already begin to feel the injuries I might sustain in the person of my wife; and tremble lest the punishment of my profligacies shall fall upon the head of my unborn posterity."[10]

Sir George's anxieties about his posterity alert us to the ways in which sentimental novels frame questions of birth and inheritance in accordance with bourgeois assumptions about the integrity of the family and property. Aristocratic libertinism is habitually opposed to cit ostentation in order to mark out a middle ground occupied by heroes and heroines whose virtue, taste, and benevolence are finally accorded the wealth that is their due. The emulative nature of middling culture in the eighteenth century, combined with the various forms of projection that novel reading encourages, ensures that these protagonists are often titled. But the recurrent stress on qualities of inwardness (the "excellent heart and refined understanding") and on a domestic order in which honor is equated with chastity (and the sottish aristocracy with venereal disease) make their class bias clear.[11]

There is, however, another range of narratives (though not necessarily of readers) in this period that represent experience, as *The Adventures of an Author* (1767) declares, in terms *"very different from the common run of languid Novels."*[12] At these further reaches from polite literature, references to venereal disease appear with some regularity, although often couched euphemistically or in coded slang. *The London-Bawd* (1711) makes use of one of the favored metaphors of fire: the eponymous protagonist was once "one of *Sampson's Foxes,* and has carried so much Fire in her Tail, as has burnt all those that have had to do with her." The same text exploits the linguistic opportunities afforded by the cant vocabulary to mock contrition after the fact: "to some notorious Wretches, she'll fix such a visible Mark in their *Faces,* as shall make 'em the Derision and the Loathing of all People; and so bring 'em to Repentance *with a Pox to 'em.*"[13] National hatreds supply an extensive fund of epithets. According to *The Tomb of Venus* (1710), each nation locates the source and name of this "ignominious Distemper" among those who are its natural enemies: to the English it is the French pox, for instance, but to the French it is the *Morbus Hispanicus.*[14]

In addition to slang derived from the disease itself, there is a rich vein of indirect references afforded by the various cures. The virtuous merchant in John Clarke's *Batchelor-Keeper* (1727) defines his son's headlong descent into vice by alluding to the spitting induced by mercury treatments: "He's fat and lean by Turns; when three Months Epicurism has swell'd him to the Size of a Porpus, a Month's Spitting reduces him to a Skeleton."[15] A "sweating illness" may also indicate infection, and references to a "month in the country" almost invariably signal withdrawal for the purposes of a private cure.[16] So standard a trope was this that John Clarke's *Virgin-Seducer* (1727) uses it ironically to make a larger moral point about the corruption of the times. The hero's friends assume that his visit to a cousin's country estate "was but a meer Excuse for his Absence, during the Time requisite to repair the damages." One of the more worldly of his circle reports that a month in the country is so transparent an excuse that, "some City Dolts excepted," those truly determined to conceal evidence of their infection prefer to claim bankruptcy as a reason for withdrawal, "they choosing rather to bear the Scandal of Insolvency, than the Disgrace of a loathed Distemper."[17]

The tacit parallel here between sex and money as equally contaminating is indicative of a larger shift over the course of this period in the interpretation of venereal disease and the narrative functions it can serve. Conventionally a sign, in seventeenth-century popular literature, of divine retribution—the wages of sin—venereal disease in the fiction of an increasingly secular age more often serves the purposes of effecting human revenge and redressing imbalances of power in relation both to class and to gender. References to the disease that depend on the residual interpretation of it as an ordained punishment manifesting the immanence of divine authority do not entirely disappear. But, increasingly, allusions to venereal disease in contemporary fiction express the imperatives of a political economy driven by consumption and emulation. Such narratives typically focus on the male urge to possess or assert property rights, an urge threatened both by the equally insistent claims of other men and by the corruptibility (or, very occasionally, the integrity) of the object of desire. That object, of course, is the female body. But given the tendency in the period to see venereal disease as exclusively the affliction of prostitutes, the infected body also carries with it a host of other negative connotations and anxieties centered on money and the exchange mode within which it operates.

Two episodes from Mary Davys's 1727 novel, *The Accomplished Rake, or Modern Fine Gentleman,* may serve as partial illustration of these larger meanings. In both, men use infected prostitutes to secure revenge against those who have invaded their property. In the first instance, a cuckolded husband, somewhat illogically given the consequences to his own person, tells a servant to

> "Go you and fetch me a fresh w———. If she proves a fire-ship, I'll carry her present to my dear wife, that she may disperse it among her multitude that so their crime may be attended with a certain punishment and everyone share alike. 'Tis a compendious revenge and reaches all, like a feast of poison to a crowd of rats." The man obeyed, brought the s———t, and conducted her to a private apartment. The consequence I never inquired after but may guess it proved as intended. [359-60]

In the second, the modern fine gentleman, Sir John Galliard, attempts to seduce the woman whom his friend Bully Bousie wishes to marry. Bully secretly substitutes for her a prostitute "that could pepper":

> This rencounter proved the very worst that ever poor Sir John was engaged in, for though he had many skirmishes with the

ladies, they had hitherto proved light ones. But in this last battle he was almost mortally wounded. And it gave him such a thorough mortification that he swore to himself if he ever got well again he would demand satisfaction of Bousie and then retire into the country where he designed to continue some time before he saw London again. [355-56]

The characteristic features of these passages are ones that the rake narratives share with the equally popular criminal and rogue biographies: the casual violence conveyed by the martial imagery, the use of idiomatic language, the satiric treatment of relationship, the episodic structure, and the tenuous relationship to the author's prefatorial claim that she has "with the utmost justice rewarded virtue and punished vice" [236].[18]

The Accomplished Rake is also typical in its depiction of women as agents of contamination rather than, equally with men, victims of venereal disease. Such agency is often construed misogynistically as a malign instance of women's ability to wield power through the body. *The Finish'd Rake, or Gallantry in Perfection. Being the Genuine and Entertaining Adventures of a Young Gentleman of Fortune* (1733) doubles the iniquity of female power by representing it as both intellectual and carnal. In this anonymous novel, the narrator's inherited fortune allows him to serve as "a most faithful and zealous Worshipper, at the Altars of the God of Wine, and the Goddess of Beauty." He tells us, "In the Course of these my Devotions, my Person sometimes came off by the Lee, and I smarted in the Flesh for them in more ways than one." But in the last recounted of these adventures, the smart inflicted by the "She-Devil" whom he fails to seduce "in some measure reveng'd the Injuries I had done her Sex."[19] In a twist on the substitutions of Davys's novel, the well-born woman whom the narrator has pursued at considerable expense cunningly betrays him with a diseased prostitute. Having "fix'd a night for the making me happy . . . she led me into her Bed-Chamber, and desired me to undress. . . . But then putting out the Candle on pretence of Modesty, she conveys into Bed in her stead, a common Whore, whom she had planted in her Closet for that Purpose, and who in return for all my Presents, gave me one, which I did not claw off in a Hurry, and which for some Time made me abhor the Sight of the whole Sex" [58-59].

While abhorrence of women most often limits the descriptive of these novels to such blunt insults as "Pocky Whore" and "Rotten Fort,"[20] writers occasionally exploit the possibilities of venereal disease with more finesse. The preface to *Entertainments of Gallantry* (1712) archly elaborates on the figure of love as a sickness in terms that rehearse the novel's subject, a courtly discussion of Ovid among a circle of witty and informed friends:

There would be no end of recounting all the Evils, Love is Cause of; *Pandora's* Box is but an *Epitome* of the Plagues *Cupid* daily torments Mankind with. A Girl thus infected, utterly rejects her *Virgin Modesty* and *Decency*: A Wife her Promises, and solemn Engagements of the *Marriage-Vow*: Soldiers their *Fortune* and *Ambition*: The Magistrate his *Justice,* and due Observance of the Laws: and the Prince his *Grandeur* and *Majesty.* . . . If then it must be indisputably agreed, that those Distempers are most dangerous, wherein the *Heart* and *Brain* share the Infection; and that this is the sure Effect, and cruel Symptom of Love: It must consequently be allow'd by all Mankind, that too great a Value, can never be set upon a Book; which contains a Remedy for so raging a Distemper. And, what ought yet more to enhance your Esteem, the Remedy, contrary to common Practice is gentle, agreeable, and to be purchas'd at an Expence, not worth naming.[21]

Thus the book, the medium used to explore love's sickness, becomes the agency of cure.

The conceit of the book as antidote, or perhaps alternative, to disease, a "Remedy" that (unlike mercury) is at once efficacious, inexpensive, and pleasurable, depends on an association of sex, money, and writing that proved suggestive to authors throughout the period. In the 1767 novel *The Adventures of an Author,* Jack Atall offers a variation on the theme with the assertion that his career as a writer (one who must "think, reason, explain, and expound for the whole nation" [1:219]) has denied him access to both sex and money. In an earthy redaction of *Tristram Shandy*'s treatment of language as a form of displacement, Jack describes how as an author he is committed to a verbal rendering of desires that poverty precludes his experiencing directly: "Appetites!—passions!—desires! strange unaccountable things to be found in beings who have not the means of gratifying them. Had I been a frog, I might have been a fortnight in the act of copulation, without my vigour, bliss, or fortune diminished—As it is, I cannot compass a shilling Venus for half an hour, without laying my estate under heavy contributions, running the risk of Cytherean scars, and wanting a dinner"[2:16].

The skeptical reading of experience afforded by a hero who sees himself as the "play-thing" of Fortune, subject to "the ingratitude and avarice of mankind in general" [2:199-200] is confirmed by the final withholding of any "moral" or "fable" at the novel's ending. His intent, he declares, has been simply to "paint after the life" and "to amuse, perhaps instruct, such of my readers as were before ignorant of those things they have found there" [2:201-2].

The picaresque elements in *Adventures of an Author* invite comparison with two of the very few canonic novels of the period that include direct references to venereal disease. The allusion in Henry Fielding's *Joseph Andrews* (1742) centers on Betty the chambermaid, once in love with an "Ensign of Foot . . . [who] did indeed raise a Flame in her, which required the Care of a Surgeon to cool."[22] She is a stock female servant of undifferentiated lust for whom the flames of love must necessarily be the literal ones provided by disease. Her relationship to Joseph and Fanny is thus a relatively uncomplicated one of contrast designed to illuminate their "higher" form of love and its domestic correlatives.

Tobias Smollett's *Adventures of Roderick Random* (1748) develops the narrative possibilities of venereal disease much more fully. In the context of Augustan satire, disease appears as the outward sign of an inner corruption which is itself generic, rather than specific: the mark of the carnal woman in *Joseph Andrews* or the dissolute aristocracy in *Gulliver's Travels*. In *Roderick Random,* the densely plotted picaresque account of "the knavery and foibles of life" is intersected by a description of the hero's venereal disease that reveals his qualities of introspection, those same qualities which will ultimately make him the appropriate heir to the recovered family estate, the loving husband to the exemplary Narcissa, and the doting father of the unborn child to whom he coyly alludes in the novel's closing lines.[23] Roderick's experience of venereal disease after his migration to London signals the lowest point of his fortunes to date: "At present my good name was lost, my money gone, my friends were alienated, my body infected by a distemper contracted in the course of an amour; and my faithful Strap, who alone could yield me pity and assistance, absent I knew not where" [114]. He is roused from a pervasive sense of misery by the greater sufferings of his neighbor, Miss Williams, whose interpolated narrative tells a history of innocence lost, imprisonment in Bridewell, and prostitution. At the conclusion of her story, Roderick's commentary asserts a seemingly necessary causal relationship between gender and class in the plot of her life. Because of the "delicacies to which her sex and rank entitled her," he assumes both that her sufferings must be more acute than his and that her "reverse of fortune" must be final [137]. As he says of himself, if "one scheme of life should not succeed, I could have recourse to another, and so to a third, veering about to a thousand different shifts, according to the emergencies of my fate, without forfeiting the dignity of my character, beyond the power of retrieving it, or subjecting myself wholly to the caprice and barbarity of the world" [136]. She, however, has "entail[ed] upon her the curse of eternal infamy!" [137].

In fact, and rather unusually for an eighteenth-century novel, Miss Williams reinvents herself and so secures another lease on respectability.[24] She later helps Roderick in his pursuit of his true love, Narcissa, and is finally rewarded with marriage to the hero's comic foil, Strap, who proclaims himself "convinced of her reformation," impressed by the "respect" shown her by Narcissa and Roderick, and unconcerned with the "censure of the world" [435].

The history of Miss Williams occupies an interesting medial position in the range from polite to popular literatures of the period. At the one extreme can be located the account of Emily Atkins in Mackenzie's *Man of Feeling;* at the other lies a conventional whore's biography such as Charles Walker's 1723 *Authentick Memoirs of the Life Intrigues and Adventures of the Celebrated Sally Salisbury;* between them is Smollett's now canonic text and another less well known one with which it has much in common, the 1766 *Genuine Memoirs of the Celebrated Miss Maria Brown. Exhibiting the Life of a Courtezan in the Most Fashionable Scenes of Dissipation.*[25]

Like Miss Williams and Maria Brown, Mackenzie's Emily Atkins is well born, her sexual seduction is foreshadowed by a verbal one (the three women all read romances), and physical suffering appears the necessary prelude to individual redemption.[26] But the extreme contrition of Emily Atkins is directed toward reinforcing traditional forms of masculine authority and not toward celebrating the possibilities of self-construction that are apparently available to Miss Williams (as they are to Maria Brown) after the chastening experience of venereal disease. Sally Salisbury, in contrast, has no pretensions to gentility (her father is a bricklayer), no reading history of which we are made aware, and no final moral reformation crowned by a successful marriage.[27] Formally, her eponymous narrative shares with Maria Brown's the distinction of a female protagonist, and in the recounting of the experiences of each we find a correspondingly full elaboration on the associations between money, disease, women, and power that appear in less detailed terms throughout contemporary popular fiction.

The differences between the two novels, however, are as illuminating as their similarities. The *Authentic Memoirs of . . . Sally Salisbury* purports to be a compilation of responses to a notice placed in the "Publick Occurences in the News-papers" for firsthand accounts of her "Life, Intrigues, and Adventures" from her mostly disaffected customers [133]. These include a range of eighteenth-century types (from nobles to squires to clergy), and their letters provide many opportunities for broad social satire, all of it directed by the male narrator who comments archly on (without analyzing) Sally's schemes of universal revenge against men. Repeatedly, her "*Repartee* and Quickness of Comprehension" [125] allow "the cunning Jilt . . . to make a Property" [99-100] of the men who pay for her favors, so reversing the more usual balance of power between the sexes.

The narrative of Caleb Afterwit is representative of the biographic notices submitted to Captain Walker. Given Sally's ability to turn even venereal disease to financial advantage, Caleb's credulous infatuation makes him the perfect gull. He tells how she mercilessly plundered him during his "Lovesick Fit" and then suddenly advised that he return to the country:

Now the Embers which had glow'd some time began to break

> out into a Flame, and I had just Reason to believe my Constitution very much impair'd by the *French-Disease*; and I found SALLY's Pretence of Retirement was only to refit and clean for a future Market. I can't tell what Favour she met with from Aesculapius's Skill, but, with Sorrow I must confess, that Part she was so kind to bestow upon me, to be beyond the Art of any of the ingenious Sons of *Galen* to master. When she was patch'd up she made me a Visit, *Damn'd me for a Son of a Bitch for giving her such an odious Distemper; [and] assur'd me of a Jail if I did not immediately discharge a pretty large Debt contracted chiefly by her self, during our Correspondence.* [137]

She has him carried "to a *Spunging-House* in a very weak Condition" and strips his lodgings of his clothes, which she passes on to her father. When he complains that she removed things "not fit" for one of her father's position, she points out that Caleb had "some few Months ago a small Estate, but that is pretty well gone" and that she intends to make her father "a Collonel, if Money can make him one: Remember, *Sirrah*, there are more rise by the Scabbard than by the Blade" [138].

As the scabbard and sword allusion suggests, the agent of the class mobility described here (Caleb's precipitous fall and the father's equally sudden rise) is Sally herself. As a conventional figure for female sexuality, the scabbard exists in a highly ironic relationship to the aristocratic connotations of the sword image. At once disease-laden and irresistible, relentlessly selfish and dynastically inclined, Sally is shown repeatedly humiliating (and infecting) a polite world whose material objects she then takes for her own. If Walker's portrayal of her is consistent with a misogynistic view of women as irredeemably debased, it also bears a strong resemblance to the contemporary attacks on the newly wealthy as the destroyers of traditional hierarchies.

The sensational and exploitative aspects of *Sally Salisbury* preclude full critical development of narrative hints that the prostitute might be read as a displaced image of fears about cultural change, fears that would see venereal disease as symptomatic of the rottenness of the new monied order. In *Maria Brown*, the attention to psychological realism, the analytical qualities of the first-person voice, and the play on the various interpretations attaching to "female commerce" all work to direct the reader's attention to the feasibility of such larger meanings.[28]

To Maria Brown and to her cohorts, the prostitute is not a marginalized or isolated figure but an emblematic one whose society exactly reproduces the political and sexual structures that underpin urban culture. Communities of the like-minded (or at least professionally affiliated) are a staple of eighteenth-century literature, but they tend to function narratively as correctives to the moral economy seen to prevail in the degenerate "real" world. The thieves' republic in Godwin's *Caleb Williams* is thus animated, at least on the part of its leader, by principles of genuine honor, whereas the community of women in Sarah Scott's *Millenium Hall* endorses forms of cooperative industry that are made available to women who exclude themselves from the corrupted masculine realm of competition. Contemporary proposals for the reform of prostitutes develop this notion of difference sociologically by suggesting that the penitents be isolated in houses of correction where a programmatic disciplining of behavior and appearance will render them indistinguishable from each other and uninterested in pursuing their former course of life.[29]

In *Maria Brown,* however, the model of community that prevails until the novel's closing pages exploits the ironies of affiliation with, rather than difference from, the real world. Prostitution becomes a figure for commerce in general, creating and then exploiting desire in terms that Madame Laborde, "one of the most celebrated bawds" [2:7] in Paris, declares are "in no way detrimental to society." She and her pensioners simply "avail ourselves of those resources with which nature has furnished us" [2:10-11]. Maria, who enlists herself under the protection of the bawd after a series of misadventures as an independent agent, comments that her new understanding of the congruity between the respectable and the "republic of fornication"

> led me to some reflections upon the conduct of the modest part of the sex, and I concluded from experience, that the women of pleasure had taught them the secret of multiplying their graces, and displaying them by foils and dress to so much advantage: I was convinced that they had borrowed our look, our gait, our air, and that every modest woman strove who should most resemble a prostitute. We are upon every occasion the objects of their attention and study. It is from us that they receive every new fashion, and all those little artifices which enchant, and which no one can define. In a word, they have but little reason to upbraid us, for they are only amiable in proportion as they know how to copy us, to tincture their chastity with coquetry, and to ape those they despise. [2:24-26]

In a world of consumption and emulation, where men and women alike have "no other object in view but interest and gain" [2:158], prostitution becomes paradigmatic.

The subversive potential of this skeptical reading of human nature operates most fully here, as in *Sally Salisbury,* when played out in the context of gender. The various communities of prostitutes with which Maria is associated are represented as consummate manipulators of men who, driven by passion and betrayed by appearance, become their dupes. The single exception to this is Mr. Williams, the great love of Maria's life. She first mentions him in an aside to an account of the venereal disease that has forced her temporarily off "Mrs. W's list . . . lest I should endanger the reputation of her house." But, she continues, "what gave me the most sensible mortification upon this occasion, was that I had communicated my disorder to a young fellow that lodged in the same house where I did" [2:123].

Considerable irony is attached to the fact that the first indication of a sexual encounter unmarked by calculation should be introduced to the reader by way of the details of the couple's shared disease. While the comic possibilities of the situation are developed in a lengthy account of a visit to a quack doctor, the history of the relationship—including her love for and plans to marry Williams, his death, and her protracted grieving—is conveyed in the sentimental mode. Maria's final conversion to the course of virtuous domesticity occurs swiftly and with virtually no preparation. Waiting at the "Asylum chapel" for an assignation, she hears a "sensible and pathetic discourse" that caused her to be "seized with all the horrors of a reproachable conscience" [2:221]. "Accident" soon after brings her to the attention of a "tradesman" able "to esteem a repenting sinner as much as a constant devotee" [2:224]; they "enter into the holy and desirable state of matrimony," which has to date produced four children.

Maria Brown's history closes, then, on a note reminiscent of Miss Williams's in *Roderick Random*: a "virtuous, honest plan of life" [2:227] eclipses the tantalizing possibilities of freedom and self-construction explored in the narrative proper. The structure of the novel, in which her independence and authority as prostitute are interrupted by the relationship with Williams and its clustering of disease, love, and death, prepares the reader for this reversion to the domesticity Maria long ago rejected when she left her parents.[30] What intrigues about this pattern is its implication that her genuine love for Williams is sufficiently alien to the plot of financial autonomy that it actually forces the novel's crisis. While venereal disease has been pragmatically regarded throughout as an unavoidable by-product of the trade, it now acquires a punitive efficacy, serving as stimulus for the conversion process completed with Maria's marriage. Emotionally and fiscally, this new "plan of life" defines her as her husband's subordinate; authorially, it entirely removes, in the absence of continuing adventures, the occasion for writing about herself.

Maria Brown indulges the prurient interests of its readers only to insist on a final retreat from the contemplation of individual pleasure. The heroine who earlier promised "to take the reader into politer scenes of action, where his curiosity, added to five guineas, could not gain him admittance," ends her narrative with the hope that some of her "fair readers should be so lucky as to gain prudence and discretion enough to escape perdition, by what they have learnt from these sheets" [2:116, 228]. The shift in gender from a complicit male reader to an educable female one is important. By casting domesticity as redemptive and venereal disease as the provocation for its recovery, *Maria Brown* allows the experiential to be superseded by the moral and then genders it female. The achievement of closure here, in other words, rehearses in peculiarly graphic terms the various kinds of subordination and sublimation present in the endings of many eighteenth-century novels.

Maria Brown can thus be seen as an exemplary instance of the textual functions served by venereal disease, whether obliquely or explicitly invoked. Maria, initially an agent of contamination but latterly of regeneration, comes to embody the moral order of the domestic realm. In our responses to her narrative, we are assumed to undergo a parallel transfiguration from questing male to "prudent and discreet" female reader. For both character and reader, venereal disease stands as the representative ailment of the dangerous world of commodity and exchange defined through powerful women, the world whose ambivalent attractions the period increasingly makes subordinate to the supposed certainties of the domestic sphere.

Notes

For their help in the preparation of this essay, I would like to thank Betty Schellenberg, Betty Rizzo, and Mark Phillips.

1. Jonathan Swift, *Gulliver's Travels*, ed. Paul Turner (Oxford: Oxford Univ. Press, 1992), 202.

2. Lawrence Stone, *The Family, Sex, and Marriage in England, 1500-1800* (New York: Harper and Row, 1977), 550.

3. Henry Mackenzie, *The Man of Feeling*, ed. Brian Vickers (London: Oxford Univ. Press, 1967), 130.

4. On the "new paradigm of dying" in which dying no longer appeared as a "Christian heroic struggle against Death but as a peaceful falling asleep," see Dorothy Porter and Roy Porter, *Patient's Progress: Doctors and Doctoring in Eighteenth-Century England* (Stanford: Stanford Univ. Press, 1989), 146-47. For a typical instance of the prostitute rendered as an object of sentimental charity, see William Dodd, *An Account of the Rise, Progress, and Present State of the Magdalen Hospital, For the Reception of Penitent Prostitutes*, 5th ed. (London, 1776).

5. See Part Four: "The Closed Domesticated Nuclear Family, 1640-1800," in Lawrence Stone, *Family, Sex, and Marriage*, 221-482. For a refinement of Stone's thesis that takes into account regional and class issues, see John R. Gillis, "Married but Not Churched: Plebeian Sexual Relations and Marital Nonconformity in Eighteenth-Century Britain" in *Eighteenth-Century Life* 9 (May 1985): 31-42 (special issue, *Unauthorized Sexual Behaviour during the Enlightenment*, ed. Robert P. Maccubbin).

6. Samuel Richardson, *Clarissa, or The History of a Young Lady*, ed. Angus Ross (Harmondsworth: Penguin Books, 1985), 1390, 1388.

7. For Gulliver's description of the "certain Malady" afflicting "prostitute Female *Yahoos*," see Swift, *Gulliver's Travels*, 257, 261.

8. Agnes Maria Bennett, *Anna, or Memoirs of a Welch Heiress. Interspersed with Anecdotes of a Nabob.* In *Four Volumes* (London, 1785), 4:194, 3:181-82.

9. Mary Ann Hanway, *Ellinor,* facsimile of 1798 ed. (New York: Garland, 1974), 4:382. I would like to thank Catherine Decker for this reference.

10. *The Fruitless Repentance, or The History of Miss Kitty LeFever,* facsimile of 1769 ed. (New York: Garland, 1974), 1:13-14.

11. Bennett, *Anna,* 4:280. The novel's closing words typically invoke the social extensions of the domestic model that has been elaborated throughout. The protagonists live "Venerated by their Children, Esteemed by their Friends, Beloved and Honoured by their Country."

12. *The Adventures of an Author. Written by himself and a friend* (London, 1767), 2:196.

13. *The London-Bawd: With her Character and Life. Discovering the Various and Subtile Intrigues of Lewd Women,* facsimile of 1711 edition, ed. Randolph Trumbach (London: Garland, 1985), 3, 6.

14. *The Tomb of Venus: or a plain and certain method, by which all people that ever labour'd under any venereal distemper may infallibly know whether they are cured or not* (London, 1710), 1-3.

15. John Clarke, *The Batchelor-Keeper. Numb. II. By Philaretus,* facsimile of 1727 edition, ed. Malcolm J. Bosse (New York: Garland, 1972), 108.

16. Mary Davys, *The Accomplished Rake, or Modern Fine Gentleman* (1727) in *Four before Richardson: Selected English Novels, 1720-1727,* ed. William H. McBurney (Lincoln: Univ. of Nebraska Press, 1963), 277.

17. John Clarke, *The Virgin-Seducer. A True History by Philaretus,* facsimile of 1727 edition, ed. Malcolm J. Bosse (New York: Garland, 1972), 95-97.

18. For a detailed consideration of rogue and criminal narratives see John J. Richetti, *Popular Fiction before Richardson: Narrative Patterns, 1700-1739* (Oxford: Clarendon Press, 1969), 23-59. For the seventeenth-century antecedents to the whore as rogue, see Roger Thompson, *Unfit for Modest Ears: A Study of Pornographic, Obscene, and Bawdy Works Written in the Second Half of the Seventeenth Century* (London: Macmillan, 1979).

19. *The Finish'd Rake, or Gallantry in Perfection,* facsimile edition of 1733 edition, ed. Josephine Grieder. (New York: Garland, 1973), 58.

20. Captain Charles Walker, *Authentic Memoirs of the Life Intrigues and Adventures of the Celebrated Sally Salisbury,* facsimile of 1723 edition, ed. Josephine Grieder (New York: Garland, 1973), 35, 33.

21. *Entertainments of Gallantry, or Remedies for Love,* facsimile of 1712 edition, ed. Josephine Grieder (London: Garland, 1973), A7v, A8.

22. Henry Fielding, *Joseph Andrews,* ed. Martin C. Battestin (Middletown, Conn.: Wesleyan Univ. Press, 1967), 86.

23. Tobias Smollett, *The Adventures of Roderick Random,* ed. Paul-Gabriel Bouce (Oxford: Oxford Univ. Press, 1979), xxxiv.

24. Smollett has Miss Williams indirectly acknowledge the uniqueness of her recovery by having her measure her own unfortunate condition against that of the more usual fate of diseased prostitutes (137-38). The contrastive technique, which reproduces Roderick's response to her story, also works, then, to establish Miss Williams as a foil to both Roderick and Narcissa.

25. In his introduction to Cleland's *Memoirs of a Woman of Pleasure* (Oxford: Oxford Univ. Press, 1985), Peter Sabor notes that the *Memoirs of Maria Brown* and *Memoirs of an Oxford Scholar* "have recently been confidently ascribed to Cleland by

their publishers, although both attributions are stylistically implausible and no evidence is offered in either case" (xi).

26. It is consistent with the more aggressive de-sentimentalizing impulse of *Maria Brown* that the "romance" which exerts a particularly deleterious influence on the heroine is Richardson's *Pamela*.

27. We are told, however, that "she Reads well, fluently, and with an admirable Grace; she writes tolerably, but Spells very indifferently. Yet it is certain, that had she been bless'd with an Education proportionable to her Natural Genius, she would have been a most accomplish'd Woman" (8).

28. *The Genuine Memoirs of the Celebrated Miss Maria Brown. Exhibiting the Life of a Courtezan in the most Fashionable Scenes of Dissipation. Published by the Author of W** of P**. In Two Volumes,* facsimile of 1766 edition (New York: Garland, 1975), 2:6.

29. See William Dodd, *Rise, Progress and Present State of Magdalen Hospital*. For a summary account of related schemes, see Vern L. Bullough, "Prostitution and Reform in Eighteenth-Century England," in *Eighteenth-Century Life* 9 (May 1985): 61-74 (special issue, *Unauthorized Sexual Behaviour during the Enlightenment*, ed. Robert P. Maccubbin).

30. The pattern is at once suggestive and very familiar. Clarissa's history, for instance, follows a parallel path: financial independence, a defining relationship with Lovelace in which her death is symbolically enacted in the rape, and the concluding representation of death as marriage to which she goes in the "all-quieting garb" of the "wedding garments" bought for the occasion (1339).

Chapter 14

Job's Curse and Social Degeneracy in Rétif de la Bretonne's *Le Paysan Perverti*

Diane Fourny

As Claude Quétel has pointed out in his admirable study on the history of syphilis, the French Enlightenment's attitude toward "la grosse vérole" marked a definitive rupture with the past in its efforts to treat the problem of sexually transmitted disease like any other illness, that is, as a legitimate object of inquiry. Confronted with the near epidemic growth of venereal disease from the seventeenth century onward, the Enlightenment's interest in its causes and cures indeed widened substantially. Yet moral valuations still weighed heavily on approaches and methods in medical research.[1] This meant that the eighteenth century's contribution toward furthering any scientific knowledge of or treatment for "le mal de Naples" would remain pitifully modest.

By the mid-eighteenth century, syphilis touches all social groups: the underclass and the nobility, rich and poor, urban as well as rural populations, the young and the old, even the unborn generation. More important, however, authorities finally begin to acknowledge that the growth of venereal infection presents a social and political calamity of incalculable proportions. Yet, these same state agencies who decry its spread (the hospitals, prisons, royal armies, and police services) do very little to control a health crisis which, they believe, threatens the nation's very moral fiber and political order.

The medical community sees the need to pronounce sexual activity, practiced within or without marriage, as now a medically dangerous human activity. This moves certain thinkers to call for a complete rethinking of the problem in terms of containment: policing social behavior, monitoring or outlawing prostitution, regulating prison populations, searching for new therapeutic technologies (the development of prophylactic ointments and baths), and finally acknowledging what we would call today the need for public education in the area of sexually transmitted diseases.[2]

The fact that venereal disease was so widespread as to become commonplace might explain how it also becomes an acceptable theme in literature; for example, three of the period's most celebrated French novels treat venereal disease in some form: *Candide, Julie, ou la Nouvelle Héloïse,* and *Les Liaisons dangereuses* (not to mention its spectacular staging in Sade's notorious *La Philosophie dans le boudoir*).[3] Once a taboo subject barely audible among medical practitioners and moralists, venereal disease is henceforth given full coverage in dictionaries of general knowledge: d'Alembert and Diderot's *Encyclopédie* includes articles on "Vénérienne" and "Vérole" (with cross-references to "Mauvais Lieux," "Brûlure," "Chaude-pisse," "Gonorrhée," "Cordée," "Bubon," "Chancre," "Salivation," and "Fumigation"). Voltaire also treats the subject in his portable *Dictionnaire philosophique* under the rubrics "Lèpre et Vérole," "Amour," and "Job."

The eighteenth century's view of venereal disease is an odd one due primarily to the fact that it still confuses the social, medical, and moral systems of human experience and knowledge on the question of human sexuality. Contemporaries might read it as part of Nature's inherent, life-giving force as well as a sure sign or consequence of the breakdown of social hierarchies, or they might read it as the demonic force subtending unbridled female sexuality. Perhaps no writer better exemplifies this odd conflation of empirical data and mythical figuration than the hopelessly underrated novelist and writer Nicolas Edmé Rétif de la Bretonne. In the lengthy epistolary novel that launched his career, *Le Paysan perverti* (1775), the topic of disease—in all its richly variegated forms—is examined through an intricate network of images and themes tying contamination and infection to the hero's story of social ascension and the author's critique of societal degeneracy. What makes Rétif's treatment of disease so unusual is precisely his ability to exploit its abundantly rich figural value, particularly that attached to sexual disease in its erotic and sacred dimensions. Rétif's text stands between a modern or "enlightened" view of disease (equating disease with economic and social disorder) and its opposite or a return to the near-medieval outlook that reads sexual disease as the outward sign of inner corruption. Furthermore, Rétif puts a personal spin on venereal disease when enlightenment and obscurantism curiously coalesce in a bizarre utopian project terminating the work, at the center of which stands the sexually diseased body.

Le Paysan perverti incorporates many styles and narrative forms. It is a novel of social ascension and libertinage that also exploits the melodramatic effects and psychological depth of novels of sensibility. Strongly influenced by Richardson and Rousseau, Rétif builds a vast, polyphonic epistolary narrative that interweaves three intimate circles of families and social arenas, from village to provincial capital to Paris. Finally, Rétif's world shares Romanticism's taste for the gothic when specters haunt cemeteries and dark alleyways of the Parisian underworld.

Le Paysan perverti recounts the story of Edmond R**, son of a rich peasant, who is sent to the city with his family's blessing to seek fortune, happiness, and self-improvement (see Pl. 15). Rétif's novel of social ascension clearly falls within a tradition of works decrying the breakdown of cultural order and social structures. In Rétif's case, the author blames this disruption on the rural exodus *en masse* toward the urban centers, which bleeds the country of its "healthy" subjects. Edmond soon falls the hapless victim of his own success and desires and of those of his two intellectual mentors: the superior-thinking libertine philosopher Gaudet, and his sometime companion, the mundane Father d'Arras. Edmond's ascent, made possible through his ever-increasing mastery of urban culture (art, philosophy, and libertinage), corresponds to his predictable, parallel descent into moral depravity, debauchery, crime, and madness. The novel ends in tragedy of seismic proportions, bringing down not only the hero but also the entire family and their circle of friends. This horrific undoing of the rétivian hero stretches interminably for hundreds of pages, slowly writing itself across his diseased body whose very scarring finally designates him as society's criminal. However, the ravages of disease also make of him, paradoxically, scapegoat and victim, and in this new role, Edmond equally functions as society's redeemer incarnate. By the end of the novel, all that remains of Edmond is a hideously deformed, one-eyed, one-armed body: a cripple covered with infectious red marks or stigmata symbolizing his sacred election. Being thus doubly branded as the guilty one and the victim of pollution, this monstrous Oedipus-Job returns to the community, drawing to him society's outcasts—the weak and the innocent—whom he has been sent to save from certain contamination and ruin. Edmond's "fall" symbolizes the purging of the body politic, laying groundwork for the arrival of a new and purified social order inscribed in the rétivian utopian project developed at the novel's close.

Thanks to the diseased sufferer's long relationship to the sacred, Rétif is able to raise a banal story of social degeneracy to a higher mythical plane where redemption of the body politic is made possible by return of the sexually diseased body, which acts like a *pharmakon*—both poison and antidote—for the purging of chaos and violence infecting the community. To follow this transformation from the social to the mythical, we shall first examine the necessary inscription of disease upon the female body: eternal origin and source of pollution. This will enable us to return to the question of disease as redemptive force when we look at its shift back to the male body (Edmond's). In a third and final section, we shall examine how venereal disease bridges the empirical world of social disease with that of the allegorical world of utopia. This will shed some light on the curious and illogical way by which Rétif chose to end his work with a utopian project of social and sexual reconstruction.

Although Rétif chooses a male protagonist to embody the morally diseased generation of late-eighteenth-century French society, the author maintains his hero in an ambiguous relation to venereal disease. We are never directly informed that Edmond has contracted syphilis, and we can only thus surmise through inference that the hero's affairs with explicitly infected female sexual partners (prostitutes) indeed leads to a venereal infection that would cause the type of ravages that later visit Edmond's body. Our suspicions are confirmed in the novel's companion work, *La Paysanne pervertie*, written several years later, in which we find Edmond's diseased state clearly pointing to syphilis.[4] However, in *Le Paysan perverti*, the infernal pox has been saved for the hero's counterpart and double, Ursule. Like her brother, Ursule migrates to the city and soon follows her brother down a similar path of social ascension and moral corruption. Sexuality and disease are thus clearly gendered in this work, collapsed into the two-headed hydra figure of the syphilitic sister/prostitute. On the one hand, Rétif merely repeats an age-old topos that couples female sexuality with the source and propagation of human evil. However, the eighteenth century lends a particularly harsh treatment to woman by designating her as primary faultmaker in the specific matter of venereal disease: she remains its source and primary vehicle of transmission.[5] While Rétif saves his hero from the moral stigmatization of venereal disease by refusing to "name" Edmond's symptoms for what they are, he marks the sister's body with a full-blown case of syphilis, which she contracts through forced and invited contacts with social outcasts and lusting misfits whose very marginality places them beyond the sphere of humanity: a filth-ridden water-carrier (for Rétif, "les porteurs-d'eau" are always certain carriers of the disease); a deformed black male servant who is ordered by Ursule's jealous and vengeful Italian lover to rape and impregnate her; a spate of perverted valets and army conscripts; and finally, any and all diseased criminal clients she perchance seduces once she has fallen to the level of a common streetwalker. Yet, if Rétif designates a secondary character as the carrier of syphilis, rather than its hero, Edmond, does the notion that venereal disease plays a significant role in the rétivian critique of society fall by the wayside? Could it not be argued that venereal disease remains of purely marginal interest here? Turning to the complicated genesis of the Edmond-Ursule cycle, we will indeed find the hero's association with venereal disease as well as locate the origins of Rétif's utopian project.

Rétif writes in a late autobiographical text that he began writing *Le Paysan perverti* in 1769, the same year he published his utopian project, *Le Pornographe*.[6] Well known to eighteenth-century scholars, *Le Pornographe* outlines a reform of prostitution by advocating nothing less than its legalization in view of more ably monitoring its activities and medical repercussions. Rétif hypothesized that the legalization of prostitution would lead to enormous progress in the control and eventual eradication of venereal disease and personal laxity.

Like the *Le Paysan perverti*, *Le Pornographe* is also written in epistolary fashion, being a monologic exchange of letters between two male friends. The project properly speaking is padded by a scantily developed love story. The author of the letters, Monsieur d'Alzan, conveniently finds himself in the home of his correspondent, who is out of town. D'Alzan is recovering from syphilis, which he contracted in London during his early years of resolute debauchery. Having returned to his native France, he carves out for himself a new life of virtue. He discovers, however, the concomitant boredom that now accompanies such an existence, which he tries to relieve by love and work. On the one side, he courts the virginal and angelic Ursule (sister of his benefactor and hostess, Mme Tianges); on the other, he whiles away the hours with his project of reform. It is obvious that D'Alzan serves as prototype for Edmond, which means that syphilis is housed within the amorous male protagonist. Also to be noted, of course, is the female protagonist, Ursule, who figures prominently in this story as a symbol of purity.

From *Le Pornographe* to *Le Paysan perverti*, syphilis moves to fix itself permanently to the female body of a different Ursule, the female protagonist having by now been transformed into the corruptible ingénue. From *Le Paysan perverti* to *La Paysanne pervertie*, published in 1784 (which is the former work all over again, told this time from Ursule's perspective), Rétif finally accords Ursule center stage (see Pl. 16).[7] Rétif saves his best descriptions of the ravages of syphilis for this third novel.

Told from the heroine's perspective of her encounter with the world of sexual and intellectual promiscuity, Rétif's fictional universe is fraught with the horrors of excess: excessive desire, beauty, wealth, and want where Ursule must confront the accompanying excesses of physical abuse, rape, humiliation, theft, hunger, and disease. From the pinnacles of fortune—having become one of Paris's most sought after courtesans—Ursule is cast down into the bowels of Paris's underworld where she turns into an unrecognizable monster of sin and disease. Here she portrays herself in the alienating voice of third-person narrative: "She is nothing. She no longer possesses either name, parents or sex; she is a monster of a nature below the human; she climbs out of it [poverty and illness], only to return, only to be the plaything of the brutes who degrade her."[8] What stands out in Rétif's feminine world becomes the hyperbolic coupling of beauty and its disfigurement, manifested through the body's scarring. Ursule's portraits emphasize the monstrous disfigurement of a past beauty:

Ursule. I am devoured by ulcers; my infected cadaver horrifies

Job's Curse and Social Degeneracy 233

even me; I grow disgusted with what I happen to touch: these exposed bones, no more fingers, are what hold my pen. Come see, at its lowest form of pain and rot, a live body, eaten, which is no longer but half of what it used to be. [*La Paysanne,* 466]
Gaudet. But what to do with this girl? Now look at her, ugly, awful, disgusting. . . . Her breath . . . that caved-in palate . . . those scarified ulcers over what she used to possess as most beautiful . . . those sunken and empty eyes . . . those sunken cheeks . . . all this makes for a monster. [*Le Paysan,* 2:48]
Edmond. Ursule has changed for the better; at present, she is bearable to look at: if her hideousness (if you'll allow me the word) continues to diminish, we will be able to take her out of her cave [= *antre,* referring to the hospital where she is receiving treatment for syphilis]. [*Le Paysan,* 2:64]
Gaudet. [Edmond] looked at her, and hurriedly raising himself, got up and ran away while turning around in fear, as if he had been chased by a ghost. [*La Paysanne,* 469]

Sander L. Gilman has duly noted how the syphilitic skin lesion was read "as a moral failing, venereal disease presented society with the overt sign of the failings of the individual." However, when marking the female body, it rejoins ancient glosses of female sexuality as deviancy and danger. Beauty is merely a mask hiding the inner bestiality, the interior pollution of Woman.[9]

In Rétif's world, venereal disease belongs not only to the woman but also to her sphere of sexual perversion, as if it had been stricken from the traditional world of bourgeois heterosexual intercourse. Ursule's relationship to the disease, the result of her sexual excesses, grows beyond the realm of "normal" heterosexual activity to embrace the category of the unnameable: bestiality, symbolized by her violent rape by the "hideous black" servant, and lesbianism. Finally, sexual excess reaches a superlative depth of depravity when it also points to incest, Ursule's lengthy and illicit affair with her own brother prompted by her seduction of Edmond.

Parallel to Ursule's sexual perversions is the highly charged homoerotic bond between Edmond and his partner in crime, Gaudet. Curiously, for all the sexual debauchery in which the two male protagonists engage, Gaudet never explicitly contracts syphilis. The figure of the noninfected homosexual of Rétif's world substantiates a claim Gilman has made that, by the eighteenth century, the replacement (i.e., guarded acceptance) of homoerotic sexuality for heterosexuality allows for the satisfaction of (male) desire without fear of contamination (moral or physical). In other words, homosexual desire was seen as a way to circumnavigate the polluted female body; homoeroticism keeps the hero at a safe distance from venereal infection in the figurative sense while the sister assumes the story of social climber to be punished for her transgression of the social order.[10] By the late sixteenth century, syphilis had become the disease of the "fog, the courtier."[11] By the close of the seventeenth century, syphilis was the affliction of the effeminate *petit-maître* attached to the court of Louis XIV.[12] At the dawning of prerevolutionary France, the male libertine seems to have found his escape through homoerotic desire.

By the conclusion of *La Paysanne,* both sister and brother are portrayed as pox-ridden, wayward souls. In the following poem, the author appears almost to enjoy describing Ursule's punishment for her crimes whereas Edmond is elevated to the role of exemplary sufferer:

Chant 26	Verse 26
Ursule, toujours plus hardie,	Ursule, always the more daring
En écarts de perversion,	In her diversions in perversions,
Gagne une laide maladie,	Traps an ugly malady,
Venant de prostitution:	From prostitution:
Défaite, difforme, ulcérée,	Haggard, deformed, ulcerated
A son frère elle fait horreur;	She horrifies her brother;
A l'hôpital elle est placée,	To the (prison) hospital she is sent
Afin d'y cacher sa laideur.	In order to hide her ugliness.

Chant 54	Verse 54
Oh! qui pourrait compter les peines	Oh! who could count the sufferings
Du pauvre et malheureux Edmond!	Of the poor and unhappy Edmond!
Tout couvert de rougeurs malsaines,	All covered with unhealthy red marks,
Aveugle et plein d'infection!	Blind and full of infection!
C'est Dieu qui prolongea sa vie	It is God who prolonged his life
Pourqu'il endurât plus longtemps	So that he endure (pain) much longer
Car elle ne lui fut ravie	For, [his life] was not taken
Qu'après les plus affreux tourments	Until after feeling the most torture.[13]

The reader's attention cannot avoid two key terms: *hôpital* and *Dieu.* Ursule's very real hell[14] stands in blatant contradistinction here to Edmond's election. Again, Ursule's exile to the "hospital," Salpêtrière, names her disease, whereas Edmond's symptoms only allude to venereal infection through the terms *rougeurs malsaines, aveugle,* and *infection.* The male syphilitic sufferer, under the protection of the deity and metaphor, thus rises to take his place at the seat of election and sacrality, bringing us to our next point and Rétif's most eccentric figuration of venereal disease.

Edmond and Ursule's common descent into moral depravity follows a parallel descent into social degeneracy. They sink into the rotting bowels of Parisian lowlife and its underworld of crime and poverty when they embark on their respective careers: swindling, prostitution, and vagrancy. They revel in self-debasement and seek its intensification at every opportunity. Edmond writes of himself as if he were a stranger: "He frequents the vilest sort of people, smoking dens, cheap bars: he only lives now among those emaciated faces that hunger and misery have dried up: idlers, swindlers, pickpockets and thieves now offer him amusing scenes.... I hid myself amongst the lowest rabble.... I soon grew disgusted with whores. I started to take girls who were even beneath that" [*Le Paysan*, 2:35-39]. Having turned to prostitution, Ursule exclaims, "My temperament has become a fury, my taste for debauchery a rage inside me; I want to annihilate myself in infamy" [*La Paysanne*, 435]. Ironically, it is from this state of depravity that they both rise again, like the Phoenix, to become the novel's redeemers.

In his seminal study on ritual sacrifice, Réne Girard has shown how the sacrificial victim embodies both the source of evil and violence plaguing a given community and the remedy for their eradication. Ritual sacrifice serves a purgatory function in the establishment and renewal of social order and cultural institutions whereby a community polarizes a maximal amount of collective violence upon a minimal quantity of victims who themselves are rendered "sacred" in the process of their expiation. Sacrifice in this respect renders the victim holy for his/her embrace of maximal evil (the violence of murder) and maximal good (the murder of an innocent). He who is identified as the community's enemy paradoxically becomes its very savior, and his violent death or expulsion merely hides, by means of the veil of the ritual, the underlying source of the purgative process: collective violence.[15]

Likewise, Edmond and Ursule's perfection in evil, the signature of which has been visibly written across their bodies in the form of the syphilitic stigmata,[16] paradoxically designates them as victims, that is, as carriers of special redemptive forces. Rétif imbues his protagonists with thaumaturgical powers that purify all who come in contact with them. Renouncing her life as a prostitute, the repentant Ursule (renamed "sister Marie") begins a new life that entails returning to the prison hospital to visit disease-stricken prostitutes or caring for those who live with her in the hospice who are still undergoing the tortuous mercurial treatment for syphilis. In one scene, the vilest of prostitutes ("back for her sixth incarceration and treatment") prostrates herself before Ursule and begs for her prayers. Afterwards, Ursule becomes an icon of saintliness and motherhood when she returns to the family farm and is reunited with her son born out of wedlock.

The earlier poetic description of the diseased Edmond (Chant 54) likens the hero to the socially cursed, yet equally revered, mythical figures of Oedipus and Job. Oedipus's pierced eyes and cleft foot are repeated in Edmond's loss of an eye and arm (the arm that murders). Similarly, the biblical Job covered with infectious sores finds his echo in Rétif's scab-and-rag-covered hero. The last books of *Le Paysan* reach gothic heights of melodrama when this monstrous one-eyed, one-armed man is spotted roaming the hero's native province at night, sleeping in graveyards, and appearing mysteriously in backyards bearing gifts for the children (his many illegitimate offspring). A towering biblical figure, Edmond finally returns to his village and like a *pharmakon*, comes to redeem the community's wayward souls and bless the righteous; his hallowed presence promises only good fortune. Ursule describes this odd phenomenon: "Today, people have gone from a state of excessive contempt to excessive veneration. I saw, and tears of emotion flowed from my eyes; in one day I saw twenty neighbors come by to apologize to him . . . so that they might marry into his family, each one hurrying to ask one of my sisters' hand in marriage. . . . The good odor of virtue makes us forget the infection of vice" [*Le Paysan*, 2:195-96].

Perhaps Rétif has not so much invented a new type of syphilitic sufferer as he has creatively drawn upon timeworn myths dealing with illness and the diseased body. Popular culture as well as "high" art had developed over centuries a stock of images and narratives to help anesthetize collective anxiety before catastrophic illnesses such as the plague, leprosy, and venereal disease. In one of Edmond's self-portraits, the hero puts a modern spin on the Old Testament narrative of Job, whose sore-covered body came to stand in for the leper during the Middle Ages: "I was less than three steps from them when I ran into Madelon and her sisters (she had been formerly betrothed to Edmond). My pallor, my bristly beard, my clothes like those of *virgines squalidae* [young girls covered in rags] of the prophet Jeremy made them turn their eyes from me. And I said: *Viderunt me, et horreurunt* [they saw me, and were filled with horror]: and with Job, *Miseremini mei, miseremini mei, saltem vos amici mei.* [Take pity on me, take pity on me, at least you who were my friends.]" [*Le Paysan*, 2:203].

The failure of Enlightenment doctors to dispel these types of myths, which only obscured the real origins and symptomology of venereal disease, was only exacerbated by the fact that some doctors themselves maintained such links between leprosy, smallpox, the plague, and syphilis. Known elements of the medical world, as well as the uneducated masses, held fast to the belief that syphilis was not a new disease at all, imported from the New World via fifteenth-century explorers, but a new form of leprosy. Voltaire devoted much of his article "Lèpre et Vérole" to dispelling the purported ties between the two diseases, and in his article on Job he ridiculed the claim that Job—"smote . . . with sore boils from the soles of his feet unto his crown" [Job 2:7]—represented the earliest historical portrait of the syphilitic sufferer. This fact demonstrates that a conflation of these diseases still prevailed at the time.[17]

As the son of pious parents (whose ancestors were renounced Huguenots), Rétif knew the Scriptures well and copiously excerpted scenes and dialogues from the Old and New Testaments. In the Edmond-Ursule cycle, biblical figures abound. Job is one of the privileged allegorical figures, and the book of Job is the favorite reading of Edmond's father and older brother (the novel's two patriarchs). Edmond's simultaneous identification with and transgression of the agrarian patriarch finds expression through the various allusions to Job, which like a template come to dominate and guide the hero's journey to the seat of election, as we have seen in the above passage or in similar passages:

> Learn from my errors, and from the terrible punishment they brought down on me: Look at me well; I am a living book upon which the Lord has written the destiny of scoundrels and the shameless; look, do not turn away your eyes. [*Le Paysan*, 2:212]

> After this confession, one day I shall dare appear before you, in order to suffer my final agony which I deserve, the indifference of my loved ones, and the disgust of my friends. [*Le Paysan*, 2:262]

The body inscribed by the outward marks of disease permits the free slippage between pure and impure, blasphemy and sacrality, and contagion and cure. Gilman has studied the iconography of this reversal in representations of syphilis in the late fifteenth and early sixteenth centuries. During this period, images of the infected individual depict him as an isolated, pox-ridden (male) sufferer, always recalling the body of the suffering Christ or martyred saint.[18] As our analysis has shown, as Rétif moves from the erotic to the religious plane, the diseased body is transformed from that of the polluted female monster, the source and carrier of the infection, to one representing the exemplary male sufferer.

In *Le Paysan perverti* the sacrificial dimension of the story comes full circle with the final staging or sacrifice of the syphilitic "scapegoats." The once infected yet now repentant Ursule is murdered (by none other than her insane brother, who is ignorant of her reform). However, through her double and substitute, Edmond, the pox-infected body also becomes the locus of healing and redemption. Rétif thus purges the community of the diseased soul and simultaneously establishes a new social order based on the return of Edmond around whom the future founders of the morally pure society will soon gather to build a new Jerusalem. Family and friends conspire to reintegrate the monstrously grotesque Edmond within their society. Infirmities and all, he is betrothed to the ever-virtuous Madame Parangon, mother of one of his many illegitimate children and the woman he had violently raped years earlier. Yet, more horrific tales befall this ill-fated family. Edmond meets his (by now) long overdue death in a freak accident, but not without first learning of the secret marriage between two of his children, Edmée-Colette and Zéphirin (who are unaware that they are siblings). As if paying for the sins of the father, the unfortunate son soon joins his dead father by succumbing to a mysterious disease. For which sins has Zéphirin been sacrificed? Rape and incest? Sexual excess or venereal infection? Or perhaps Rétif had in mind to stage the most scandalous effects of venereal disease: congenital syphilis.

The author was certainly aware of the dangers facing the unborn child whose parents had contracted syphilis, as is amply evidenced in Rétif's *Le Pornographe*. In fact, it is this threat to future generations that drives Rétif's obsession with prostitution and venereal disease.

Despite its many imperfections, Rétif's *Le Paysan perverti* remains one of the eighteenth century's most original novels for daring to combine speculative ideas on society's reform with imaginative narrative. Yet his work borders on the eccentric when he transforms an otherwise naughty erotic epistolary novel into a utopian platitude. How and why would an author choose to mix such an odd duo?

What this study has not been able to emphasize for lack of space is that Rétif's massive epistolary narrative equally turns around the actions of Gaudet, the libertine, whose quest for knowledge and power is insatiable. His mastery of human desire both fascinates and terrifies the naively impressionable pupils, Edmond and Ursule.[19] The interminable exchanges between mentor and pupil on every metaphysical and aesthetic subject imaginable read like a compendium of Enlightenment secular dogma. Ursule becomes his prized pupil; Edmond becomes the wayward prodigal son who always returns to the father for forgiveness and guidance. What Gaudet offers them is knowledge, and the libertine's knowledge is, of course, synonymous with self-empowerment: the power to dominate and transform. Yet, to transform what or whom and to what end? As I already explained, the novel ends in a debacle that confirms Rétif's vitriolic denunciation of the urbane and cultured world of Parisian society. Paris's power to dominate becomes a seduction of the rural masses, the pernicious flight of human labor from the country to the urban center of immense wealth for the elected few and certain poverty for the ignorant many. In this context, the two versions of the Edmond-Ursule cycle read as a novelized form of Rousseau's "Discourse on the Sciences and Arts."

By the second half of the eighteenth century, social upheaval expressed as the physical degeneracy of the nation's population is perhaps a well-worn leitmotif of Enlightenment literature. In the rétivian universe, upheaval occurs not only in the socioeconomic sphere but also, and more significantly, in the world of intellectual inquiry. The perversion of knowledge that places itself solely in the service of self-interest—Reason's blind spot—finds its image returned in the reflection of the syphilitic's poxed-eaten eye: the eye of inquiry of a blinded Edmond, of Pangloss or Madame de Merteuil, or symbolically, of the Sadean mother's genitalia.

By the end of *Le Paysan perverti*, villains and dupes alike have either disappeared or repented. This return to order is staged as a grand cleansing: the snuffing out of the diseased body and mind in preparation for the return to the "lost garden." Rétif's journey back indeed mimics Rousseau's regressive turn toward a society modeled on a mythical agrarian form of social organization. Rétif's utopia—like all utopias—proves to be disappointingly predictable. Unsurprisingly, the "siege" mentality dominates Rétif's program, obsessed with control, contamination, and invasion from without. The dream of retrieving Adam's lost garden expresses all too clearly the unsubtle desire to rid the community of its unclean—requisite sacrifice for the fertilization and development of the future generations. Once purged, the land, its inhabitants, and their culture are cut off, immured in an atemporal and hermetically sealed space. Details of Rétif's perfect society are spelled out in the list of statutes that terminates the novel. The community's government is ideologically totalitarian, economically agrarian, and socially patriarchal. An all-knowing, all-loving, omnipotent father guarantees the moral direction of the community and sees to it that "our children [are forever preserved] from the inevitable contagion of the cities, and guarded from misery."[20]

Rétif's use of the word *contagion* is to be taken literally and figuratively, since the novel's direct filiation has been established to the author's earlier utopian project, *Le Pornographe*. In this earlier work, contagion means much more than venereal infection; it represents what Rétif perceived (and he was not alone in this) to be a great social and political threat to France. As *Le Pornographe* explains, prostitution is not simply an evil in itself. (Rétif was of the same opinion as Diderot on this point, that is, that sexuality was a natural, hence amoral, human activity.) Rather, it represents the single greatest source for the *depopulation* of the nation. Rétif never envisaged the eradication of prostitution as a whole but only that of the venereally diseased prostitute whose polluted body was a catastrophic curse on the properly "male" house of France. Venereal disease weakened the male constitution in its reproductive functions, rendering the man impotent or simply beyond cure. Worse, it blatantly passed down to future generations (who are always, curiously, males in this text) the very seeds of degeneracy in the form of a sickly, effeminate character or certain infantile death. In the year of *Le Pornographe*'s publication (1769), questions surrounding the depopulation theory were on the minds of many. France was only eleven years from the founding of its first hospital for "newborns attacked by venereal disease" (1780) and another fifteen years from the establishment of its first public hospital reserved solely for the care of the venereally diseased adult population.[21]

Once placed in this context, that is, within the prevailing discussions bordering on collective hysteria over the problem of depopulation, the *Paysan(ne)* cycle reveals its deep involvement with the Enlightenment projects of reform. Underlying every utopia is the problem of evil, understood as the source of social disharmony and unrest. In Rétif's world, evil is the child of thought, culture, and aesthetic refinement that thrives among the degenerate subjects of urbane French society. Furthermore, Rétif has chosen to express evil metaphorically as a contagious disease spread by the notorious "other" of society: the venereally diseased female. However, as the story of Edmond's diseased body also shows, contagion may reverse into its sacred election to become the source of renewal and cure. In other words, Rétif's novel arrives at utopia since, by definition, utopian thought invariably returns to the archaic logics of sacrifice. Projects of social reconstruction must forcibly build their new societies upon the sacrifice of a few to ensure the healthy future of the many.

It comes as no surprise that these utopias emerge during the troubled decades of prerevolutionary France. Nor should it surprise us that French society at the time associated some of their uneasiness concerning social and economic turmoil with disease—more specifically, with venereal contamination. Even the physician who wrote the *Encyclopédie*'s article on "Vérole" in 1785 predicted that "one can thus be assured that this illness will finish with the human species, and that it will one day represent the cause of a revolution in Europe . . . similar to the one which occurred in the fifth century, when the Roman monarchy fell into the abyss because of its weakness, its luxury, and its debauched mores."[22]

We should also not lose sight of Voltaire's Pangloss, whose pox-riddled face ties venereal disease not only to the "sin" of knowledge but also to that of greed. Behind Pangloss's burlesque story explaining how chocolate made its way to Europe by the same route taken by venereal disease, Voltaire hides his scathing condemnation of the New World's rape by greedy Europeans. As Gilman has suggested, sexual disease became Europe's punishment for having destabilized the placid "Old World Order." During the Renaissance, the overbearing reality of sexual disease was tied to the notion of punishment for "disruption of the clear though already crumbling boundaries of nationality and class, in allowing the marginal and disaffected a place of their own."[23]

The punishment Rétif meted out to his hero and heroine in the *Paysan(ne)* cycle confirms Gilman's theory and demonstrates that the figure of the sexually diseased body remains mythically charged two hundred years later; the difference for Rétif is that the "disruption" and "crumbling boundaries" fester within France's borders, having been transformed into the great migratory waves of human labor toward the cities. Although the Enlightenment may have shed little useful light on a better medical understanding of and cure for venereal disease, venereal disease—as it figures in the literature of the period—teaches us much about the way in which French society expressed its collective fears before profound social and economic change.

Notes

1. Claude Quétel, *Le Mal de Naples: Histoire de la syphilis* (Paris: Seghers, 1986), 95-108.

2. On prostitution and venereal disease in France, consult Erica Marie Benabou, *La prostitution et la police des mœurs au XVIIIe siècle* (Paris: Librairie Académique Perrin, 1987); on medical, philosophical, and literary expressions of the sexually diseased body, see Sander L. Gilman's *Sexuality: An Illustrated History Representing the Sexual in Medicine and Culture from the Middle Ages to the Age of AIDS* (New York: Wiley, 1989); on the separation of hospital and prison populations and the emergence of prophylactic technologies, see Quétel, *Le Mal de Naples*, 108-19.

3. In *Candide*, Voltaire uses Pangloss's infection (by way of Paquette, the servant girl) to develop a biting commentary on Europe's economic and social rape of the New World. The despicable Madame de Merteuil of *Les Liaisons dangereuses* is horribly disfigured by the novel's end—fitting punishment for a life of debauchery. Sade's Eugénie in *La Philosophie dans le boudoir* orders her mother to be raped by an infected valet, which ensures certain death of future offspring (once the mother is also "sewn shut"). Though readers may be surprised to find Rousseau's Julie listed here among the "vérolés," it is my contention that Julie's contraction of "la petite vérole" (smallpox) is merely a smoke screen for venereal disease. If only by way of allusion, the "pox" still leaves her noticeably disfigured; furthermore, she contracts the disease because of her illicit sexual relationship with Saint-Preux, who has fathered the unborn child she loses through miscarriage. Julie's disease, or "fault," cannot be separated from the eighteenth century's obsession with sexually transmitted disease and sexuality in general. Illicit sex, feminine sexuality, pregnancy, and monstrosity (the aborted foetus) form a network of interrelated themes that transcribe Julie and Saint-Preux's tragic fault in terms of moral and social disease. Proof of these connections remains the fact that, at this time, medicine had still not isolated syphilis from other venereal diseases, and certain doctors still believed that the "grosse vérole" (Grand Pox) was related to smallpox and leprosy. Given that the *Encyclopédie*'s article on vérole claimed as totally false any connection between the two poxes, people probably continued to confuse the two diseases. Hence, Rousseau's rendering of sexuality's ravages upon the heroine readily belongs to the same semantic field of sexually transmitted infection and moral disease. For other literary references to venereal disease in the eighteenth century, consult the essay by Patrick Wald Lasowski, "Syphilis et littérature," in *Peurs et Terreurs face à la contagion*, ed. J.-P. Bardet et al. (Paris: Fayard, 1988), 296-313.

4. In a letter to Gaudet, Edmond recounts his unseemly visit to a prostitute, which sours his newly acquired taste for lowly brands of sexual debauchery. After a casual embrace ending in coition, the prostitute abruptly proceeds to douch herself with the famous "eau de Préval" bath, a bogus mercurial treatment intended to stop venereal infection. She invites Edmond to use some himself. See *Le Paysan perverti*, 2 vols. (Paris: Union Générale d'Edition [10/18], 1978), 1:412. All subsequent quotations and references are taken from this edition of the novel unless indicated otherwise.

5. It is more than telling that the woman is perceived to be more closely attached, if not highly receptive, to venereal infection when we read in the *Encyclopédie*'s article, "Vérole," that men may hope for total recovery from syphilis (though in most

cases, the cure is less than full); however, it adds, a woman will never be completely cured. Furthermore, women's symptomology points to a more profound contamination than that of men. Not only does she contract all the horrible "outward" symptoms that men do, she also rots more intensely from within, which doctors tried to demonstrate from autopsies revealing the rotting of ovaries, uterus, vagina, and breast and gland tumors.

6. He writes about the genesis of his novel in *Mes Oeuvres*, cited in *Le Paysan perverti*, 2:308. *Le Pornographe* is reprinted in the collection *L'Enfer de la Bibliothèque Nationale*, 2, *Oeuvres érotiques de Rétif de la Bretonne* (Paris: Fayard, 1985). The original title of this second work is *Le Pornographe ou Idées d'un honnête homme sur un projet de règlement pour les prostituées, Propre à prévenir les malheurs qu'occasionne le publicisme des femmes avec des notes historiques et justificatives* (1769).

7. Rétif also published a new edition of *Le Paysan perverti* in 1787, which incorporates first editions of both works, *Le Paysan* and *La Paysanne*. In this version, the libertine philosopher, Gaudet, and his companion, Father d'Arras, have been collapsed into one and the same villainous hero: the libertine philosopher, Gaudet d'Arras.

8. Translated from the French edition of *La Paysanne pervertie* (Paris: Garnier-Flammarion, 1976), 433. All translations are mine.

9. Gilman, *Sexuality*, 203. Also see Gilman's remarks on the face, mask, and disease (ibid., 85).

10. See Gilman's provocative development of this idea in his chapter on "Goethe's Touch" (ibid., 221-30).

11. Ibid., 88.

12. Quétel, *Le Mal de Naples*, 95-96.

13. *La Paysanne pervertie*, 551, 558.

14. Although all the secondary works cited in this essay document the horrors of Paris's various prison hospitals, see esp. Quétel, *Le Mal de Naples*, 127-31, for a particularly "Dantesque" description.

15. René Girard, *Des Choses cachées depuis la fondation du monde* (Paris: Grasset, 1978).

16. Ursule writes: "I wish only to live in a state of penitence and wailing, in order to erase, by the power of my tears, the marks which vice has imprinted upon me" (*La Paysanne*, 471).

17. "Dictionnaire philosophique," *Oeuvres complètes de Voltaire* (Paris: Fortic, 1828), 6:239-44 and 345-49.

18. Gilman adds: "The image [of] the male sufferer is portrayed as the primary victim of the disease, rather than as its harbinger": *Sexuality*, 80. See *Sexuality*, chap. 3, particularly the subsection on "Disease and Sexuality," 77-88.

19. On Gaudet Edmond writes: "I want to believe that this man is a real friend, but he is too dangerous. What surprises me with him is that he is without principles: he has devised for himself a system of loose living, monstrous in truth, yet which possesses all the same, a certain harmony" (*Le Paysan*, 2:154).

20. Quoted from the last paragraph of the "Statutes" establishing the covenant of Rétif's utopian enclave, which comprises Edmond's family (or what remains of it): "Ouden, composed of the R** Family, living in community." Rétif closes the novel with this sentence (*Le Paysan*, 2:303).

21. Quétel, *Le Mal de Naples*, 130.

22. Quétel quoting the doctor Sanchez (Antoine Numes Ribeiro), "Observations sur les maladies vénériennes" (Paris, 1785), ibid., 22.

23. Gilman, *Sexuality*, 22.

Chapter 15

Contagion and Containment

Sade and the Republic of Letters

Julie Candler Hayes

It is hardly surprising that the Marquis de Sade should include venereal disease among the scenarios of a literary project aimed at achieving encyclopedic thoroughness in the exploration of the darker side of the sexual imaginary. He succeeded to such an extent that it is such works as *Justine, Juliette,* and *Les 120 Journées de Sodome* that have come to stand for another form of venereal contagion, as purveyors of pornography's textual "disease." Sade's texts mobilize both dimensions of diseased embodiment in a representation of syphilitic infection and in a meditation on the relation of pornographic representation to action in the world.

At first glance, Sade's view appears similar to that of the feminist lawyer and antipornography activist Catharine MacKinnon, who argues that in pornography, word and act become the same, that the consumer of pornography is "having sex."¹ Or as Sade puts it as he explains the importance of the pornographic narratives recounted for the pleasure of the libertine characters in *Les 120 Journées,*

> Il est reçu parmi les véritables libertins, que les sensations communiquées par l'organe de l'ouïe sont celles qui flattent davantage et dont les impressions sont les plus vives.²

> ⟨It is understood among true libertines that the sensations communicated by the organ of hearing are those which produce the greatest pleasure and the liveliest impressions.⟩

Sade's other texts also stress the erotic possibilities of narration and exemplification and their role in libertine pedagogy. In Sade's writings and in the discourse of the antipornography campaign there are two sorts of bodies: the body of the reader/viewer/listener, and the body of the text/image. (For brevity's sake I shall be referring to readers and texts, although I think it probable that the different media are differently cathected by their audiences.) The textual body is a contagious body: its scenes and scenarios replicate themselves, viruslike, in the body of the reader. The reader's body is passive; once acted upon, invested, infested, it becomes capable, according to some, of reenacting the scenarios of violence and domination on the body of another. The body of the reader is like the body of the eventual victims in its penetrability, its availability to assault or contagion from without. Only within the pornographic body—text or image—reside true agency and originality.

In this chapter I am going to question this model of infection and replication, partly through a questioning of the familiar metaphoric glide between the domains of perception, morality, and disease, but primarily through a consideration of how "contagion" functions in and around the writings of the marquis de Sade. I will look first at specific representations of venereal disease in Sade's works, then turn to various condemnations of pornographic "contagiousness," particularly Catharine MacKinnon's *Only Words* and the transcript of the Sade trial of 1956, in order to analyze their contending notions of "embodiment." Sade is of interest for several reasons here. From the publication of *Justine* and *La Philosophie dans le boudoir* in the 1790s, to Catharine MacKinnon's pronouncements in the 1990s, Sade is consistently singled out as the author of exemplary dangerous, contagious texts.[3] Foucault singles him out as exemplary in another respect: as one whose texts embody epistemic rupture and the absolute limit of *la pensée classique*. In this view, Sade's texts are implicated in the construction of the modern natural body, the disciplinary body. It is this body that the antipornography campaign strives to defend. And yet, as I will argue, Sade's understanding of contagion and his own "contagiousness" both enable and undermine the disciplinary drive of normalization.

Sade's writings, like the pornography debate itself, offer two versions of contagion, which for simplicity's sake one might categorize as "biological" and "psychological." At first sight it would appear that there is less attention given to the former. The destruction wrought on the body in these texts is almost invariably brought about not through "contagion" as such but through torture, mutilation, and rape, and even these physical acts derive much of their significance from the superimposition of various semiotic grids, notably kinship structures and religious practices.[4] On occasion, Juliette and other master libertines have recourse to poison, but this too is a foreign substance introduced into the body, which it disrupts more in the manner of a knife than that of a disease,

Contagion and Containment 245

despite the systemic effects, for it remains the inert instrument of a poisoner. Venereal disease also tends to be portrayed, on one level, as a weapon for the voluntary invasion of the victim's body.

The infectious disease that leaves the most visible mark in the eighteenth-century French novel is smallpox, which occasions a moment of sublime devotion in Rousseau's *Julie,* when the hero receives "l'inoculation de l'amour" at his lover's bedside, and one of dire retribution in Laclos's *Liaisons dangereuses,* when the marquise de Merteuil's disfiguring illness leaves "her soul written on her face." Syphilitic infection understandably makes fewer appearances in nonclandestine literature, although a notable exception occurs when Voltaire's Pangloss recounts the illustrious genealogy of his illness in one of *Candide*'s scenes of rueful comedy. A lingering suspicion that the two diseases were related remains in the language (*petite vérole* and *grosse vérole*), however: the *Encyclopédie* speculates that they may be distinct, but it refrains from definitively pronouncing on the question.

Pockmarked characters make occasional appearances in Sade's novels, as in those of other writers, but the "great pox" is not especially privileged as an accident of sexual life. It is true that Sade's libertine communities—the chateau of Silling in *Les 120 Journées,* the monastery of Sainte-Marie-des-Bois in *Justine,* and the Society of the Friends of Crime in *Juliette*—restrict their sexual economies to exchange within a controlled group. But libertines do not as a rule limit their sexual activity to members of these groups, and in any event the elaborate screening procedures detailed in *Les 120 Journées* do not single out "health" as an issue.[5] Indeed, one of the members of the group, the "duenna" Fanchon, has what appears to be a syphilitic chancre.

> Elle avait soixante-neuf ans, elle était camuse, courte et grosse, louche, presque point de front, n'ayant plus dans sa gueule puante que deux vieilles dents prêtes à choir; un érésipèle lui couvrait le derrière, et des hémorroïdes grosses comme le poing lui pendaient à l'anus; un chancre affreux dévorait son vagin et l'une de ses cuisses était toute brûlée. [*OC* 13:43]

> ‹She was sixty-nine years old, flat-nosed, short, fat, squinting, with scarcely any forehead and in her stinking mouth only two old teeth ready to fall out; her ass was a running sore and hemorrhoids large as a fist hung from her anus; a horrible canker ate at her vagina and one of her thighs was burned.›

Fanchon's genital sores and a notable lack of sphincter control provide the culminating moment in the series of descriptions of the members of the Silling seraglio, which range from the indescribable loveliness of the boys and girls to Fanchon. This portrait is introduced by a well-known passage arguing that, for the true libertine, ugliness has more appeal than beauty: "La beauté, la fraîcheur ne frappent jamais qu'en sens simple; la laideur, la dégradation portent un coup bien plus ferme, la commotion est bien plus forte, l'agitation doit donc être plus vive" [OC 13:41-42]. ‹Beauty and youth only affect one in a single manner; ugliness and degradation strike a firmer blow and produce a livelier agitation.› Fanchon's chancre, a symptom of mortal illness, functions as an element of a portrait meant to evoke the maximum shudder of disgust, even horror, but her illness plays no further role in the action (unlike the sphincter problem). Thus, even though it appears to be the referent of a natural biological body, the chancre's function is "semiotic" rather than "biological," a signifier and not a symptom. All the libertines have sex with Fanchon to no ill effect, and she is eventually massacred along with most of the other members of the household.

A brief scene occurs in *Juliette* [OC 8:135-36], where Juliette narrowly avoids becoming infected during her career as a prostitute (she turns around just in time to see her client's chancres). Here, the disease functions to provide yet another novel "passion" for the catalog. The frustrated client explains, "Payerais-je les femmes aussi cher, si ce n'était pas pour le plaisir de leur communiquer mon venin? C'est là mon unique passion, la seule cause qui fait que je ne me fais point guérir." ‹Would I pay as much for women if it weren't for the pleasure of communicating my venom to them? It's my only passion, the only reason that I don't get myself cured.›

A more significant instance of venereal contagion occurs in the final scene of *La Philosophie dans le boudoir,* a set of "philosophical dialogues" that detail the education of young Eugénie de Mistival at the hands of a group of libertines. In the last scene, when her mother comes to retrieve her, the accomplished pupil is able to demonstrate what she has learned by overseeing the abuse and rape of her mother. At last the libertine Dolmancé calls in his syphilitic valet:

> J'ai là-bas un valet muni d'un des plus beaux membres qui soient peut-être dans la nature, mais malheureusement distillant le virus et rongé d'une des plus terribles véroles qu'on ait encore vues dans le monde. [OC 3:545]

> ‹Outside I've a valet armed with what is perhaps one of the finest members that Nature has produced, but which is unfortunately running with virus and eaten away by one of the worst cases of pox the world has ever seen.›

The valet Lapierre is made to infect Mme de Mistival, whose vagina and anus Eugénie promptly sews up using a thick red thread, so that the infection will better "concentrate," according to one of the libertines:

> Je crois qu'il est maintenant très essentiel que le venin qui circule dans les veines de madame ne puisse s'exhaler; en conséquence, il faut qu'Eugénie vous couse avec soin le con et le cul, pour que l'humeur virulente, plus concentrée, moins sujette à s'évaporer, vous calcine les os plus promptement. [*OC* 3:546]

> ‹I believe that it is now essential that the venom presently circulating in my lady's veins be prevented from evaporating; as a consequence, Eugénie must carefully sew up your cunt and ass, so that the virulent humor, more concentrated, less likely to evaporate, will scorch your bones all the more promptly.›

Dolmancé administers syphilis to Mistival as part of a carefully calculated and controlled performance. In this parody of medical practice, the disease is ironically associated with medicine when Dolmancé suggests to Lapierre that having sex with Mistival might cure him. Later Dolmancé quips that the "inoculation" is hardly like anything produced by Tronchin [*OC* 3:546].

This *pharmakon* is actually considered a poison, of course. The interchangeability of disease and poison is reflected in the Latin meaning of the word *virus*, "poison." In Sade's day, medical understanding had not yet clearly distinguished virus from bacteria or organic from inorganic "*venin.*" As Claude Quétel has observed, in the late eighteenth century, French chemical theories of venereal contagion competed with parasitic theories as well as with notions of "sympathetic" inflammation of disease from one part of the body to another.[6] Speculations regarding "tiny animals swimming in the blood" had been current since midcentury, but Sade's implicit model seems more akin to the other theories. "Sympathy" functions as an explanatory model insofar as it describes the resonance of a material body, as in Diderot's work. In particular, however, Saint-Ange's concern with the evaporation of "l'humeur virulente" harks back to earlier humoral theory as well as to more current work suggesting that venereal disease occurred by means of "an ethereal and fermentative phlogistic principle, which by its communication infects the other fluids of the human body."[7] Sade here reverses the direction or meaning of such "exhalations," and what had been viewed as the agent of contagion now offers a potential for dissipation. The evocation of the disease in *La Philosophie dans le boudoir* would seem to participate in several overlapping, loosely connected, and evolving sets of beliefs about the body and bodily communicability, a point to which I shall return.

Other issues are at work in the outrage done on Mistival, including such typical Sadean elements as Eugénie's desire to be unique (sewing her mother up "so that you won't give me any brothers or sisters" [*OC* 3:546]), a horror of maternity, and the odd *frisson* (so appreciated by Barthes) produced by the gratuitous physical detail of the thread. What is not commented on, of course, is that the sewing-up prevents Mme de Mistival from infecting another libertine (such as her husband, who is in league with her torturers). Contagion is effectively contained, both by its enclosure within Mistival's body and by Dolmancé's total control of his valet, who performs precisely as ordered.

More dangerous in its disseminating effects is the libertine word. Much of the fascination that Sade has exercised on twentieth-century writers and critics, from the surrealists to *Tel Quel* and beyond, stems from his reiterated insistence that language is the true body of desire; representation, the most arousing of crimes. The entire elaborate combinatory structure of *Les 120 Journées* is built on the systematic recitation and replication of carefully graduated acts or "passions"; in the pedagogical *Philosophie dans le boudoir*, the libertine attentiveness to speech is underscored when Dolmancé sends Augustin out of the room during the reading of a political pamphlet—no revolution in front of the servants, please.

In short, Sade proposes a communicative model that is very much that of those who have wanted to control and contain his writings from his day to ours. Two classic attacks on his writings—the novelist Rétif de la Bretonne's 1798 *Anti-Justine,* and critic Jules Janin's 1834 essay on Sade for the *Revue de Paris*—offer key scenes in which a character reads a text of Sade's and finds himself driven in one case to erotic violence—

> Or, de toutes les lectures la plüs entraînante, est celle des Ouvrages Erotiques, surtout lorsqu'ils sont accompagnés de Figures expressives. Blasé sur les Femmes depuis longtemps, la *Justine* de Dfds me tomba sous la main. Elle me mit en feu; je voulus jouir; ét ce fut avec fureur: je mordis les seins de ma Monture; je lui tordis la chair des bras.[8]

> ‹Now, the most compelling reading of all is that of Erotic Works, especially when accompanied by expressive Figures. I had been bored with women for a long time when Dfds's *Justine* came into my hands. It inflamed me; I wanted to experience pleasure, and did so in a furor: I bit the breasts of my Mount and twisted the flesh of her arms.›

and in the other, to insanity.

> Je vous laisse à penser ce que devint ce jeune homme ignorant,

timide et frêle, à la lecture d'un livre qui suffirait à ébranler les organisations les plus solides.... Comme tout entier le pauvre petit Julien succombe sous le souffle empoisonné du marquis de Sade! comme il retirait en ployant en deux son corps si frêle pour n'être pas touché par cette lueur pestilentielle! [Janin, in Laugaa-Traut, 130]

‹I leave you to imagine what became of this ignorant, timid, and frail young man while reading a book capable of unsettling the most solid of temperaments.... Poor little Julien, how he succumbs to the poisonous breath of the marquis de Sade! how he draws back, his frail body bent double so as not to be touched by the pestilential light!›

Rétif, as Jean-Marie Goulemot has pointed out, is given to hyperbolic depictions of texts' effects on readers; he participates in a gradual "medicalization" of the act of reading that accompanies the increasingly materialist preoccupations with the psychobiological conditions of "sympathy," *sensibilité,* and the like.[9] Janin's fervid imagery, on the other hand, appears rather to bespeak the fears instilled by the Parisian cholera epidemic of the early 1830s and a persistent belief in contagion through "miasma."

I wish to call particular attention to two aspects of these texts. One is the double mechanism whereby the act of reading can either incite the reader to violence or work violence on the reader; the second is the way that the language of contagion or poison furnishes the explanatory medium for the reader's cathexis. Rétif calls *Justine* "un poison" (and *L'Anti-Justine* "le contrepoison"); for Janin the key terms (other than *frêle!*) are *poison* and *pestilence.* He is echoed in an 1842 piece by Joseph Joubert, who refers to "the odor of this foul [*infect*] book" in speaking of *Justine,* but refuses to cite the title, "for fear that the air might be soiled." Interestingly, this reference to Sade arises in the context of a discussion of Staël's *Delphine* and others marked by the Revolution, or as Joubert puts it, "born in the same atmosphere and during the same plague" [Laugaa-Traut, 135].

The twin effects imputed to Sade's texts, inciting some readers to violence and doing violence to others, are also attributed to pornography in Catharine MacKinnon's book *Only Words.* Like Rétif, MacKinnon envisions strong forms of reading wherein the text's representations of violence suborn and invest the desires of the reader. Many of her examples are meant to build a case for this "causative" feature of pornographic representation: "George Fisher was convicted of the murder and attempted rape of Jean Kar-Har Fewel, an eight-year-old adopted Chinese girl found strangled to death hanging from a tree in 1985. Mr. Fisher testified that he went to an adult bookstore on the day of the murder to watch movies" [MacKinnon, 125-26n. 62]. MacKinnon goes farther, however, in that, like Janin, she also attributes to the pornographic text the capacity to oppress, silence, and victimize (female) readers. Just as courts have recognized the aggression and asymmetrical relations produced by sexual and racial harassment, so, she argues, pornography needs to be recognized as a form of hate speech aimed at silencing women and keeping them in a subordinate place [MacKinnon, 9-10, 108, passim].

Sade, it might be noted, also provides examples of both kinds of textual work in *La Philosophie dans le boudoir*. Dolmancé and Saint-Ange are careful to let theory precede practice, and they actually begin Eugénie's education with a language lesson: "Ces mouvements se nomment *pollution* et, en terme de libertinage, cette action s'appelle *branler*" [*OC* 3:385]. ‹These motions are called *masturbation* and the action is called, as the libertines say, *jerking off*.› Thus, the "causative" aspect of obscene representation is amply demonstrated in the dialogues' pedagogical narrative, in which Eugénie is already crying out, "Je voudrais une victime," well before her mother arrives [*OC* 3:471]. The victimization of Mme de Mistival is so blatant, however, that it can distract us from noticing the effective silencing of two male characters in the final scene. In contrast to his earlier earthy volubility, the gardener Augustin never speaks after having been recalled following Dolmancé's reading of the pamphlet "Français, encore un effort si vous voulez être républicains." One wonders if he had previously "gone too far" in expressing a preference for having sex with Eugénie rather than Dolmancé. While Augustin's silence may represent the restrictions and impositions of class hierarchy, the case of the chevalier, a social equal, is striking. The brother of Saint-Ange and an enthusiastic participant in the education of Eugénie, the chevalier responds to "Français, encore un effort" with an unexpected attempt at rebuttal. He does not defend traditional morality as such, but rather makes a typically "enlightened" appeal to civic virtue guided by reason and "heart." Dolmancé scoffs [*OC* 3:527], neither Eugénie nor Saint-Ange is swayed, and the chevalier speaks less and less in the final scenes. His final utterances express his resignation as he joins in the orgy surrounding Eugénie's mother: "Obéissons, puisqu'il n'est aucun moyen de persuader ce scélérat que tout ce qu'il nous fait faire est affreux" [*OC* 3:544]. ‹Let's obey, since there is no way of persuading this villain that everything he makes us do is abominable.›[10]

What does it mean to observe that the models of linguistic effect and affect denounced by pornography's critics are already contained in Sade's text? In the first analysis, it might be said that Sade justifies the critics by providing them with examples and appearing to agree with them. The clear, unilateral functioning of libertine pedagogy, the upholding of class privilege, and the extinction of any opposition point to a well-regulated, disciplined, "disenchanted" world of hierarchy, exclusion, and control, of clear and distinct bodies and identities. We are not surprised to find such strictures in the conservative critic Janin, nor even in the more plebeian Rétif, whose opposition to Sade and whose vaunted sexual fetishism rely on similar strategies of exclusion, distinction, and possession.

The case of MacKinnon is more complex. On the one hand, she skillfully points out the absurdities in the American legal system's dogged efforts to distinguish "content" and "expression," "ideas" and "acts." On the other hand, her own distinctions and conflations seem no less forced. Pornography is viewed in exclusively heterosexual terms[11] in which there is one possible subject position for the male, one for the female, in their relation to or consumption of the text. Female pleasure could only be understood as false consciousness. MacKinnon nods briefly in the direction of classical speech-act theory, but she dismisses more recent inquiries into language, meaning, and the social as "elitist."[12] She makes no reference to the work of feminist film theorists who have analyzed the complex ways in which women interact with pornographic representation.[13] The flat demarcations of objects, persons, and schools of thought are carried out by an identitarian logic that manifests itself everywhere: "pornography is no less an act than the rape and torture it represents" [MacKinnon, 24]. No less an act, no doubt, but it is not *the same* act.

"Sameness" is the law of *Only Words*, whose rhetorical energies constantly work to align heterogenous examples, corral them into place, and produce guilt by association. The essentializing gesture creates some logical tensions. MacKinnon is skeptical that even the most "clinical" therapeutic or academic setting can divest pornography of its innate capacity to harm (female) spectators or incite (males) to violence.[14] But if this is so, what are we to make of MacKinnon's own dramatic examples? They range from the memorable second-person opening pages of *Only Words* ("You grew up with your father holding you down," etc.) to innumerable cases and precedents, to the quotation *in extenso* of a letter sent by a man to a woman (actually, three women) in which he details the (inelegantly expressed, but fairly standard) sexual acts he hoped to perform with her, ending with the threat that made the letter something other than a valentine that misfired: "I am going to fuck you even if I have to *rape* you" [MacKinnon, 133-34, n. 47]. Elizabeth MacArthur has argued that if MacKinnon is right, then there is no difference in the letter's interpellation of its addressee, "Sandy," who found it waiting on her desk one day, and its effect on the (female) reader of *Only Words*, and that the would-be abolitionist, whether Catharine MacKinnon or Jules Janin, cannot escape replication, cannot escape being pornography's purveyor.[15] This odd "epistolary moment" in *Only Words*, consigned to the footnotes, does remind us that letters find themselves in odd destinations, that the itineraries and acts of reading produced along the way remain as various as they are turbulent and unpredictable.

Is reading "dangerous"? In the "Français, encore un effort" section of

La Philosophie dans le boudoir, Sade—more precisely, the authorial "I" of the pamphlet—produces a defense that MacKinnon could use as well, in which he denies any "perverse intention":

> Tant pis pour ceux que ces grandes idées corrompraient, tant pis pour ceux qui ne savent saisir que le mal dans les opinions philosophiques, susceptibles de se corrompre à tout! Qui sait s'ils ne se gangrèneraient peut-être pas aux lectures de Sénèque et de Charron? Ce n'est point à eux que je parle: je ne m'adresse qu'à des gens capables de m'entendre, et ceux-là me liront sans danger. [*OC* 3:494]
>
> ⟨So much the worse for those whom great ideas corrupt, who can see only evil in philosophical opinions, who can be corrupted by anything! Who knows but that they might be infected by reading Seneca and Charron? It is not to them that I speak: I address only those people who are capable of understanding me, and they will read me without danger.⟩

The word *danger* derives from Old French *dangier* (to be at someone's mercy), which is from Latin *dominiarium* (the ability to dominate). Despite its often disembodied contemporary usage, then, the word's etymology involves personal relations, an aspect that is reinforced by the phrase used by Chrétien de Troyes and other medieval writers: *an son dangier* (to be in her power). *Danger* evokes a (male) fear of powerlessness and the (female) power of sex.

The danger in reading is a common refrain in debates over what the eighteenth century called *mauvais livres,* a category that included licentious works as well as antireligious or politically suspect books. Danger is also the operative term in the "Sade trial" of 1956. In this trial, similar in certain respects to the landmark judicial reviews of Joyce and Lawrence, publisher Jean-Jacques Pauvert was brought to court for publishing the first serious, generally available editions of Sade's works, officially categorized as "contraires aux bonnes moeurs." Pauvert called France's leading intellectuals to his defense—and lost. The transcript of the trial[16] reveals curious moments of "contagiousness" among the arguments of the prosecution and the defense. (It also bears an uncanny structural resemblance to *La Philosophie dans le boudoir:* seven "scenes," mostly dialogued sections, and longer exhortatory set pieces by the lawyers.)

The first three witnesses were Pauvert himself, Jean Paulhan, and Georges Bataille. The judge's skepticism and aggressivity are evident in the first exchange, where he interrupts Pauvert to remind him of "le caractère et le danger de ce livre" [*L'Affaire Sade,* 44]. Pauvert argues that his relatively expensive, limited-run edition aimed at specialists ("des philosophes, des professeurs") does not constitute a public "danger," but in effect he has already lost his case by leaving open the possibility that a more widely diffused edition would indeed be "dangerous." Subsequent scenes do little to change the situation. In his interrogation of Jean Paulhan, the judge uses the words *danger* and *dangerous* seven times; Paulhan does little good to Pauvert's case by making a reference to Saint-Just and turning the judge's language on its head:

> Président. Vous trouvez que la pureté de cette destruction n'est pas dangereuse pour les moeurs?
> J. Paulhan. Elle est dangereuse. J'ai connu une jeune fille qui est entrée au couvent après avoir lu les oeuvres de Sade.
> Président. Vous trouvez que c'est un mauvais résultat que d'être entrée au couvent?
> J. Paulhan. Je constate que c'est un résultat. [*L'Affaire Sade*, 49-50].

> ‹Judge. You believe that the purity of this destruction is not dangerous for morality?
> Paulhan. It is dangerous. I once knew a young girl who went into a convent after reading the works of Sade.
> Judge. You believe that entering a convent is a bad consequence?
> Paulhan. I merely observe that it is a consequence.›

Finally, Georges Bataille, after a sombre evocation of Sade's "contemplation de la mort et de la douleur," makes a disconcerting—given the circumstances—admission:

> Il est certain en effet que la lecture de Sade ne peut être que réservée. Je suis bibliothécaire; il est certain que je ne mettrai pas les livres de Sade à la disposition de mes lecteurs sans aucune espèce de formalité. [*L'Affaire Sade*, 56]

> ‹Certainly the reading of Sade must be controlled. I am a librarian; certainly I will not put Sade's books at my readers' disposal without any sort of formality.›

Even André Breton's erudite written deposition (which begins by citing the *Philosophie dans le boudoir* passage on readers who can read "sans danger") uses the language of "poison" to claim that Sade's very excesses provide their own "antidote."

Even the prosecution appears to change sides, however, when the prosecuting attorney begins his summation by describing the unenviable plight of his predecessor who argued the Flaubert and Baudelaire obscenity trials of the nineteenth century and thereby earned himself an ignominious place in literary history. For the lawyer, the whole business is not so much "dangerous," perhaps, as "delicate" [*L'Affaire Sade,* 69]. The "danger" most prevalent in the Sade trial, apparently, is making the other side's case one's own.

That "danger" emanates from certain profound fears, rather than causing them, is suggested not only in the history of the word but also in Mary Douglas's classic study of pollution, disorder, and contagion, *Purity and Danger.* Much of her analysis underscores the degree to which "pollution danger" arises in proportion to the degree of formal structure in a given society.[17] There exist several kinds of dangers or threats to the system, of which the human body is often the fantasmatic map. Prominent among these threats is pressure on the system's "external boundaries." Most dangers, however, reside within: dangers from the margins, from crossed "internal lines," from inconsistency and self-contradiction [Douglas, 94-122, passim].

It is not difficult to imagine scenarios in which these types of threat become related, as when the social body projects its own internal tensions and disruptions onto a conveniently externalized other: illegal aliens, AIDS patients, "foreign" terrorists. It is simpler to mobilize political and intrapsychic energies against a focused, distinct, external agent. Thus diseases are construed in terms of foreign origins: "French sickness," "maladie de Naples," etc. The same work of rationalization and externalization is carried out in military metaphors, which, as Susan Sontag points out in her essay on the cultural construction of AIDS, draw together a number of compatible narratives of "alien takeover" in science fiction, disease management, and politics.[18] So too pornography. To the extent that it can be identified, isolated, and banned, there is the illusion that some dangerous incursion in the body politic might be arrested. During the Sade trial, the judge and Bataille exchange words over whether or not the purchasers of Pauvert's edition might be moved by "unhealthy curiosity" [*L'Affaire Sade,* 58], but neither stops to address the issue of the *prior* existence of such "curiosity" before the encounter with a "dangerous" book.

In a rather more thoughtful discussion of transgression elsewhere, Bataille meditates on the way in which "transgression" is proportionately related to "law." Like Douglas, he also considers how the blurring of the identities and internal lines afforded by law produces acute anxiety: "Nous ne serions pas terrifiés ... par la violence si nous n'avions conscience, obscurément, qu'elle pourrait nous porter nous-mêmes au pire" ⟨We would not be terrified ... by violence if we weren't in some way aware that we ourselves could be drawn to the worst.⟩[19] The truly dangerous moment is that of uncanny recognition, the moment of "the system against itself," in Douglas's phrase, the moment of the dissolution of distinctions that opens out onto what Bataille calls in *L'Érotisme* "la transgression indéfinie."

Contagion and Containment 255

Sade might well be "dangerous" in this way. For if, as I have said, he appears to "justify his critics," working within a purely rationalized system of controlled and controllable transmissions and exchanges—thereby revealing the violent potential in "enlightened" operations, as Horkheimer and Adorno once argued[20]—in other ways various refractory elements of his writing continue to suggest that, as in mathematics, the formal system must be either incomplete or inconsistent.[21] The crucial instability in his work accounts for its continuing to be privileged as particularly "dangerous," whether or not one classifies it as "pornographic."[22]

Let us then return to Sade. *Les 120 Journées de Sodome* stages the disappearance of "clear and distinct bodies" despite what appears to be a paroxistic exercise in classification and control, where competing and asymmetrical sets of familial, affective, ideological, and erotic relational systems criss-cross the categories until, as Buffon said, there are only individuals. And yet each individual-in-relation bears little resemblance to the classical liberal notion of the "bourgeois individual." As for *La Philosophie dans le boudoir,* consider those moments when various forms of "contagion" offer a countermodel to rationalized procedures for transmission. As we have seen, the moment of Mistival's infection is already the site for some odd reversals: remedy/disease, intensification/dissipation. Communication is an occult phenomenon and takes place out of sight. The final passage of the pamphlet "Français, encore un effort" makes the argument for a radical political isolationism *so that* the republican model imagined in the text might spread beyond the nation's borders: the contagiousness of the exemplar. In an earlier passage, however, the "spread" of ideas is accompanied by a reference to the spread of disease.

> S'il règne, je suppose, une influence malsaine à Hanovre, mais que je ne doive courir d'autres risques, en m'exposant à cette inclémence de l'air, que de gagner un accès de fièvre, pourrai-je savoir mauvais gré à l'homme qui, pour m'empêcher d'y aller, m'aurait dit qu'on y mourait dès en arrivant? Non, sans doute; car, en m'effrayant par un grand mal, il m'a empêché d'en éprouver un petit. La calomnie porte-t-elle au contraire sur un homme vertueux? qu'il ne s'en alarme pas: qu'il se montre, et tout le venin du calomniateur retombera bientôt sur lui-même. [*OC* 3:495]
>
> ‹Let us imagine that there is an unhealthy wind in Hanover but that the only risk I run in exposing myself to this inclement air is to catch a sudden fever; should I bear a grudge against the man who in order to prevent me from going told me that I would die as soon as I set foot there? Certainly not: for by fright-

ening me with a great ill he prevents me from suffering a lesser one. And if a virtuous man finds himself the object of calumny? Let him not be alarmed: let him reveal himself, and all the venom will fall back on the slanderer himself.⟩

This defense of calumny comes just after the passage previously referred to on reading *sans danger*. It is an incongruous passage, redirecting the idea of contagion or poison away from its traditional analogous relation with calumny and attributing to the latter a remarkable dichotomizing power. Calumny casts both vice and virtue into sharp relief in contrast to the argumentative weight of most of *La Philosophie dans le boudoir* but in keeping with the Rousseauist dreams of "transparency" in the revolutionary republic. The passage on calumny also points to Sade's unquestioning assimilation of the belief current in his day that disease was communicated by the air, by unhealthy "exhalations" and "miasmas."[23]

It is not my purpose here to follow up all the implications and ramifications of these many discursive filaments. I only note their multiplicity and observe that they bear uneven and varying relations to the text's arguments, which some support, others contradict, and to which others seem indifferent. These fragments—I am thinking particularly of the floating references to contagion, air, evaporation, and openness—form a not fully articulated group of beliefs about corporeal existence that, by their fragmentariness, say something about the status of "systematic" thought in Sade and that, as part of a generalized somatic unconscious, suggest an alternative to the disciplined models of communication that we have seen in the pornography debate from his day to ours.

In his analysis of "corruption" in *La Philosophie dans le boudoir*, Claude Lefort discusses the ways in which the *disjecta membra* of the discourse of civic humanism contribute to the vision of profound social disintegration.[24] "Corruption" bespeaks both the discourse of political failure and that of bodily decay, tissue breakdown, fetid exhalation, contagion, dissolution, dispersion, and dissipation. Mistival's sewn-up orifices notwithstanding, the body imagined by the text is not an intact, distinct, or autonomous body. Rather it is a "dissipative" body, susceptible to change. Above all, it is open, porous. We might take as emblematic of the body's enigmatic openness the curious notion that Mistival's syphilis might somehow "evaporate," as well as the realization that, far from closing off her body, the sewing is only a pretext for gratuitously puncturing the flesh, perforating its surfaces, letting blood flow freely.

In his history of cleansing practices in France, Georges Vigarello offers a look at the evolution of cultural constructions of the body in the early modern period. Although he sees significant changes, particularly in terms of the body's relative "passivity" or "autonomy," it is still striking to observe the durability of an image of the body as open and permeable through its myriad pores. Water and steam were shunned in the sixteenth and seventeenth centuries for fear of the plague, for example: "the skin being, as a result of the heat, more easily opened, pestilential air gets in."[25] Even as bathing became more accepted in the eighteenth century, it was still understood that water penetrated the body throughout, insinuating itself "into every interstice," according to the *Encyclopédie*. In the words of a 1756 source, "The force with which water enters the pores is immense. Its limits are unknown" [Vigarello, 95]. In the late eighteenth century, an increasingly medicalized view of cleanliness contributed to an ever more rigorously normative regulation of the pores and severe social measures aimed at controlling dangerous "exhalations" and "emanations." This "open" body is not the same as the disciplined, rationalized "penetrable body" of the antipornography campaigns. The penetrable body exists insofar as its identity and that of the other can be said to remain rigorously distinct; there is no possibility for exchange or cross-identification that is not categorized as aberrant. The open or porous body is a site for infusion, evaporation, and change; in its mobility it cannot be said to maintain a distinct, intact, or unified subject.

I have not attempted to claim that the changing state of medical knowledge from Sade's day to ours results in a specific change in our construals of bodily communicability. Therefore, rather than arguing that an epistemic break occurred in the move toward definition and regulation of the "natural body," I tend to see smaller-scale shifts within an ineluctably fissured hegemony, a tesseract of residual and emergent practices. Sade can figure as a prophet of modernity for Paulhan, Bataille, and, for that matter, MacKinnon, but as I have argued here, his revolutionary moment is closely implicated in a historically locatable form of body-consciousness. The porous body, particularly when considered in terms of Sade's materialist view of life forms as evanescent permutations of matter in motion, offers an understanding of mutable, permeable embodiment far removed from the models of bodily communication that subtend much of the contemporary rhetoric of "danger," whether in the context of disease control or in that of the antipornography movement. Abandoned for a time by "normal science" in the wake of the bacterial revolution's intensification of the dichotomies of body and disease, inside and outside, attack and defense, this "older" form of embodiment finds echoes in the contemporary discourse of the body as "ecology."[26] The open body may provide a useful site for psychosocial imagining, offering complexity without hierarchy, identity without exclusion, and communication without contagion.

Notes

I am grateful to Ladelle McWhorter, Linda Merians, and Charles Stivale for their helpful comments and criticisms at various stages of this project.

1. "In other words, as the human becomes thing and the mutual becomes one-sided and the given becomes stolen and sold, objectification comes to define femininity, and one-sidedness comes to define mutuality, and force comes to define consent as pictures and words become the forms of possession and use through which women are actually possessed and used. In pornography, pictures and words are sex. At the same time, in the world pornography creates, sex is pictures and words. As sex becomes speech, speech becomes sex." Catharine MacKinnon, *Only Words* (Cambridge: Harvard Univ. Press, 1993), 26.

2. D.A.F. de Sade, *Les 120 Journées de Sodome*, in *Oeuvres complètes*, ed. Gilbert Lely (Paris: Cercle du livre précieux, 1967), 13:27. Further references to Sade's works will be to this edition, indicated by the abbreviation *OC*. All translations are mine. I am indebted to Elizabeth J. MacArthur for having pointed out the parallels between MacKinnon's and Sade's accounts of textual effect, in her paper "Extreme Reading: Ultimate Sade and the Censor's Ultimatum," presented at the meeting of the Modern Language Association, Toronto, December 1993.

3. "For example, if a professor were to force students to read some of the work of the Marquis de Sade as part of a course on French society, 'it would be actionable,' she said." "[Catharine] MacKinnon Leaves Yale Grads with Tough Talk on Sex Abuse," *National Law Journal*, 1989, cited by Carolyn J. Dean, *The Self and Its Pleasures: Bataille, Lacan, and the History of the Decentered Subject* (Ithaca: Cornell Univ. Press, 1992), 123.

4. Roland Barthes's reading of Sade offers the most thorough such analysis: "Pour le reste, tout est remis au pouvoir du discours. Ce pouvoir, on n'y pense guère, n'est pas seulement d'évocation, mais aussi de négation. Le langage a cette faculté de dénier, d'oublier, de dissocier le réel: écrite, la merde ne sent pas; Sade peut en inonder ses partenaires, nous n'en recevons aucune effluve, seul le signe abstrait d'un désagrément. Tel apparaît le libertinage: un fait de langage." *Sade, Fourier, Loyola* (Paris: Seuil, 1971), 140-41. For an analysis of the ways in which Sade confounds the kinship categories constitutive of society, see Josué V. Harari, *Scenarios of the Imaginary: Theorizing the French Enlightenment* (Ithaca: Cornell Univ. Press, 1987), 172-87.

5. In contrast, Sade's contemporary (and enemy) Rétif de la Bretonne envisages careful disease control in the state-run brothels he proposes in *Le Pornographe* (1769). Similar institutions proposed in the "Français, encore un effort" section in Sade's *La Philosophie dans le boudoir* involve no such hygienic measures.

6. Claude Quétel, *The History of Syphilis*, trans. Judith Braddock and Brian Pike (Baltimore: Johns Hopkins Univ. Press, 1990), 73-81.

7. *James's Medical Dictionary*, translated by Diderot in 1747. Cited by Quétel, *History of Syphilis*, 78.

8. Rétif de la Bretonne, *L'Anti-Justine* (Paris: J-C Lattès, 1980), 1. This preface also appears in Françoise Laugaa-Traut, *Lectures de Sade* (Paris: Colin, 1973), 89.

9. Jean-Marie Goulemot, *Ces livres qu'on ne lit que d'une main* (Aix-en-Provence: Alinéas, 1991), 48-51.

10. There is also an instance of a form of "self-silencing" on Dolmancé's part. In spite of his role as master of the libertine "word," he refuses to explain what he wants to do with Augustin when the two leave the room briefly ("cela ne peut pas se dire"), leaving the chevalier to whisper his intentions to Eugénie and Saint-Ange out

of the reader's "hearing" (*OC*, 3:532). Despite the powerful clarity of definitions and examples, it seems that language derives force from what is left unsaid, from its own (momentary) lapses and wells of oblivion. The contrast between Dolmancé's silences and the defiant words of his pamphlet, "N'avons-nous pas acquis le droit de tout dire?" (*OC*, 3:513), should be seen as one of the principal conflicts running through the work.

11. The Dworkin/MacKinnon Model Ordinance is framed in terms of the "subordination of women" presumably by or at the very least *for* men. The brief proviso that one can substitute "men, children, or transsexuals in the place of women" only reifies the assigned roles through the insistence on women's "place" (MacKinnon, *Only Words*, 121-23, n. 32).

12. See MacKinnon, *Only Words*, 31 (and 123n. 41) for a blanket condemnation of "postmodernism" as oblivious to social stratification, or see her scathing allusion to contemporary concerns with "representation" (MacKinnon's quotation marks) as "non-reality" (ibid., 28-29).

13. See, among many, Linda Williams, *Hard Core: Power, Pleasure, and the "Frenzy of the Visible"* (Berkeley: Univ. of California Press, 1989), especially chap. 7 on the issue of women's possible "multiple identifications" in sadomasochistic pornography (184-228).

14. "Many believe that in settings that encourage critical distance, its showing does not damage women as much as it sensitizes viewers to the damage it does to women. My experience, as well as all the information available, makes me think that it is naive to believe that anything other words can do is as powerful as what pornography itself does.... Tom Emerson said a long time ago that imposing what he called 'erotic material' on individuals against their will is a form of action that 'has all the characteristics of a physical assault'" (MacKinnon, *Only Words*, 108).

15. In "Extreme Reading," Elizabeth MacArthur discusses the dilemma of replication in *Only Words* and in Janin's "Julien" sequence.

16. Jean-Jacques Pauvert, ed., *L'Affaire Sade: Compte-rendu exact du procès intenté par le ministère public, aux Editions Jean-Jacques Pauvert* (Paris: Pauvert, 1957). Reprinted in Pauvert, *Nouveaux (et moins nouveaux) visages de la censure* (Paris: Les Belles Lettres, 1994).

17. Or, as she pragmatically puts it: "Where there is dirt there is system. Dirt is the by-product of a systematic ordering and classification of matter, insofar as ordering involves rejecting inappropriate elements." Mary Douglas, *Purity and Danger: An Analysis of the Concepts of Pollution and Taboo* (London: Routledge and Kegan Paul, 1966), 35.

18. Susan Sontag, *AIDS and Its Metaphors* (New York: Farrar, Straus and Giroux, 1989), 18.

19. Georges Bataille, *L'Erotisme* (1957; Paris: Union Générale des Editions, 1975), 71.

20. Max Horkheimer and Theodor Adorno, *Dialectic of Enlightenment*, trans. John Cummings (German orig., 1949; trans. 1972; New York: Continuum, 1987). See esp. "Juliette, or Enlightenment and Morality," 81-119.

21. As Jane Gallop puts it, "Sade's work seems to be a long, concerted effort to subsume the body, sexuality, desire, disorder into the categories of philosophy, of thought. But there is always some disorderly specific which exceeds the systematizing discourse": "The Immoral Teachers," *Yale French Studies* 63 (1982): 122.

22. In the Sade trial, both prosecution and defense tend to agree that Sade is "boring" (*L'Affaire Sade*, 62). On the difficulty of classifying Sade as "pornographic," see Goulemot, *Ces livres qu'on ne lit que d'une main*, 90-91, among others. Lynn Hunt

sees in Sade the "culmination" of the early modern pornographic tradition of social and political commentary, but she also sees him as something of an anomaly in the revolutionary decade. "Pornography and the French Revolution," in *The Invention of Pornography*, ed. Lynn Hunt (New York: Zone Books, 1993), 331-32.

23. See Alain Corbin, *The Foul and the Fragrant: Odor and the French Social Imagination* (Cambridge: Harvard Univ. Press, 1986).

24. Claude Lefort, "Sade: Le Boudoir et la Cité," in *Ecrire: A l'épreuve du politique* (Paris: Calmann-Lévy, 1992), 91-111. Lefort's account of the politics in *La Philosophie dans le boudoir* complements that of Michel Delon, for whom the text's inconsistencies point to "cynisme indicible" in "Sade Thermidorien," in *Sade, écrire la crise*, ed. Michel Camus and Philippe Roger (Paris: Belfond, 1983), 99-117.

25. N. Houel, *Traité de la peste* (1573), cited by Georges Vigarello, *Concepts of Cleanliness: Changing Attitudes in France since the Middle Ages*, trans. Jean Birrell (Cambridge: Cambridge Univ. Press, 1988), 9.

26. Francisco Varela and Mark Anspach discuss immunological research that rejects inside/outside dichotomies and the reliance on "defense" as a guiding principle, in favor of a theory of "autonomous immune networks": "autonomous" and engaged in "self-production," rather than determined by incursions from the "outside"; "networks" or "ecologies" suggesting decentered complexity, rather than strategically hierarchized "systems." See "The Body Thinks: The Immune System and the Process of Somatic Individuation," in *Materialities of Communication*, ed. Hans U. Gumbricht and K.L. Pfeiffer, trans. W. Whobrey (Stanford: Stanford Univ. Press, 1994), 273-85.

Contributors

Susan P. Conner is a professor and chairperson of History at Central Michigan University. She has published articles on women in the French Revolution, marginality, crime, and medical issues in *Journal of Women's History, Journal of Social History, Eighteenth-Century Life,* and *Eighteenth-Century Studies.* A book-length study, tentatively titled *Artisans of the Street: Prostitution in Revolutionary Paris,* is in progress.

Barbara J. Dunlap is head of Archives and Special Collections of the Library of the City College of the City University of New York. She is currently working on an edition and translation of Marie Angelique Anel Lerebours's *Avis aux meres qui veulent nourrir leurs enfants.*

Diane Fourny is an associate professor of French at the University of Kansas. She has published articles on the eighteenth-century French novel, Rousseau, Diderot, and René Girard.

Leon Guilhamet is the author of two books in eighteenth-century studies: *The Sincere Ideal: Studies on Sincerity in Eighteenth-Century English Literature* and *Satire and the Transformation of Genre.* He is professor of English at the City College of New York.

Julie C. Hayes is an associate professor of French at the University of Richmond. She is the author of *Identity and Ideology: Diderot, Sade, and the Serious Genre* (1991) and a number of articles on eighteenth-century topics. She is currently completing a book project on systemization, rationalization, and critical consciousness in the French Enlightenment.

April London teaches English at the University of Ottawa. She has written on early women writers, the Tradescants, Samuel Richardson, Henry Fielding, Ann Radcliffe, Jane West, and Henry Mackenzie.

Fred Lowe lectures at the Royal College of Surgeons in Ireland and at Trinity College Dublin and University College Dublin. He has published articles on Jonathan Swift, Mary Wollstonecraft, William Hogarth, and Samuel Beckett.

Marie E. McAllister has taught at Villanova University and Naussau Community College. She is currently working on women's travel writing and the novel and on the literature of the 1790s. She has published articles on Samuel Richardson and Hester Thrale.

Linda E. Merians is an associate professor of English at La Salle University. She has published articles on eighteenth-century primary-source research, representations of the so-called 'Hottentot' in British literature, Mary Astell, Colley Cibber, John Abell, and Matthew Prior, and on teaching South African literature. She is completing a book on the figure of the 'Hottentot' in British literature from the Renaissance through the nineteenth century.

Kathryn Norberg is an associate professor of History at UCLA. She is the author of *Rich and Poor in Grenoble, 1600-1814*, and, with Philip Hoffman, has edited *Fiscal Crises and Representative Government*. She has published articles on prostitution in France and Europe, the poor in eighteenth-century France, and women in seventeenth- and eighteenth-century France. A book on prostitution and its representation in seventeenth- and eighteenth-century France is forthcoming from the University of California Press.

Roy Porter is a professor in the Social History of Medicine at the Wellcome Institute for the History of Medicine. He is currently working on a general history of medicine. His most recent books include *London: A Social History* (1994) and, with Lesley Hall, *The Facts of Life: The Creation of Sexual Knowledge in Britain, 1650-1950*.

Betty Rizzo is a professor of English at the City College of New York and the Graduate Center of the City University of New York. She is the author of books and articles on Christopher Smart and eighteenth-century women writers. Her most recent books are *Companion without Vows: Relationships among Eighteenth-Century British Women* (1994) and an edition of Sarah Scott's *The History of Sir George Ellison* (1996).

Mary Margaret Stewart is a professor of English at Gettysburg College. She has published articles on Boswell, Collins, Smart, and Fielding.

Philip K. Wilson is an assistant professor of the History of Science at Truman State University. He has recently edited a five-volume work entitled *Childbirth: Changing Ideas and Practices in Britain and America, 1600 to the Present* and *Medicine In the Enlightenment*. His articles have appeared in *Annals of Science*, *London Journal*, and *Journal of the Royal Society of Medicine*.

Rose Zimbardo is a SUNY Distinguished Professor at Stony Brook and teaches at the University of San Francisco. Her best known books are *Wycherley's Drama: A Link in the Development of English Satire* and *A Mirror to Nature: Transformations in Drama and Aesthetics 1660-1732*. Her latest book is *At Zero Point: Politics, Discourse, and Satire in Restoration England* (forthcoming).

Index

Abelove, Henry, 188
Account of the Institution of the Lock Asylum (1788), 141
Account of the Nature and Intention of the Lock Hospital (1796), 143
Account of the Proceedings of the Governors of the Lock Hospital (1751), 134
Addison, Joseph, 177, 190; *Spectator* #50, 177-78
adultery, venereal consequences of, 105-6, 155-56, 159. See also *Trials for Adultery*
Adventures of an Author, 216, 219-20
AIDS and venereal disease, 10-11, 35, 42, 50 nn 62, 68, 254
animals, as symbols of sexuality, 170, 172, 176, 178, 180, 191
antipornography debate, 244, 249-55, 259 nn 11, 12. See also pornography
Antoinette, Marie, 2
Armstrong, John, 121; *Oeconomy of Love*, 121-22
associationism, 190
Astruc, Jean, 8, 18, 23, 36, 116, 172-73, 174, 175, 176, 177; *De Morbis Veneris Libri Sex*, 1, 5, 6, 7, 8
Avison, Charles, 136; *Ruth*, 136
Ayloffe, John, 204; "Advice to a Painter," 203-4

Balfour, Francis, 6; *Dissertation medica inauguralis de gonorrhoea virulenta*, 6
Barry, Spranger, 135
Barrymore, Lord, 153
Bataille, Georges, 252, 253, 254, 257
Battie, William, 181; *Treatise on Madness*, 181

Baylis, Dr., 91-92
Beauclerk, Topham, 159-61, 162
beauty spots, 178-80
Becket, William, 5, 11 n 9
Bell, Benjamin, 6; *A Treatise on Gonorrhea Virulenta*, 6
Belloste, Augustine, 72
Benabou, Erica Marie, 9, 19-20, 47 n 13, 49 n 34
benefit performances, 135-36
Bennett, Agnes Maria, 215; *Anna*, 215, 226 n 11
Benoit, Madame, 37
Bible: story of Job, 235-37; Book of John, 130
Bienville, 44; *Fureurs utérines*, 44
bills of mortality, 150, 164 n 2
Blackmore, Richard, 194
Blake, William, 103, 209; "London," 103, 209
Blankaart, Steven, 77; *Venus Belegert en Ontset*, 77
Blumenberg, Hans, 183
Bolingbroke, Lord "Bully," 155-64
Boswell, James, 7, 11 n 12, 52, 156, 157, 199; *London Journal*, 7
Boucher, François, 170, 171; *La Toilette*, 170
Bouverie, Mrs., 139
Boyveau, Paul, 24
breast-feeding, 115, 117-18
Brest, Vincent, 72
Breteuil, Minister of the Interior, 27
Breton, Andre, 253
Brief Account of the Institution of the Lock Asylum (1802), 143
Bromfield, William, 12 n 15, 129, 131, 136, 145 n 15, 155

Bryson, Norman, 168
Buchan, William, 88-89, 95
Bunbury, Lady Sarah, 158
Burrows, John, 6, 10, 85-99, 129, 150, 152; *A Dissertation on the Nature and Effects of a New Vegetable Remedy*, 94-99, 100 n 9, 101 n 26, 150; *A New Practical Essay on Cancers*, 93-94, 101 n 26; *Remarks on Certain Passages*, 90
Butler, Samuel, 201-2, 206-7; *Hudibras*, 201-2, 207
Bynum, W.F., 6, 9, 52, 64 n 9, 81, 96
Byron, George Gordon, 199

Cadogan, William, 122
Carnegie, Robert, earl of Southesk, 204
Carter, Elizabeth, 139
Carteret, Mrs., 139
Carteret, Robert, 156
case histories:
—British: Barrymore, 153; Belcher, 156; Bolingbroke, 156-64; Chudleigh, 152, 165 n 9; Cibber, 152, 163-64, 165 n 9; Dewars, 106; Folkestone, 152, 165 n 9; Heatley, 155; Morpeth, 153; Robinson, 155-56; Sandwich, 152, 165 n 9; Siddons, 105, 152, 165 n 9; Spencer, 157-64; Thrale, 103-4; Williams, 106-10, 156; Worgan, 155
—French: Dubuisson, 28; Guerchy, 153; Henriette, 26, Marianne, 15-16, 17, 25; Marie, 26; Marie Elisabeth, 26; Sabot, 28. *See also* periodical press
Cavendish, Mrs. Anne Isabella, 139
Charles II (England), 203
Charles VIII (France), 5
Chicoyneau, François, 69, 72, 79-80
children: attacks on, 134-35, 145 n 12; congenital syphilis, 118, 125 n 2, 174-75, 182 n 12; venereal disease in, 9, 19, 25, 42, 115-27, 152, 173-76, 193, 215. *See also* Foundling Hospital; hospitals
Chudleigh, Elizabeth, 152
Churchill, Charles, 197, 210; *The Ghost*, 208-9
Cibber, Colley, 185; *Love's Last Shift*, 185

Cibber, Susannah, 152, 163
City Politiques (Crowne), 185-86
Clarke, John: *The Batchelor-Keeper*, 216; *The Virgin-Seducer*, 216
Clowes, William, *Morbus Gallicus*, 95
Cobb, Samuel, 116; translation of *Callipaedia*, 117
Cockburn, William, 69, 73, 76
College, Stephen, 204; "An Historical Poem," 204-5
Collier, Jeremy, 198
Copp, Dr., 152
Coram, Thomas, 122, 126 n 28
Cotes, Charles, 129
Country Wife, The (Wycherley), 185
Coventry, Lady, 157-58
Cowley, Robert, 173-74, 175, 176, 177, 180
Cuisin, Pierre-François, 45; *Les femmes entretenues*, 45-46
Cullerier, Michel, 17, 27-28
cured, eighteenth-century notions of, 71, 73-74, 132, 144 n 7

Dabydeen, David, 179
Dartmouth, countess of, 139
d'Aucour, Godard, 37; *Thermidore*, 37
Davenant, Charles, 189; *Essay upon the Probable Methods*, 189
Davys, Mary, 217; *The Accomplished Rake*, 217-18
de Bachaumont, Louis Petit, 36
De'Coetlogon, Rev. Charles, 137
Defoe, Daniel, 69, 114, 115, 117, 125 n 2, 189, 207; *Moll Flanders*, 114, 117; *Reformation of Manners*, 207
de Horne, 16, 25-26, 32 n 38, 36
de Knorr, Lewis Wilhelm, 172; *Venus à la mode*, 172
de la Chanterie, Madamoiselle, 38
de La Mettrie, Julien Offroy, 35
de la Morandière, Turmeau, 39
Delaney, Mary, 110
Delasalle, Claude, 123
Delaunay, Paul, 9, 24
de Marsilly, Raffart, 24
Denman, Thomas, 117-18, 121
Desault, Pierre, 69, 72, 80

Index 265

de Velno, 89-91
Dickinson, Robert, 89
Diderot, Denis, 19, 34, 35, 46, 229, 239, 247; *Encyclopédie*, 34, 46, 46 n 1, 116, 229, 240, 241 nn 3, 5, 257
divorce, 159. *See also Trials for Adultery*
Donne, John, 197, 210 n 5
Dorset, "A Faithful Catalogue of our Most Eminent Ninnies," 205
Douglas, John, 69, 72, 73, 74, 80-81, 84 nn 38, 39
Douglas, Mary, 254; *Purity and Danger*, 254
Dover, Thomas, 69, 76, 80, 83 n 28
Downman, Hugh, 117; *Infancy, or the Management of Children*, 117
Dryden, John, 184; "The Medal," 202-3
DuBarry, Madame, 43
Duncan, Andrew, the elder, 6; *Observations on the operation and use of mercury in the venereal disease*, 6
Dunn, Edward, 73
D'Urfey, Thomas, 186; *The Fond Husband*, 186

Earle, John, 200-201, 209
Entertainments of Gallantry, 218
Erasmus, 197, 198, 199, 209; *A Marriage in Name Only*, 197-98
Evangelicalism, 4, 136-37

Farington, Joseph, 152, 164 n 2, 165 n 10, 167 n 43
Farquhar, George, 197, 199
Fauchery, Pierre, 37
Ferne, James, 72
Fettiplace, George, 129
Fielding, Henry, 220; *Joseph Andrews*, 220
Finish'd Rake, The, 218
Fitzgerald, Lady Mary, 139
Foederé, 46
Folkestone, Lady, 152, 165 n 9
Foote, Samuel, 135
Forrest, Alan, 124-25
Foucault, Michel, 21, 35; *Folie et deraison*, 21
Foundling Hospital (London), 122, 135

Foundling Hospital (Paris), 123, 124
Fox, Henry, 106, 108, 109, 111 n 16, 112 nn 17, 28, 113 n 29
Fracastoro, Girolamo, 198; *Syphilis*, 198
Franks, Dr., 152
Frederick, duke of York, 139
Fredrick, Jonathan, 135
Fruitless Repentance, The, 215-16

Gardane, J.J., 17-18, 24-25, 26
Garrick, David, 135
Garrick, Eva Maria, 135, 139
Garth, Samuel, 205; *The Dispensary*, 205
Genuine Memoirs of the Celebrated Miss Maria Brown, 221, 222, 223-25, 227 n 26
George III (England), 136
Giardini, Felice, 136; *Ruth*, 136
Gilman, Sander, 233, 237, 240, 241 n 2
Godwin, William, 223; *Caleb Williams*, 223
gonorrhea: complications of, 7; symptoms of, 7, 70; treatment of, 7-8, 53. *See also* venereal disease
Gould, Robert, 202; "Love Given O'er," 202
Goulemot, Jean-Marie, 249
Granville, George, 105; "Cleora," 105-6
Green, Joseph, 52
Grover, Jan Zita, 35
Guerin, Maynard, 129
Guillemeau, Jacques, 115; *The Manual of Nursing and Bringing Up of Children*, 115-16

Hall, Joseph, 199, 200; *Virgidemiarum*, 199
Hamilton, Sir William, 157
Handel, George Frideric, 135; *Judas Maccabeus*, 135-36
Hanway, Jonas, 122
Hanway, Mary Ann, 215; *Ellinor*, 215
Hardy, S., 16
Hecquet, Philippe, 23; *Traité de la Peste*, 23
"Hodge," 204
Hodson, Dr., 91, 92
Hogarth, William, 168-81, 213; *A*

Harlot's Progress, 168, 190-94; *A Rake's Progress*, 178-79; *Enthusiasm Delineated*, 178-179; *The Four Times of Day*, 179; *Marriage à la Mode*, 172-73, 180
homoeroticism, 233-34
hospitals (that treated venereal disease), 4, 20;
—French: Bicêtre, 20-22, 25, 27, 36, 37, 47 n 14; Hospice de Vaugirard, 4, 25, 26; Hospice des Vénériens, 17, 25, 26, 27-28, 29; la Petite Pologne, 15, 25; La Salpêtrière, 20, 36-37, 47 n 14
—British: Lock (Southwark), 73; London Lock, 4, 128-36, 162; St. Thomas's, 72-73
Hunt, Lynn, 2; *Eroticism and the Body Politic*, 11 n 3
Hunter, John, 5-6, 7, 8, 9, 91; *Treatise on the Venereal Disease*, 5, 6, 91
husbands, infected by wives, 152, 155-56

James, Robert, 153; *James's Medical Dictionary*, 19, 153
James II (England), 203-5
James IV (Scotland), 5
Janin, Jules, 248, 249, 250, 251
Johnson, Samuel, 161, 198, 206; *Dictionary*, 150; "London," 206
Jonson, Ben, 206; "An English Monsieur," 206
Joubert, Joseph, 249

Kildare, Lady, 106, 107
Kneibler, Yvonne, 44

Laclos, Pierre Choderlos de, 245; *Liaisons Dangereuses*, 47 n 16, 229, 239, 245
Lalouette, Pierre, 23-24
Leake, John, 151-52; *A Dissertation on the Properties and Efficacy of the Lisbon Diet Drink*, 152
Lecointe, Jourdain, Dr., 41; *La santé de Mars*, 41
Lee, Sir George, 159

Le Fébure de Saint-Ildepont, 24
Lefort, Claude, 256
LeNoir, Jean-Charles-Pierre, 120
Lerebours, Marie Angelique Anel, 120-21
Linguet, Simon Nicolas Andre, 36
Lloyd, Vaughan, 129
Lock Asylum for Women, 136-43; establishment of, 136-39; outcomes, 140-42; rules of, 139-40
Locke, John, 198, 211 n 10
London-Bawd, The, 216
Louyer-Villermay, M., 44
Lyttleton, Sir Richard, 92-93, 129

MacArthur, Elizabeth, 251
MacKenzie, Henry, 214; *The Man of Feeling*, 214, 221
MacKinnon, Catherine, 243, 244, 249-50, 251-52; *Only Words*, 244, 249-50, 251, 258 nn 1, 3, 259 nn 11, 12, 14
Macklin, Charles, 135
Madan, Rev. Martin, 128, 134-35, 136; *A Collection of Psalms and Hymns*, 136
madness, as symptom of venereal disease, 156, 158. See also Battie, William
Mandeville, Bernard, 114-15; *A Modest Defense of Public Stews*, 114-15
Manuel, Pierre, 43, 49 n 44
marriage, dangers of, 105-6, 152-53, 162
Marston, John, 199, 202; *The Metamorphosis of Pigmalion's Image*, 199-200; *The Scourge of Villains*, 200
Marten, John, 52-63, 69; *Attila of the Gout*, 52; *The Dishonour of the Gout*, 52; *Gonsologium Novum*, 53, 57, 59-60, 62; *Treatise of all the Degrees and Symptoms*, 52, 63
Ménétra, Jacques-Louis, 18
Mengel, Elias, 204
Mercier, Louis-Sébastian, 20, 34, 89, 90
mercury, attacks on, 25, 74-75, 80-81, 87, 90
Mesmer, 19
Mettler, Cecilia, 115, 125 n 4
Middleton, Charles, 137-38
Middleton, Lady, 139

Index

Mildmay, Henry, 205
misogyny. *See* women, expressions against
Mittié, Jean Stanislaus, 25
Montagu, Lady Mary Wortley, 153, 197
Mordant, Lady Mary, 105
More, Hannah, 137, 139
More, Thomas, 197; *Utopia*, 197
Morpeth, Lord, 153
Morris, James, 129
Moulsdale, Dr., 91-92
Murray, Fanny, 129

Needham, Elizabeth, 171, 177
Nègre de Mondragon, 16, 22
Neisser, Albert, 6
newspapers. *See* periodical press
Nicolson, Malcolm, 70
Nicolson, Marjorie, 78
Nougaret, Pierre-Jean-Baptiste, 36, 38

Oldfield, Dr. J., 107, 109, 110, 113 n 29
Orford, Lord, 156
Osborn, Sarah Byng, 153

Packe, Edmund, Dr., 74, 79
Palmer, Samuel, 73
Pancoucke, 43, 46; *Dictionnaire des sciences médicales*, 46; *Encyclopédie méthodique*, 43
Paracelsus, 88
Parent-Duchâtalet, Alexandre, 35, 39-40, 43, 45, 50 n 66; *De la prostitution*, 50 nn 61, 66
Paul, Josiah, 72
Paulhan, Jean, 252, 253, 257
Paulson, Ronald, 168, 180
Pauvert, Jean-Jacques, 252-53, 254
Pembroke, Lord, 158, 160, 161, 166 n 39, 167 n 50
Percy, Lord, 154
periodical press: advertisements in, for cures, 1-2, 22, 149, 150, 151-52; gossip gazette (French), 38, 42-43, (British), 153-54, 156, 158, 162, 165 n 7
Perry, Ruth, 4
Petit, Jean Louis, 72

Petit, John, 152
Peuchet, Jacques, 43-44
pharmakon, 230, 236, 247
Pidding, James, 92
Pitt, William Morton, 137
Plenck, Joseph James, 151
Pomfret, Lord, 156
Pope, Alexander, 150, 197, 208, 210 nn 4, 5
pornography, 243, 254, 258 n 1. *See also* antipornography debate
Porter, Roy, 9, 100 n 4
Powell, William, 135
Powys, Sir Thomas, 105
Prévost, Abbé, 37; *L'Histoire du Chevalier des Grieux et de Manon Lescaut*, 37, 39
Profily, Dr. John, 6, 104-5, 106, 108; *Easy and Exact Method of Curing the Venereal Disease*, 6, 104-5, 111 nn 6, 9, 112 nn 21, 23
prostitutes and prostitution: in art, 169, 170-71, 177, 178, 190-94; depictions of, in novels, 37-39, 214-15, 217, 222-23, 246; as figures of blame, 4, 20, 34-36, 39-40, 42-46, 47 n 7, 121-22, 137-38, 232, 239-40; policing of, 28-30, 38-40, 44-46

quackery, 59-61, 74, 76, 81, 100 n 4, 176-177, 189-90
Quétel, Claude, 2, 9, 100 n 13, 114, 118, 228
Quillet, Claude, 116; *Callipaedia*, 116

Raulin, Joseph, 118
reading, as a dangerous activity, 190, 248, 249-54, 255-57
religion, 4, 171, 199; invocation of Christian sensibility, 62, 130-31, 143, 235, 236-37
Rétif de la Bretonne, 34, 39-40, 41, 48, 229-41, 248-49; *Anti-Justine*, 248, 249; *Le Paysan Perverti*, 229-41, 242 nn 7, 19; *Le Pornographe ou les idées d'un honnête homme sur un projet de règlement pour les prostituées*, 39, 41, 231-32, 238, 239, 242 n 6, 258 n 5

Rich, John, 135
Richardson, Samuel, 214-15; *Clarissa*, 214-15, 227 n 30; *Pamela*, 227 n 26
Ricord, Phillipe, 6, 31 n 11
Robinson, Martha, 155-56
Rochester, 196, 197, 199
Rock, Dr., 151, 165 n 7, 179
Rousseau, Jean-Jacques, 119, 229, 239, 245; "Discourse on the Sciences and Arts," 238; *Julie*, 229, 245
Roussel de Vauzesme, 16
Rowlandson, Thomas, 86; "Mercury and His Advocates defeated," 86
Rowley, Dr. William, 152
Royer, 24, 25

Sade, marquis de, 229, 243, 244, 246, 249, 257; *Juliette*, 246; *La philosophie dans le boudoir*, 229, 247-48, 250, 252, 253, 255-56; *Les 120 Journées*, 243, 245-46, 255
"Sade trial" of 1956, 252-54, 259 n 22
Saffory, Henry, 90
Saint Léger, 16
salivation: debate over, 84 n 42; description of, 108-9, 112 nn 21, 23. *See also* syphilis; venereal disease.
Sandwich, Lady, 152
satire, 150, 169-71, 173, 176, 181, 184, 186, 190, 193, 197, 199, 203, 207, 212 n 40, 213, 220
Saunders, William: *A New and Easy Way of Giving Mercury*, 151
Schaudinn, Fritz, 6
Scott, Sarah, 223; *Millenium Hall*, 223
Scott, Rev. Thomas, 137
Scroope, Sir Carr, 196
Selwyn, George, 153, 160
Shadwell, Thomas, 186; *The Humourists*, 186-88
Shaw, Peter, 129
Sheppard, Edward, 129
Sheratt, John, 92-93
Shesgreen, Sean, 175, 179
Siddons, Sarah, 110-11, 152, 165 n 9
Sloane, Hans, 122
smallpox, 37, 115, 197, 241 n 3, 245
Smart, Christopher, 156, 165 n 19

Smith, Virginia, 87
Smollett, Tobias, 150, 220, 226 n 24; *The Adventures of Roderick Random*, 220, 224
Smythe, Lady, 139
Sontag, Susan, 10-11, 254; *AIDS and Its Metaphors*, 10-11, 50 n 68
Spencer, Lady Diana, 157-64
Spinke, John, 60; *Quackery Unmasked*, 60; *Venus's Botcher*, 60
Staël, Germaine de, 249; *Delphine*, 249
Steele, Richard, 174; *Spectator* #246, 174-75
Stone, Lawrence, 1, 9, 156, 214, 225 n 5
Swainson, Isaac, 85, 89, 90, 91, 92; *Mercury Stark Naked*, 90, 94
Swift, Jonathan, 172, 175, 198, 206-7, 209, 213; *Gulliver's Travels*, 206-7, 213, 220, 225 n 7; "Phyllis, or The Progress of Love," 208; "The Progress of Marriage," 207
syphilis, symptoms of, 8-9, 15, 17-18, 70; treatment of, 8-9, 74-80, 107-8, 111 n 15, 112 nn 21, 23 *See also* mercury; salivation; venereal disease

Temkin, Oswei, 88
testimonials, 58-59, 66 n 27, 96-98, 141-42
Thornton, Henry, 137
Thornton, Robert, 137
Thrale, Henry, 103-4, 111 nn 6, 12
Thrale, Hester, 103-5, 110, 111 nn 6, 12, 150
Tomb of Venus, The, 216
Torella, Gaspara, 115, 125 n 4
Town and Country: Tête-à-Têtes, 153-54, 158, 162, 165 n 20
Trevor, Mary, 107
Trials for Adultery, 155, 156, 161
Trumbach, Randolph, 119, 121; *The Rise of the Egalitarian Family*, 121
Turner, Daniel, 36, 68-81, 179, 189; *The Modern Quack*, 189-90; *Syphilis*, 70-76, 172, 178

Vandeput, George, 129
Van Swieten, Gerhard, 118

vegetarianism, 22, 87-88
venereal disease: acquisition and transmission theories, 6, 19-20, 31 n 11, 53, 55, 70, 115, 118, 247; in children *(see* children); and the city, 20, 40, 48 n 32, 170, 180, 190-91, 230-31, 238-39; debate over origins, 5, 17, 87-88, 115, 197, 236, 240; fear of depopulation, 35, 40-42, 114, 116, 173-76, 180, 206-7, 213, 239; as metaphor, 2, 170-72, 176, 181, 185-86, 192, 198, 202-5, 209-10, 216-17, 239; as moral impurity, 21, 42, 44, 70, 128, 168, 184, 189, 198, 208-9, 233, 235; names for, 1, 17, 150-51, 172, 197, 216, 229; and nationalism, 40-41, 59, 114, 117-18, 124, 138, 183-84, 188-89, 197, 206-7, 239-41; remedies and modes of treatment, 6, 15-17, 22-25, 32 n 33, 42-43, 49 n 43, 55-56, 75-76, 82 n 19, 83 nn 21, 28, 29, 84 nn 37, 41, 85-89, 91-92, 94-95, 100 n 13, 131-32, 151, 186; rivalry between physicians and surgeons, 23, 52, 59-60, 71-73; unicist and dualist theories, 5-6, 17-18, 150. *See also* gonorrhea; mercury; salivation; syphilis
Venette, Nicolas, *Le Tableau de l'Amour Conjugal*, 53
Vernon, Lydia, 106
Vertue, George, 168
Vigarello, Georges, 256-57
Virey, J.J., 44
Voltaire, 16, 229, 240, 245; *Candide*, 16, 229, 239, 240, 241 n 3, 245

von Hutten, Ulrich, 82 n 13, 88; *De Morbo Gallico*, 82 n 13

Wagner, Peter, 96
Walker, Charles, 221; *Authentick Memoirs ... Sally Salisbury*, 221-22, 223
Walpole, Horace, 110, 153, 157, 160, 162
Walpole, Robert, 129
Ward, Joshua, 69, 78-79, 80, 83 n 31
Warner, John, 163
Watteau, Antoine, 169, 170; *La Toilette du Matin*, 169
West, George, 157
West, Liveth G., 1, 2
wet-nursing, 118-21, 122, 123-25; attacks on, 120-21
Wilberforce, William, 136-37
Williams, Carolina, 132, 144 n 9. *See also* Lock Asylum for Women
Williams, Charles Hanbury, 106-10, 111 n 6, 156
Williams, Frances, 106-10
Williams, Thomas, 129
Willoughby, C., 84 n 42
Winckler, Jean Benoit: *"Le transport des filles de joye à l'hopital,"* 29
Windham, William, 129
wives: as caregivers to infected husbands, 103-4; infected by husbands, 103-6, 110-11, 152-53, 155, 200
women, expressions against, 4, 11 n 12, 19-20, 44 130, 137-38, 149, 199, 210, 217-18, 231, 240
Worgan, Dr. John, 155